This report contains the collective views of an international group of experts and does not necessarily represent the decisions or the stated policy of the United Nations Environment Programme, the International Labour Organization or the World Health Organization.

Environmental Health Criteria 236

PRINCIPLES AND METHODS FOR ASSESSING AUTOIMMUNITY ASSOCIATED WITH EXPOSURE TO CHEMICALS

First draft prepared by the World Health Organization Collaborating Centre for Immunotoxicology and Allergic Hypersensitivity at the National Institute for Public Health and the Environment (RIVM), Bilthoven, The Netherlands, in conjunction with an international group of experts.

Published under the joint sponsorship of the United Nations Environment Programme, the International Labour Organization and the World Health Organization, and produced within the framework of the Inter-Organization Programme for the Sound Management of Chemicals.

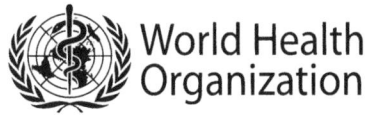

The **International Programme on Chemical Safety (IPCS)**, established in 1980, is a joint venture of the United Nations Environment Programme (UNEP), the International Labour Organization (ILO) and the World Health Organization (WHO). The overall objectives of the IPCS are to establish the scientific basis for assessment of the risk to human health and the environment from exposure to chemicals, through international peer review processes, as a prerequisite for the promotion of chemical safety, and to provide technical assistance in strengthening national capacities for the sound management of chemicals.

The **Inter-Organization Programme for the Sound Management of Chemicals (IOMC)** was established in 1995 by UNEP, ILO, the Food and Agriculture Organization of the United Nations, WHO, the United Nations Industrial Development Organization, the United Nations Institute for Training and Research and the Organisation for Economic Co-operation and Development (Participating Organizations), following recommendations made by the 1992 UN Conference on Environment and Development to strengthen cooperation and increase coordination in the field of chemical safety. The purpose of the IOMC is to promote coordination of the policies and activities pursued by the Participating Organizations, jointly or separately, to achieve the sound management of chemicals in relation to human health and the environment.

WHO Library Cataloguing-in-Publication Data

Principles and methods for assessing autoimmunity associated with exposure to chemicals.

(Environmental health criteria ; 236)

1.Autoimmunity. 2.Autoimmune diseases - diagnosis. 3.Organic chemicals - adverse effects. 4.Inorganic chemicals - adverse effects. 5.Environmental exposure. I.World Health Organization. II.Inter-Organization Programme for the Sound Management of Chemicals. III.Series.

ISBN 92 4 157236 1   (NLM classification: WD 305)
ISBN 978 92 4 157236 1
ISSN 0250-863X

©World Health Organization 2006

All rights reserved. Publications of the World Health Organization can be obtained from WHO Press, World Health Organization, 20 Avenue Appia, 1211 Geneva 27, Switzerland (tel: +41 22 791 3264; fax: +41 22 791 4857; e-mail: bookorders@who.int). Requests for permission to reproduce or translate WHO publications — whether for sale or for noncommercial distribution — should be addressed to WHO Press, at the above address (fax: +41 22 791 4806; e-mail: permissions@who.int).

The designations employed and the presentation of the material in this publication do not imply the expression of any opinion whatsoever on the part of the World Health Organization concerning the legal status of any country, territory, city or area or of its authorities, or concerning the delimitation of its frontiers or boundaries. Dotted lines on maps represent approximate border lines for which there may not yet be full agreement.

The mention of specific companies or of certain manufacturers' products does not imply that they are endorsed or recommended by the World Health Organization in preference to others of a similar nature that are not mentioned. Errors and omissions excepted, the names of proprietary products are distinguished by initial capital letters.

All reasonable precautions have been taken by WHO to verify the information contained in this publication. However, the published material is being distributed without warranty of any kind, either express or implied. The responsibility for the interpretation and use of the material lies with the reader. In no event shall the World Health Organization be liable for damages arising from its use.

The named authors alone are responsible for the views expressed in this publication.

This document was technically and linguistically edited by Marla Sheffer, Ottawa, Canada, and printed by Wissenschaftliche Verlagsgesellschaft mbH, Stuttgart, Germany.

CONTENTS

ENVIRONMENTAL HEALTH CRITERIA ON PRINCIPLES AND METHODS FOR ASSESSING AUTOIMMUNITY ASSOCIATED WITH EXPOSURE TO CHEMICALS

PREAMBLE	xi
ACRONYMS AND ABBREVIATIONS	xxii
1. SUMMARY	1
2. INTRODUCTION AND DEFINITIONS OF AUTOIMMUNITY AND AUTOIMMUNE DISEASE	5
3. INTRODUCTION TO THE IMMUNE SYSTEM: FOCUS ON AUTOIMMUNE MECHANISMS	9
3.1 Introduction	9
3.2 The innate immune response	10
3.3 The adaptive immune response	11
3.3.1 Function	11
3.3.2 Aberrant function	14
3.3.3 Ageing	15
3.4 Mechanisms of self-tolerance	16
3.5 Immunopathogenesis of autoimmune disease	18
3.5.1 Mechanisms of induction	18
3.5.2 Effector mechanisms	21
3.6 Summary	22
4. INTRINSIC FACTORS IN AUTOIMMUNITY	24
4.1 Genetic factors involved in the induction of or susceptibility for autoimmune diseases	24
4.1.1 Probable monogenic autoimmune syndromes	24
4.1.2 Multigenic autoimmune diseases	26
4.1.2.1 Immune deficiencies	27

		4.1.2.2	Defects and dysregulation in apoptosis pathways and cell cycle regulation	29
		4.1.2.3	Associations with MHC alleles or haplotypes	31
		4.1.2.4	Polymorphisms in genes coding for regulatory and effector molecules of the immune system	35
		4.1.2.5	Hormones and genes	37
		4.1.2.6	Genetic polymorphisms of xenobiotic-metabolizing enzymes	38
		4.1.2.7	Genes coding for autoantigens	39
		4.1.2.8	Genes coding for enzymes involved in post-translational modification of autoantigens	40
		4.1.2.9	DNA methylation	41
	4.1.3	Problems and perspectives		41
4.2	Hormonal influence on autoimmunity			42
	4.2.1	Pregnancy		42
		4.2.1.1	Suppression of autoimmunity	42
		4.2.1.2	Stimulation of autoimmunity	43
	4.2.2	Psychological stress		46

5. CLINICAL EXPRESSION OF HUMAN AUTOIMMUNE DISEASES   47

5.1	Introduction	47
5.2	Addison disease	50
5.3	ANCA-associated vasculitis	51
5.4	Antiphospholipid syndrome	52
5.5	Coeliac disease	53
5.6	Diabetes mellitus	54
5.7	Goodpasture disease	55
5.8	Guillain-Barré syndrome	56
5.9	Autoimmune haemolytic anaemia	57
	5.9.1 Warm autoimmune haemolytic anaemia	57
	5.9.2 Cold autoimmune haemolytic anaemia	58
	5.9.3 Drug-induced autoimmune haemolytic anaemia	59
5.10	Autoimmune hepatitis	59
5.11	Inflammatory bowel disease	61
	5.11.1 Crohn disease	61

		5.11.2 Ulcerative colitis	62
	5.12	Multiple sclerosis	63
	5.13	Myasthenia gravis	64
	5.14	Myocarditis	66
	5.15	Autoimmune myositis	66
	5.16	Paraneoplastic neurological syndromes	67
	5.17	Pemphigus/pemphigoid	68
		5.17.1 Pemphigus	69
		5.17.2 Pemphigoid	70
	5.18	Pernicious anaemia	70
	5.19	Autoimmune polyglandular syndromes	71
		5.19.1 APGS type 1	71
		5.19.2 APGS type 2	72
		5.19.3 APGS type 3	72
	5.20	Primary biliary cirrhosis	72
	5.21	Psoriasis	73
	5.22	Rheumatoid arthritis	74
	5.23	Scleroderma (systemic sclerosis)	75
	5.24	Sjögren syndrome	77
	5.25	Systemic lupus erythematosus and lupus syndrome	78
		5.25.1 Systemic lupus erythematosus	78
		5.25.2 Lupus syndrome	79
	5.26	Autoimmune thrombocytopenia	80
		5.26.1 Immune thrombocytopenic purpura	80
		5.26.2 Thrombotic thrombocytopenic purpura	81
		5.26.3 Drug-induced thrombocytopenia	81
	5.27	Autoimmune thyroid diseases	82
		5.27.1 Graves disease	83
		5.27.2 Hashimoto thyroiditis	83
		5.27.3 Iodine and thyroid disease	84
	5.28	Diseases with autoimmune components	85
6.	EPIDEMIOLOGY		87
	6.1	Descriptive epidemiology	87
		6.1.1 Demographic patterns	89
		6.1.2 Co-morbidity of autoimmune diseases	91
	6.2	Epidemiology of autoantibodies	92
		6.2.1 Prevalence of autoantibodies in the general population	92

| | | 6.2.2 | Associations between antibodies and environmental exposures | 94 |

7. MECHANISMS OF CHEMICAL-ASSOCIATED AUTOIMMUNE RESPONSES 96

    7.1 General 96
    7.2 Induction of antigen-specific responses 98
        7.2.1 Formation of neoantigens 98
        7.2.2 Cross-reactivity 99
        7.2.3 Release of non-tolerant epitopes 100
        7.2.4 Interference with central tolerance 101
        7.2.5 Signal 2 increasing mechanisms 102
            7.2.5.1 Importance of signal 2 102
            7.2.5.2 Induction of signal 2 103
        7.2.6 Immunoregulation 104
    7.3 Other mechanisms 106

8. CHEMICAL/PHYSICAL AGENTS AND AUTOIMMUNITY 107

    8.1 Toxic oil syndrome 107
        8.1.1 Clinical features of toxic oil syndrome 108
        8.1.2 Immune markers in toxic oil syndrome 109
        8.1.3 Experimental studies of toxic oil syndrome 111
    8.2 TCDD (dioxins) 114
    8.3 Pesticides 115
        8.3.1 General 115
        8.3.2 Hexachlorobenzene 117
            8.3.2.1 Accidental poisoning in Turkey 118
            8.3.2.2 Adverse immune effects of hexachlorobenzene 118
    8.4 Ultraviolet radiation 122
    8.5 Silica 122
        8.5.1 Introduction to epidemiological studies of silica exposure 122
        8.5.2 Occupational silica exposure and systemic autoimmune diseases 124
        8.5.3 Experimental studies of immune- and autoimmune-related effects of silica 127
        8.5.4 Summary 130
    8.6 Heavy metals 131

		8.6.1 Mercury	131
		8.6.2 Gold	135
		8.6.3 Cadmium	135
		8.6.4 Other heavy metals	136
	8.7	Solvents	138
	8.8	Tobacco smoke	141
	8.9	Ethanol	145
	8.10	Iodine	148
	8.11	Therapeutic agents	149
		8.11.1 General	149
		8.11.2 Hydralazine	150
		8.11.3 Procainamide	151
		8.11.4 D-Penicillamine	152
		8.11.5 Zimeldine	153
		8.11.6 Gold drugs	153
		8.11.7 Biopharmaceuticals	155
		8.11.8 Diethylstilbestrol	156
		8.11.8.1 Diethylstilbestrol-induced immune alterations	156
		8.11.8.2 Immune effects of diethylstilbestrol in humans	157
		8.11.8.3 Conclusion	159
	8.12	Silicones	159
		8.12.1 Introduction	159
		8.12.2 Silicone breast implants and systemic disease	160
		8.12.3 Conclusion	162
9.	NON-CHEMICAL FACTORS IN AUTOIMMUNITY		163
	9.1	Infections: cause of autoimmunity, and immune programming	163
		9.1.1 Streptococcus and rheumatic fever	165
		9.1.2 Hepatitis C virus	166
		9.1.3 Epstein-Barr virus	167
		9.1.4 Other infections	167
		9.1.5 Absence of infections: the hygiene hypothesis	168
	9.2	Vaccine-related factors	169
		9.2.1 Vaccines themselves	169
		9.2.2 Vaccine additives	170
	9.3	Dietary factors	171
		9.3.1 Caloric restriction and leptin	172

		9.3.2 Dietary fat and fatty acid content	172
		9.3.3 Antioxidants	174
		9.3.4 Vitamin D	174
		9.3.5 L-Tryptophan and eosinophilia myalgia syndrome	175

10. ANIMAL MODELS TO ASSESS CHEMICAL-INDUCED AUTOIMMUNITY   178

    10.1 Introduction   178
    10.2 Rat models   180
        10.2.1 The Brown Norway rat model   180
            10.2.1.1 Metals   181
            10.2.1.2 D-Penicillamine   182
            10.2.1.3 Hexachlorobenzene   182
        10.2.2 Other rat models   183
    10.3 Mouse models   183
        10.3.1 Metals   184
        10.3.2 Drugs   184
        10.3.3 Pristane   185
    10.4 Genetically predisposed animal models   186
        10.4.1 Systemic lupus erythematosus-prone strains of mice   186
    10.5 Other species   187
    10.6 Local and popliteal lymph node assays   188
        10.6.1 Introduction   188
        10.6.2 Primary, secondary, and adoptive popliteal lymph node assays and the lymph node proliferation assay   188
        10.6.3 Reporter antigen popliteal lymph node assay   189
        10.6.4 Popliteal lymph node assay as predictive assay   191
    10.7 Testing strategy   191

11. HUMAN TESTING FOR AUTOIMMUNE DISEASE   193

    11.1 Introduction   193
    11.2 Methods of human autoantibody detection   195
        11.2.1 Indirect immunofluorescence technique   195
        11.2.2 Counter-immunoelectrophoresis   195
        11.2.3 Haemagglutination   196

| | | 11.2.4 Enzyme-linked immunosorbent assay/ | |
| | | fluorescent enzyme immunoassay | 197 |

	11.2.4 Enzyme-linked immunosorbent assay/ fluorescent enzyme immunoassay	197
	11.2.5 Radioimmunoassay	198
	11.2.6 Immunoblotting	199
	11.2.7 Multiplex analysis	199
11.3	Selection of detection method	200
	11.3.1 Autoantigens	200
	11.3.2 Anti-immunoglobulin reagents	202
11.4	Clinical interpretation	203
11.5	Human immunoglobulins	204
	11.5.1 Autoimmune disease and human immunoglobulin levels	204
	11.5.2 Quantification of human immunoglobulins	205
11.6	Testing in the diagnosis of delayed-type chemical hypersensitivity	207
11.7	Conclusions	208
12. RISK ASSESSMENT		**211**
12.1	Introduction	211
12.2	Hazard identification of chemical-induced autoimmune disease (animal models)	212
12.3	Exposure assessment (animal models)	213
12.4	Mode of action	213
12.5	Epidemiological issues	215
12.6	Susceptibility factors	216
12.7	Burden of autoimmune disease	217
13. CONCLUSIONS AND RECOMMENDATIONS		**219**
13.1	Conclusions	219
13.2	Recommendations	220
TERMINOLOGY		**222**
REFERENCES		**256**
RESUME		**325**
RESUMEN		**330**

NOTE TO READERS OF THE CRITERIA MONOGRAPHS

Every effort has been made to present information in the criteria monographs as accurately as possible without unduly delaying their publication. In the interest of all users of the Environmental Health Criteria monographs, readers are requested to communicate any errors that may have occurred to the Director of the International Programme on Chemical Safety, World Health Organization, Geneva, Switzerland, in order that they may be included in corrigenda.

Environmental Health Criteria

PREAMBLE

Objectives

In 1973, the WHO Environmental Health Criteria Programme was initiated with the following objectives:

(i) to assess information on the relationship between exposure to environmental pollutants and human health, and to provide guidelines for setting exposure limits;
(ii) to identify new or potential pollutants;
(iii) to identify gaps in knowledge concerning the health effects of pollutants;
(iv) to promote the harmonization of toxicological and epidemiological methods in order to have internationally comparable results.

The first Environmental Health Criteria (EHC) monograph, on mercury, was published in 1976, and since that time an ever-increasing number of assessments of chemicals and of physical effects have been produced. In addition, many EHC monographs have been devoted to evaluating toxicological methodology, e.g. for genetic, neurotoxic, teratogenic, and nephrotoxic effects. Other publications have been concerned with epidemiological guidelines, evaluation of short-term tests for carcinogens, biomarkers, effects on the elderly, and so forth.

Since its inauguration, the EHC Programme has widened its scope, and the importance of environmental effects, in addition to health effects, has been increasingly emphasized in the total evaluation of chemicals.

The original impetus for the Programme came from World Health Assembly resolutions and the recommendations of the 1972 UN Conference on the Human Environment. Subsequently, the work became an integral part of the International Programme on Chemical Safety (IPCS), a cooperative programme of WHO, ILO, and UNEP. In this manner, with the strong support of the new partners, the importance of occupational health and environmental effects was

EHC 236: Principles and Methods for Assessing Autoimmunity

fully recognized. The EHC monographs have become widely established, used, and recognized throughout the world.

The recommendations of the 1992 UN Conference on Environment and Development and the subsequent establishment of the Intergovernmental Forum on Chemical Safety with the priorities for action in the six programme areas of Chapter 19, Agenda 21, all lend further weight to the need for EHC assessments of the risks of chemicals.

Scope

Two different types of EHC documents are available: 1) on specific chemicals or groups of related chemicals; and 2) on risk assessment methodologies. The criteria monographs are intended to provide critical reviews on the effect on human health and the environment of chemicals and of combinations of chemicals and physical and biological agents and risk assessment methodologies. As such, they include and review studies that are of direct relevance for evaluations. However, they do not describe *every* study carried out. Worldwide data are used and are quoted from original studies, not from abstracts or reviews. Both published and unpublished reports are considered, and it is incumbent on the authors to assess all the articles cited in the references. Preference is always given to published data. Unpublished data are used only when relevant published data are absent or when they are pivotal to the risk assessment. A detailed policy statement is available that describes the procedures used for unpublished proprietary data so that this information can be used in the evaluation without compromising its confidential nature (WHO (1990) Revised Guidelines for the Preparation of Environmental Health Criteria Monographs. PCS/90.69, Geneva, World Health Organization).

In the evaluation of human health risks, sound human data, whenever available, are preferred to animal data. Animal and in vitro studies provide support and are used mainly to supply evidence missing from human studies. It is mandatory that research on human subjects is conducted in full accord with ethical principles, including the provisions of the Helsinki Declaration.

The EHC monographs are intended to assist national and international authorities in making risk assessments and subsequent risk management decisions and to update national and international authorities on risk assessment methodology.

Procedures

The order of procedures that result in the publication of an EHC monograph is shown in the flow chart on p. xiv. A designated staff member of IPCS, responsible for the scientific quality of the document, serves as Responsible Officer (RO). The IPCS Editor is responsible for layout and language. The first draft, prepared by consultants or, more usually, staff from an IPCS Participating Institution, is based on extensive literature searches from reference databases such as Medline and Toxline.

The draft document, when received by the RO, may require an initial review by a small panel of experts to determine its scientific quality and objectivity. Once the RO finds the document acceptable as a first draft, it is distributed, in its unedited form, to well over 100 EHC contact points throughout the world who are asked to comment on its completeness and accuracy and, where necessary, provide additional material. The contact points, usually designated by governments, may be Participating Institutions, IPCS Focal Points, or individual scientists known for their particular expertise. Generally, some four months are allowed before the comments are considered by the RO and author(s). A second draft incorporating comments received and approved by the Coordinator, IPCS, is then distributed to Task Group members, who carry out the peer review, at least six weeks before their meeting.

The Task Group members serve as individual scientists, not as representatives of any organization, government, or industry. Their function is to evaluate the accuracy, significance, and relevance of the information in the document and to assess the health and environmental risks from exposure to the chemical or chemicals in question. A summary and recommendations for further research and improved safety aspects are also required. The composition of the Task Group is dictated by the range of expertise required for the subject of the meeting and by the need for a balanced geographical distribution.

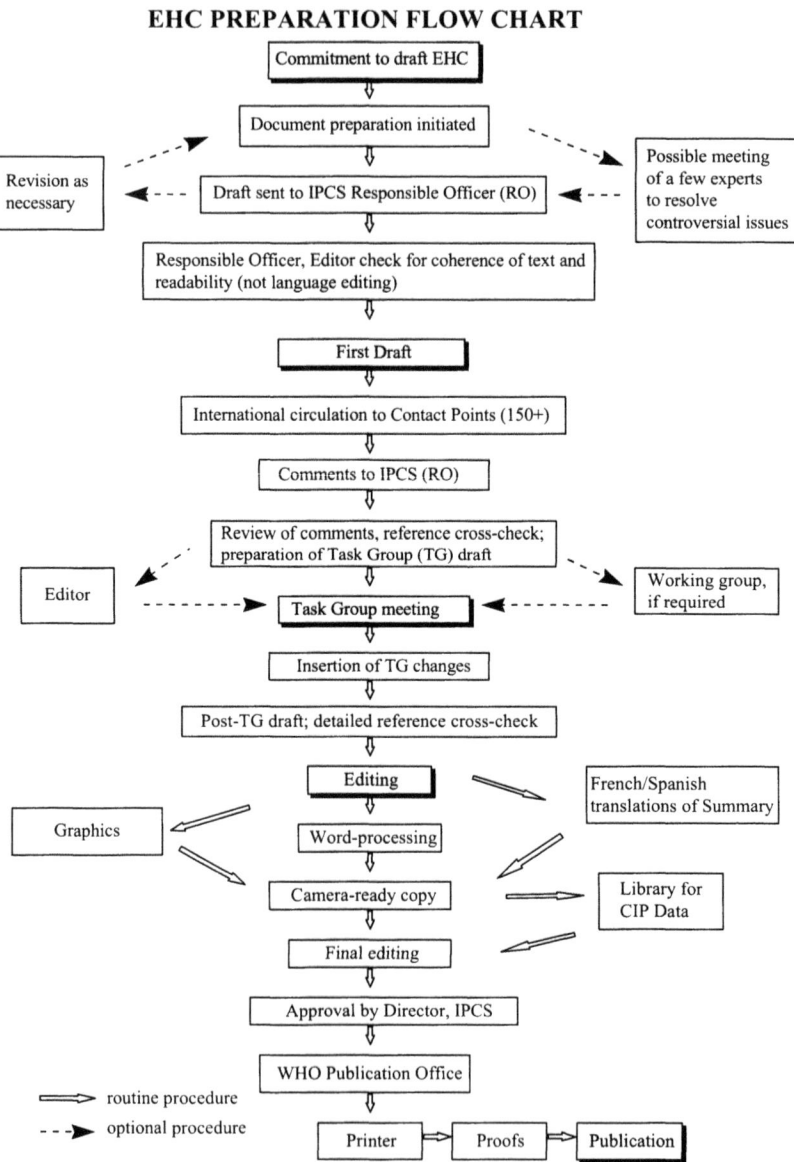

Preamble

The three cooperating organizations of the IPCS recognize the important role played by nongovernmental organizations. Representatives from relevant national and international associations may be invited to join the Task Group as observers. Although observers may provide a valuable contribution to the process, they can speak only at the invitation of the Chairperson. Observers do not participate in the final evaluation of the chemicals; this is the sole responsibility of the Task Group members. When the Task Group considers it to be appropriate, it may meet in camera.

All individuals who as authors, consultants, or advisers participate in the preparation of the EHC monograph must, in addition to serving in their personal capacity as scientists, inform the RO if at any time a conflict of interest, whether actual or potential, could be perceived in their work. They are required to sign a conflict of interest statement. Such a procedure ensures the transparency and probity of the process.

When the Task Group has completed its review and the RO is satisfied as to the scientific correctness and completeness of the document, it then goes for language editing, reference checking, and preparation of camera-ready copy. After approval by the Coordinator, IPCS, the monograph is submitted for printing.

It is accepted that the following criteria should initiate the updating of an EHC monograph: new data are available that would substantially change the evaluation; there is public concern for health or environmental effects of the agent because of greater exposure; an appreciable time period has elapsed since the last evaluation.

All Participating Institutions are informed, through the EHC progress report, of the authors and institutions proposed for the drafting of the documents. A comprehensive file of all comments received on drafts of each EHC monograph is maintained and is available on request. The Chairpersons of Task Groups are briefed before each meeting on their role and responsibility in ensuring that these rules are followed.

WHO TASK GROUP ON ENVIRONMENTAL HEALTH CRITERIA ON PRINCIPLES AND METHODS FOR ASSESSING AUTOIMMUNITY ASSOCIATED WITH EXPOSURE TO CHEMICALS

The first draft of the Environmental Health Criteria (EHC) monograph was prepared for the International Programme on Chemical Safety (IPCS) by the World Health Organization (WHO) Collaborating Centre for Immunotoxicology and Allergic Hypersensitivity at the National Institute for Public Health and the Environment (RIVM), Bilthoven, The Netherlands. To prepare the first draft, the Collaborating Centre convened two drafting group meetings of experts in Bilthoven, the first in December 2002 and the second in June 2004.

The draft was widely distributed by IPCS for international peer review for approximately two months from mid-June to late August 2005. A revised proposed draft document, taking into account comments received, was prepared by Professor Henk van Loveren of the WHO Collaborating Centre. An EHC Task Group was convened from 1 to 4 November 2005, in Bilthoven, to further develop and finalize the document.

Ms C. Vickers, WHO, was responsible for production of the monograph.

The efforts of all who helped in the preparation and finalization of the monograph are gratefully acknowledged.

* * *

Risk assessment activities of IPCS are supported financially by the Department of Health and Department for Environment, Food & Rural Affairs, United Kingdom; Environmental Protection Agency, Food and Drug Administration, and National Institute of Environmental Health Sciences, USA; European Commission; German Federal Ministry of Environment, Nature Conservation and Nuclear Safety; Health Canada; Japanese Ministry of Health, Labour and Welfare; and Swiss Agency for Environment, Forests and Landscape.

Preamble

Participants at December 2002 Preparatory Meeting

Professor R.S. Chauhan, Department of Pathology, College of Veterinary Sciences, G.B. Pant University of Agriculture & Technology, Pantnagar, India

Professor J.W. Cohen Tervaert, Department of Clinical and Experimental Immunology, University Hospital Maastricht, Maastricht, The Netherlands

Professor K. Conrad, Institute of Immunology, Medical Faculty, Technical University of Dresden, Dresden, Germany

Dr G.S. Cooper, National Institute of Environmental Health Sciences, National Institutes of Health, Research Triangle Park, NC, USA

Professor M.L. de Souza Querioz, Department of Pharmacology, Faculty of Medical Sciences, State University of Campinas, Campinas, SP, Brazil

Dr D.R. Germolec, National Institute of Environmental Health Sciences, National Institutes of Health, Research Triangle Park, NC, USA

Professor A.J. Hall, Immunology and Epidemiology Group, London School of Hygiene & Tropical Medicine, London, England

Professor M. Ohsawa, Department of Toxicology and Environmental Health, Faculty of Pharmaceutical Sciences, Teikyo University, Sagamiko, Kanagawa, Japan

Dr R.M. Philen, Centers for Disease Control and Prevention, Atlanta, GA, USA

Dr R.H.H. Pieters, Institute for Risk Assessment Sciences — Immunotoxicology, Universiteit Utrecht, Utrecht, The Netherlands

Professor N.R. Rose, Center for Autoimmune Disease Research, Johns Hopkins University, Baltimore, MD, USA

Professor H. van Loveren, Laboratory for Pathology and Immunobiology, National Institute for Public Health and the Environment, Bilthoven, The Netherlands

Dr J.G. Vos, Laboratory for Pathology and Immunobiology, National Institute for Public Health and the Environment, Bilthoven, The Netherlands

Secretariat

Ms C. Vickers, International Programme on Chemical Safety, World Health Organization, Geneva, Switzerland

* * *

Participants at June 2004 Meeting of Chapter Authors

Professor R.S. Chauhan, Joint Director, Centre for Animal Disease Research and Diagnosis, Indian Veterinary Research Institute, Izatnagar, India

Professor J.W. Cohen Tervaert, Department of Clinical and Experimental Immunology, University Hospital Maastricht, Maastricht, The Netherlands

Professor K. Conrad, Institute of Immunology, Medical Faculty, Technical University of Dresden, Dresden, Germany

Dr J. Damoiseaux, Department of Clinical and Experimental Immunology, University Hospital Maastricht, Maastricht, The Netherlands

Dr W.H. de Jong, Laboratory for Toxicology, Pathology and Genetics, National Institute for Public Health and the Environment, Bilthoven, The Netherlands

Professor M.L. de Souza Querioz, Department of Pharmacology, Faculty of Medical Sciences, State University of Campinas, Campinas, SP, Brazil

Dr D.R. Germolec, National Institute of Environmental Health Sciences, National Institutes of Health, Research Triangle Park, NC, USA

Professor M. Ohsawa, Department of Toxicology and Environmental Health, Faculty of Pharmaceutical Sciences, Teikyo University, Sagamiko, Kanagawa, Japan

Dr R.H.H. Pieters, Institute for Risk Assessment Sciences — Immunotoxicology, Universiteit Utrecht, Utrecht, The Netherlands

Professor N.R. Rose, Department of Molecular Microbiology and Immunology, School of Hygiene and Public Health, Johns Hopkins University, Baltimore, MD, USA

Professor H. van Loveren, Laboratory for Toxicology, Pathology and Genetics, National Institute for Public Health and the Environment, Bilthoven, The Netherlands

Dr J.G. Vos, Laboratory for Toxicology, Pathology and Genetics, National Institute for Public Health and the Environment, Bilthoven, The Netherlands

Secretariat

Ms K. van Londen, International Programme on Chemical Safety, World Health Organization, Geneva, Switzerland

Ms C. Vickers, International Programme on Chemical Safety, World Health Organization, Geneva, Switzerland

* * *

Final Task Group Members

Professor J.W. Cohen Tervaert, Department of Clinical and Experimental Immunology, University Hospital Maastricht, Maastricht, The Netherlands

Dr C. Colosio, International Centre for Pesticides and Health Risk Prevention, University Hospital Luigi Sacco, Milan, Italy (*Co-Rapporteur*)

Dr G.S. Cooper, National Institute of Environmental Health Sciences, National Institutes of Health, Research Triangle Park, NC, USA

Dr E. Corsini, Laboratory of Toxicology, Department of Pharmacological Sciences, University of Milan, Milan, Italy (*Co-Rapporteur*)

Dr J. Damoiseaux, Department of Clinical and Experimental Immunology, University Hospital Maastricht, Maastricht, The Netherlands

Professor J. Descotes, Centre Antipoison, Centre de Pharmaco-vigilance, Lyon, France (*Co-Rapporteur*)

Dr D.R. Germolec, National Institute of Environmental Health Sciences, National Institutes of Health, Research Triangle Park, NC, USA

Dr/Professor M. Løvik, Division of Environmental Medicine, Norwegian Institute of Public Health, and Department of Environmental Immunology, Norwegian University of Science and Technology, Oslo, Norway

Dr M.I. Luster, National Institute for Occupational Safety and Health, Morgantown, WV, USA (*Co-Rapporteur*)

Professor M. Ohsawa, Department of Toxicology and Environmental Health, Faculty of Pharmaceutical Sciences, Teikyo University, Sagamiko, Kanagawa, Japan

Professor M. Pallardy, INSERM UMR-S 461, Faculté de Pharmacie Paris-Sud, Châtenay-Malabry, France (*Co-Rapporteur*)

Dr R.H.H. Pieters, Institute for Risk Assessment Sciences — Immunotoxicology, Universiteit Utrecht, Utrecht, The Netherlands

Professor N.R. Rose, Department of Pathology, Molecular Microbiology and Immunology, School of Medicine and Public Health, Johns Hopkins University, Baltimore, MD, USA

Professor H. van Loveren, Laboratory for Toxicology, Pathology and Genetics, National Institute for Public Health and the Environment, Bilthoven, The Netherlands (*Chairman*)

Secretariat

Mrs S. Kunz, International Programme on Chemical Safety, World Health Organization, Geneva, Switzerland

Ms C. Vickers, International Programme on Chemical Safety, World Health Organization, Geneva, Switzerland

ACRONYMS AND ABBREVIATIONS

AChR	acetylcholine receptor
ADH	alcohol dehydrogenase
AIDP	acute inflammatory demyelinating polyneuropathy
AIH	autoimmune hepatitis
AIHA	autoimmune haemolytic anaemia
AIRE	autoimmune regulator
ALDH	aldehyde dehydrogenase
ALPS	autoimmune lymphoproliferative syndrome
AMAN	acute motor (and sensory) axonal neuropathy
ANA	antinuclear antibody
ANCA	antineutrophil cytoplasmic antibody
AnolA	antinucleolar antibody
APECED	autoimmune polyendocrinopathy with candidiasis and ectodermal dysplasia
APGS	autoimmune polyglandular syndrome
APS	antiphospholipid syndrome
ATPase	adenosine triphosphatase
BTK	Bruton's tyrosine kinase
CI	confidence interval
CIE	counter-immunoelectrophoresis
CREST	calcinosis, Raynaud phenomenon, oesophageal dysmotility, telangiectasias
CRH	corticotropin-releasing hormone
CTLA-4	cytotoxic T lymphocyte antigen-4
CVID	common variable immunodeficiency
CYP	cytochrome P450
DALD	Dianzani autoimmune lymphoproliferative disease
DCM	dilated cardiomyopathy
DEPAP	1,2-di-oleyl ester of 3-(N-phenylamino)-1,2-propanediol (PAP)
DHA	docosahexaenoic acid
DM	dermatomyositis
DNA	deoxyribonucleic acid
DNMT	DNA methyltransferase

DRESS	drug rash with eosinophilia and systemic symptoms
ds	double-stranded
Dsg	desmoglein
dSSc	diffuse systemic sclerosis
EAE	experimental allergic encephalomyelitis
EBT	ethylidenebis[L-tryptophan]
EHC	Environmental Health Criteria
ELAM-1	endothelial leukocyte adhesion molecule-1
ELISA	enzyme-linked immunosorbent assay
ELISPOT	enzyme-linked immunosorbent spot
EPA	ecoisapentaenoic acid
ERK	extracellular signal-regulated kinase
FcγR	receptors of the Fc portion of immunoglobulin G
FEIA	fluorescent enzyme immunoassay
GABA	gamma-aminobutyric acid
GAD	glutamic acid decarboxylase
GBM	glomerular basement membrane
GBS	Guillain-Barré syndrome
GM-CSF	granulocyte–monocyte colony stimulation factor
HIGM	hyper IgM syndrome
HIT	heparin-induced thrombocytopenia
HIV	human immunodeficiency virus
HLA	human leukocyte antigen
Hp	haptoglobin alpha
HPA	hypothalamic–pituitary–adrenocortical
HSP	heat shock protein
IA2	insulinoma antigen 2
IAA	insulin autoantibodies
IBD	inflammatory bowel disease
ICA	islet cell antibodies
ICAM-1	intercellular adhesion molecule-1
IDDM	diabetes mellitus type 1 or insulin-dependent diabetes mellitus
IFN	interferon
Ig	immunoglobulin
IIF	indirect immunofluorescence

IL	interleukin
ILO	International Labour Organization
iNOS	inducible nitric oxide synthase
IPCS	International Programme on Chemical Safety
IPEX	immunodysregulation, polyendocrinopathy, enteropathy, X-linked syndrome
IRF	interferon regulatory factor
ITP	immune (idiopathic) thrombocytopenic purpura
KLH	keyhole limpet haemocyanin
LFA-1	lymphocyte function-associated antigen-1
LKM1	liver–kidney microsome type 1
lSSc	limited systemic sclerosis
LTE	leukotriene
LTT	lymphocyte transformation test
MBP	major basic protein
MEPAP	3-oleyl-ester of 3-(N-phenylamino)-1,2-propanediol (PAP)
MFS	Miller Fisher syndrome
MG	myasthenia gravis
MHC	major histocompatibility complex
MICA	MHC class I chain related gene A
MOG	myelin oligodendrocyte glycoprotein
MPO	myeloperoxidase
mRNA	messenger ribonucleic acid
MS	multiple sclerosis
MuSK	muscle-specific kinase
NK	natural killer
NOD	non-obese diabetic
nRNP	nuclear ribonucleoproteins
OR	odds ratio
oxLDL	oxidized low-density lipoproteins
PAA	3-(phenylamino)-L-alanine
PADI	peptidylarginine deiminase
pANCA	perinuclear antineutrophil cytoplasmic antibody
PAP	3-(N-phenylamino)-1,2-propanediol
PBC	primary biliary cirrhosis

PCB	polychlorinated biphenyl
PCDD	polychlorinated dibenzo-p-dioxins
PCDF	polychlorinated dibenzofurans
PD-1	programmed cell death 1
PF	pemphigus foliaceus
PF4	platelet factor 4
PGE	prostaglandin
PHA	phytohaemagglutinin
pia	pristane-induced arthritis
PM	polymyositis
PR3	proteinase 3
PSC	primary sclerosing cholangitis
PV	pemphigus vulgaris
PWM	pokeweed mitogen
RA	rheumatoid arthritis
RIA	radioimmunoassay
RID	radial immunodiffusion
RO	Responsible Officer
RR	risk ratio
SIgAD	selective IgA deficiency
sIL-2R	soluble IL-2 receptor
SLE	systemic lupus erythematosus
Sm	Smith (antigen)
SSc	systemic sclerosis
ssDNA	single-stranded DNA
T1D	diabetes mellitus type 1
T3	triiodothyronine
T4	thyroxine
TAP	transporters associated with antigen processing
TBM	tubular basement membrane
TCDD	2,3,7,8-tetrachlorodibenzo-p-dioxin
TCR	T cell receptor
TCRB	T cell receptor β
TGF	transforming growth factor
Th	T cell helper
TLR	Toll-like receptor

TNF	tumour necrosis factor
TNP	trinitrophenol
TNP-OVA	trinitrophenol-ovalbumin
tRNA	transfer ribonucleic acid
TSH	thyroid-stimulating hormone
TSHR	thyroid-stimulating hormone receptor
tTG	tissue transglutaminase
TTP	thrombotic thrombocytopenic purpura
UN	United Nations
UNEP	United Nations Environment Programme
VNTR	variable number of tandem repeats
WHO	World Health Organization
XLA	X-linked agammaglobulinaemia

1. SUMMARY

Autoimmunity is characterized by the reaction of cells (autoreactive T lymphocytes) or products (autoantibodies) of the immune system against the organism's own antigens (autoantigens). It may be part of the physiological immune response ("natural autoimmunity") or pathologically induced, which may eventually lead to development of clinical abnormalities ("autoimmune diseases"). Many different autoimmune diseases can occur, but all are characterized by the inappropriate or excessive immune response against autoantigens, leading to chronic inflammation, tissue destruction, and/or dysfunction. To date, more than 60 diseases have a proven or strongly suspected autoimmune etiology.

Generally, autoimmune diseases are perceived to be relatively uncommon. However, when all autoimmune diseases are combined, the estimated prevalence is high (3–5% of the general population), which underlines their importance to public health. Because of difficulties in diagnosis and in designing and standardizing epidemiological studies, limited data are available, and the prevalence may actually be underestimated. Nonetheless, there is epidemiological evidence of increasing prevalence of certain autoimmune diseases in highly industrialized countries, which cannot be attributed to better diagnosis alone. Furthermore, there is growing evidence that autoimmune mechanisms may play a role in many other diseases (atherosclerosis, for instance).

Autoimmune diseases are multifactorial. Both intrinsic factors (e.g. genetics, hormones, age) and environmental factors (e.g. infections, diet, drugs, environmental chemicals) may contribute to the induction, development, and progression of autoimmune diseases. Environmental factors are believed to be a major factor responsible for their increased prevalence. Environmental factors operating in a genetically susceptible host may directly initiate, facilitate, or exacerbate the pathological immune process, induce mutations in genes coding for immunoregulatory factors, or modify immune tolerance or regulatory and immune effector pathways.

Drug-induced autoimmune or autoimmune-like disorders and hypersensitivity are of major concern and often the reason for withdrawing drugs from the market or restricting their use. Systemic allergy is not well understood and is often considered idiosyncratic, but it may be of an allergic or autoimmune nature. We have learned much about the mechanisms of idiosyncratic autoimmune diseases by studying the autoimmune phenomena that result from exposure to therapeutics. In addition, there have been several "point source" outbreaks of autoimmune diseases due to environmental exposures to chemicals such as Spanish toxic oil and L-tryptophan that have advanced our knowledge substantially.

There is now considerable epidemiological evidence pertaining to the association between occupational exposure to crystalline silica dust (quartz) and the risk of several systemic autoimmune diseases (specifically, systemic sclerosis, systemic lupus erythematosus, rheumatoid arthritis, and systemic small vessel vasculitis). Epidemiological studies also support a role of occupational exposure to solvents in the development of systemic sclerosis, but a clear consensus has not developed on the specific exposures or classes of chemicals involved and whether this association extends to other diseases. Some autoimmune diseases (e.g. Graves disease, rheumatoid arthritis) have been associated with tobacco use, particularly among current smokers, but only weak or no associations have been seen with other diseases. Additional experimental research examining the effects of these and other chemical and physical agents, using exposure routes relevant to the human experience in occupational settings or in environmental contamination, is needed to advance our understanding of the pathogenesis of autoimmune diseases. In contrast to the available studies concerning silica, solvents, and smoking, there are relatively few epidemiological data pertaining to the effect of dioxins, pesticides, or heavy metals on the development or progression of autoimmune diseases.

There is also some research on the influence of dietary factors on autoimmune diseases. This is a broad area that includes caloric intake, specific nutrients and foods, and dietary supplements. Coeliac disease is an example of an autoimmune disease with a clear dietary link in which an immunological response to specific proteins in wheat, barley, and rye produces autoantibodies directed against tissue transglutaminase, causing mucosal damage in the small intestine.

Summary

It is highly likely that infection plays a role in many autoimmune disorders, although the infectious agent and mechanism by which it causes disease may differ from one disorder to another. Most hypotheses relating infection to autoimmunity have assumed that infection plays a direct causal role, although it may simply serve as a predisposing factor. Infectious agents may play a role due to sequence homology with endogenous proteins, resulting in "molecular mimicry", and also may act as "priming" agents due to non-specific/polyclonal stimulation of immune factors such as cytokines and co-stimulatory molecules. Hygienic status, resulting in a lack of infectious stimuli, may have an impact on autoimmunity. Chemical agents may play an important role in interacting with infections, an area that has been poorly studied.

There exist a variety of methods to detect enhanced antibody formation and autoantibodies in humans and experimental animals following environmental exposure. In contrast, tests available for measuring the potential of chemicals or environmental factors to produce autoimmune disease or augment existing autoimmune disease are not readily available.

A large number of animal models exist that have been used primarily to explore basic mechanisms and therapeutic possibilities for certain autoimmune diseases. Etiology in the various models is based on genetic predisposition, induction with specific antigens (mostly in combination with an adjuvant), or challenge with infectious agents. Chemical-induced autoimmune disease models are less common. In addition, autoimmunogenic and allergenic effects of compounds are usually not identified in routine toxicity studies, in part because outbred animals are used and relevant parameters are not studied. In addition, outliers are usually discarded from the experiment, whereas in fact outliers may indicate unexpected and idiosyncratic immune effects.

A general strategy to assess the autoimmunogenic potential of chemicals is lacking. One promising approach is the popliteal lymph node assay. This represents a straightforward and robust animal test model that may be used to link direct lymphocyte node reactions to local application of potentially immunoactive chemicals. However, these assays may be predictive of the sensitizing potential, but not necessarily of the autoimmunogenic potential, of agents and do not represent a systemic route of exposure.

The burden on health and heavy costs of autoimmune diseases highlight their importance with regard to risk assessment. Risk assessment of autoimmunity associated with chemical or physical agents should consider available epidemiological data, hazard identification and dose–response data derived from animal and human studies, data related to mode of action, and susceptibility factors. The risk assessment process may eventually help to calculate the cost of autoimmune disease associated with exposure to chemical and physical agents. Currently, the risk assessment for agents that are suspected of inducing or exacerbating autoimmunity or autoimmune diseases is hampered by the fact that appropriate information is not available, particularly validated animal models. Because of the individual- and population-level burden of autoimmune disease, risk assessment with respect to this group of diseases assumes special importance.

2. INTRODUCTION AND DEFINITIONS OF AUTOIMMUNITY AND AUTOIMMUNE DISEASE

Normal functioning of the immune system prevents serious illnesses, such as infections, tumours, and allergic and autoimmune diseases. Exposure to chemicals and drugs may lead to abnormalities in the immune system, such as partial or severe immunosuppression, resulting in reduced defences against microorganisms, virus-infected cells, as well as premalignant and malignant cells. The International Programme on Chemical Safety (IPCS) Environmental Health Criteria monograph 180: *Principles and Methods for Assessing Direct Immunotoxicity Associated with Exposure to Chemicals* (IPCS, 1996) reviewed the cause, consequences, and detection of disorders mediated by "immunotoxicity". The mechanisms, as well as the clinical aspects, epidemiology, hazard identification, and risk assessment of allergy, another type of adverse effect on health produced by harmful immune responses following exposure to certain chemicals or therapeutics, are described in the IPCS Environmental Health Criteria monograph 212: *Principles and Methods for Assessing Allergic Hypersensitization Associated with Exposure to Chemicals* (IPCS, 1999).

Chemical-associated autoimmunity and autoimmune disease represent a third type of adverse effects on health produced by harmful effects of chemicals on the immune system. Kimber & Dearman (2002) reviewed the immunological basis for autoimmunity, including adaptive immunity and maintenance of self-tolerance. Autoimmunity is characterized by the reaction of cells (autoreactive T lymphocytes) or products (autoantibodies) of the immune system against the organism's own antigens (autoantigens). This does not necessarily imply a harmful consequence. Autoimmunity may be part of the physiological immune response ("natural autoimmunity") or pathologically induced without ("autoimmune responsiveness"; subclinical disease) or with ("autoimmune disease") development of clinical abnormalities.

Autoimmune diseases are characterized by the inappropriate or excessive immune response against autoantigens, leading to chronic inflammation, tissue destruction, and/or dysfunction. Autoimmune disease may be defined as a clinical syndrome caused by the activation of T cells or B cells, or both, in the absence of an ongoing infection or other discernible cause. The main measurable feature of an autoimmune disease is the production and long-lasting expression of disease-specific autoantibodies and/or autoreactive T cells. However, the classification of autoimmune disease demands additional evidence, which may be direct, indirect, or circumstantial (Rose, 1996). *Direct evidence* of the autoimmune nature of an autoantibody- and/or cell-mediated disease includes (i) dysfunction producing circulating autoantibodies (target cell damage, receptor stimulation or inhibition, interaction with an enzyme or hormone), (ii) autoantibodies localized to the site of the lesion, (iii) immune complexes containing autoantibodies localized to the site of the lesion, (iv) reproduction of disease by passive transfer of autoantibodies (maternal–fetal transfer producing congenital autoimmune disease, animal models), (v) proliferation of T cells in vitro in response to self-antigen or autoantigen, (vi) induction of disease by xenotransplantation of human target tissue plus injection with sensitized T lymphocytes to immunodeficient mice, and (vii) in vitro cytotoxicity of T cells with cells of the target organ. Much *indirect evidence* is shown by different kinds of animal models, such as experimental immunization, development of spontaneous autoimmunity, and animal models produced by manipulation of the immune system. Other characteristic features (*circumstantial evidence* for the presence of an autoimmune disease) are the association with other autoimmune diseases, the association with major histocompatibility complex (MHC) haplotypes, the lymphocytic infiltration of target organ(s), and the favourable response to immunosuppression. The so-called classical autoimmune disease fulfils at least three criteria of direct evidence as well as almost all of those of the indirect and circumstantial evidence.

Generally, autoimmune diseases are perceived to be rare; however, when all autoimmune diseases are combined, the estimated prevalence of 3–5% is not rare, which underlines their importance in the public health sector. Because of problems in designing and standardizing epidemiological studies and because of the fact that only limited data are available, this prevalence may be underestimated (Jacobson et al., 1997). There is epidemiological evidence of increasing prevalence of some autoimmune diseases (e.g. diabetes mellitus type 1, multiple sclerosis), although the rates for other diseases (specifically, rheumatoid arthritis, or RA) appear to be decreasing (Jacobson et al., 1997; Cooper & Stroehla, 2003). Environmental factors (e.g. exposure to pathogen, components of food, chemicals) may play an important role in this process.

According to the clinical manifestation, autoimmune diseases may be classified as systemic (e.g. systemic lupus erythematosus, or SLE) or as organ-specific (e.g. Graves disease). However, this clinically useful classification does not correspond to the underlying pathogenetic mechanisms. Despite progress in the research of autoimmune processes, the etiologies and pathological mechanisms involved in the development of autoimmune disease are incompletely understood. A multifactorial genesis, including immunological, genetic, endocrine, and environmental factors, is suggested by evidence from both human and animal studies (Shoenfeld & Isenberg, 1990). Different mechanisms, which are not mutually exclusive, may be involved in the induction and progression of pathological autoimmunity; these include genetic or acquired defects in immune tolerance or immunoregulatory pathways, molecular mimicry to viral or bacterial proteins, an impaired clearance of apoptotic cell material, the generation of autoimmunity to cryptic or modified self, adjuvant-like activity, and susceptibility of target organ(s) for the autoimmune attack (Oldstone, 1987; Wick et al., 1989; Flescher & Talal, 1991; Fox et al., 1992; Casciola-Rosen et al., 1997; Vaishnaw et al., 1997; Magistrelli et al., 1999; Andrade et al., 2000; Dean et al., 2000; Asseman & von Herrath, 2002; Filaci & Suciu-Foca, 2002; Grodzicky & Elkon, 2002; Pittoni & Valesini, 2002; Vogel et al., 2002). In most cases, exogenous factors (e.g. radiation, infections, chemicals, foodstuff components, drugs) may play a role in inducing or modulating those or other not yet identified mechanisms. Environmental factors operating in a genetically susceptible host may directly initiate, facilitate, or exacerbate the pathological immune process, induce mutations in genes coding for immunoregulatory factors, or modify immune tolerance or regulatory and immune effector pathways. The search for such factors and the elucidation of their action are therefore of great importance for better understanding the pathogenesis of autoimmune disease as well as for improving the prophylaxis and therapy of these diseases.

The goal of this documentation is to provide a framework for the evaluation of the role of chemical risk factors in the development of autoimmune diseases.

3. INTRODUCTION TO THE IMMUNE SYSTEM: FOCUS ON AUTOIMMUNE MECHANISMS

3.1 Introduction

This chapter introduces the general reader to the fundamental strategies employed by the immune system in carrying out its primary function of protecting the host against infection. In evolutionary terms, the immune response of vertebrate animals represents a consolidation of two systems. The more ancient innate immune system response is shared, to some degree, by all multi-cellular animals. It includes a number of physical, chemical, and biological barriers that combine to prevent or control microbial invasion; together, they stand guard on an immediate and constant basis.

The second, more recently evolved, system provides vertebrates with the acquired or adaptive immune response. Although it requires more time to mount, in terms of several days, adaptive immunity is aimed at a particular pathogen. It is more powerful, but more restricted in its effects. Since the variety of pathogens is increasing and constantly changing, the adaptive immune response needs an extensive capacity for recognition and so has evolved a unique system of gene recombination. At the same time, the adaptive response reconfigures and reuses many of the components of the innate immune response to produce its effects.

Because the adaptive immune response requires the generation of such broad diversity in recognition capabilities, it also recognizes molecules found in the body of the host itself. The self-directed immune response can potentially cause autoimmune disease. In an effort to avoid this harm, the body carefully shapes, regulates, and controls the adaptive immune response. These mechanisms are described in the second half of the chapter.

The fundamental concepts of how immunity develops form the basis for an understanding of how environmental agents can interact with the immune system to trigger autoimmune disease.

3.2 The innate immune response

The word immune derives from the Latin *immunis*, meaning free of burden or free from taxes. During the Middle Ages, it took on a derived meaning of free from disease, and the term now refers to the many strategies employed by the body to avoid or limit infectious (and perhaps malignant) disease. Initial defence is provided by the natural or innate immune response, which provides immediate, non-pathogen-specific resistance to disease. Innate immune defences are inherited and, therefore, generally present from birth. They include external chemical and physical barriers provided by the skin and mucous membranes, as well as various internal defence mechanisms, such as inflammation and phagocytosis.

The skin and mucous membranes represent the first line of defence. The skin provides a formidable physical barrier that very few, if any, microorganisms can penetrate. If, however, the skin is damaged, pathogens can invade, penetrating other parts of the body. The mucous membranes represent much less of a physical barrier, but can call upon a number of defensive devices. These include mucus itself, which entraps many microorganisms, the hair-like cilia of the respiratory passages, which propel inhaled organisms towards locations where they can be expelled by coughing or sneezing, and specific antimicrobial agents, such as the enzyme lysozyme in saliva and tears. The flow of urine retards microbial colonization of the urinary system, and the normal microbial population of the large intestine retards the overgrowth of pathogenic organisms. The strong acidity of gastric juice destroys many ingested microorganisms.

When pathogens penetrate the barriers of skin and mucous membranes, they encounter internal inborn defences. Inflammation is a stereotypic defensive response of the body to most forms of tissue injury, whether chemical, physical, or infectious. The cardinal signs of redness, pain, heat, and swelling serve to localize the infection and recruit cells of the innate immune response. They include the major circulating phagocytic cells, neutrophils, which leave the blood and migrate to inflamed areas. The process involves, first, adherence of the cells to the vascular endothelium of vessels near the damaged tissue site, followed by passage through the endothelial lining and chemotactic attraction to the site of damage. Tissue phagocytes, macrophages, also migrate to the site of inflammation. The phagocytes ingest and, in most cases, destroy the invading pathogens. A subpopulation of lymphocytes, the natural killer (NK) cells, arrives with the ability to kill infectious microorganisms that have taken up residence within tissue cells. In addition to direct action, these cells — the neutrophils, NK cells, and macrophages — secrete a number of cell products (cytokines). They include the interferons (IFN), which interfere with viral reproduction, tumour necrosis factors (TNF), which kill tumour cells and inhibit growth of certain bacteria, and interleukins (IL), which facilitate communication among cells. A group of normally inactive proteins in the blood plasma also becomes activated by inflammatory reactions. They make up the complement system, which may directly destroy certain bacteria and may also promote the later development of adaptive immunity.

Recent studies have shown that pathogens share molecular patterns that activate the innate immune response and influence the later adaptive reaction. For example, many Gram-negative bacteria express lipopolysaccharides on their outer membranes. Lipopolysaccharides interact with Toll-like receptors (TLR) on dendritic cells, macrophages, and neutrophils to induce production of TNF-α and other cytokines.

3.3 The adaptive immune response

3.3.1 *Function*

The innate immune response is broad, nonspecific in the range of pathogens it attacks, and often of limited effectiveness. More potent protection of the body against particular invading pathogens relies upon the subsequent development of adaptive, or acquired, immunity. A substance that provokes a specific immune response is called an antigen. In practice, any foreign material of sufficient size can act as an antigen, be it pathogenic or harmless, living or inanimate. Most antigens are large, complex molecules, such as proteins or carbohydrates. Complete antigens usually have a molecular weight in excess of 10 000 daltons, but even smaller substances, termed haptens, can activate the adaptive immune response if they are complexed with a larger carrier molecule. Adaptive immune responses can be beneficial when they protect against invading pathogens. Sometimes, however, immune responses to seemingly innocuous material can lead to deleterious or even disastrous consequences. Such harmful responses are termed allergies or hypersensitivities.

The two cardinal features of the adaptive immune response are specificity and memory. Specificity is exemplified by the ability of the immune response to distinguish one foreign antigen from another, as well as to distinguish autoantigens from non-autoantigens. Memory is seen when a second encounter with an antigen prompts a more rapid and vigorous immune response to the same antigen. The job of the adaptive immune response, then, is to sort out the virtually limitless array of possible antigens. The task is accomplished by expressing a large number of recognition structures on the surface of lymphocytes. These specialized white blood cells are responsible for immunological specificity and memory. In principle, each of the body's 10^{12} lymphocytes bears a distinctive recognition structure or receptor, providing a sufficient diversity of receptors so that any possible antigenic determinant, or epitope, will find a lymphocyte with a corresponding receptor. In order to generate a sufficient diversity of receptors on their surface, lymphocytes employ a unique system of genetic shuffling and recombination. When they encounter an appropriately configured portion of an antigen, usually in the form of a small sequence of amino acids in a large protein molecule or a few monosaccharide units in a large carbohydrate, the lymphocyte binds the antigenic determinant. The initially small, quiescent lymphocyte then springs into action. It enlarges, becomes metabolically active, and divides repeatedly. Each of the progeny bears the same specific receptor as its progenitor lymphocyte. In a few days, a large clone of lymphocytes emerges, each being the specific receptor. Some of these lymphocytes proceed to provide the specific protection against the invader. Other lymphocytes return to their normal quiescent state in which they persist for long periods of time. On second exposure to the same antigen, a larger number of lymphocytes bearing the specific receptor is available to respond, producing the rapid, vigorous response associated with immunological memory.

Lymphocytes all develop from pluripotential stem cells located in the red bone marrow. Most B cells complete their development in the bone marrow, whereas precursor T cells migrate from the bone marrow to the thymus, where they mature. When mature B cells encounter their corresponding antigen, they proliferate and transform into plasma cells that synthesize and secrete specific antibodies. These are soluble globular proteins (immunoglobulins, Ig) found in blood and other body fluids that bear the same recognition structures as the original lymphocyte. T cells, on the other hand, recognize antigen only when the large antigenic molecule has been cleaved into fragments and incorporated into glycoproteins located on cell surfaces, referred to as MHC products. The MHC differs from one individual to another. Some of the T cells that have matured in the thymus bear a surface marker called CD4, whereas others carry a CD8 marker. CD4 T cells can recognize fragments of antigen complexed with its own type of MHC. The MHC recognized by CD4 T cells, called MHC class II, is displayed on specialized populations of cells, referred to as antigen-presenting cells. They include the same cells mentioned previously. Another population of very important antigen-presenting cells comprises dendritic cells, which are strikingly proficient in taking up soluble molecules. These cells have the ability to cleave antigenic molecules and to incorporate the fragments into the MHC class II structure, so that even naive CD4 T cells can recognize their corresponding antigenic determinants in the company of its identical MHC. The CD4 T cells then enlarge and replicate to produce a clone. Some T cells become memory cells, whereas others initiate a number of important functions of the adaptive immune system. CD4 T cells can interact with antigen-specific B cells, so that the latter become more effective producers of antibody. Without help from T cells, B cells usually produce only the largest, macroglobulin form of antibody, IgM. With T cell help, class switching occurs, so that B cells secrete a different class of antibody, the smaller IgG molecules that can more readily distribute themselves across the tissues or pass through the placenta. At the same time, B cells go through a selective process whereby antibodies of increasing affinity for their respective antigenic determinants are produced, a process referred to as affinity maturation. In this way, antibodies of greater binding capabilities are gradually produced over time. Sometimes, class switching proceeds further to the production of IgA antibodies. These antibodies are especially prominent in secretions, such as saliva or mucosal fluid, where they are in a position to provide an early defence against invading microorganisms.

Finally, as described above, there are subpopulations of CD4 helper T cells that are involved primarily in cell-mediated immunity or antibody-mediated immunity. They are designated Th1 and Th2, respectively. In instances where autoimmune diseases are due primarily to the inflammatory damage, they are associated with Th1 responses, whereas in situations such as immediate hypersensitivity reactions, Th2 responses are predominant.

3.3.2 Aberrant function

In some genetically predisposed individuals, T cell-directed class switching leads to the overproduction of IgE antibodies. This population of antibodies has a particular affinity for mast cells and basophils, cells that contain granules rich in histamine, serotonin, heparin, and other mediators of immediate allergic reactions. The release of these mediators can give rise in animals to anaphylactic reactions characterized by loss of vascular integrity, escape of intravascular fluids, hypovolaemic shock, and sometimes respiratory embarrassment and death. Similar reactions in humans can take the form of asthmatic attacks, hives, rhinitis, or gastrointestinal distress. The reactions are characterized by high levels of antigen-specific IgE and can be demonstrated on humans by the appearance of a wheal and flare response to the particular antigen (or allergen) injected into the skin. The reaction occurs within minutes and is called an immediate skin reaction.

Other adverse reactions can be produced when antibody binds to its counterpart antigen in the bloodstream. Immune complexes may form. If not immediately taken up by phagocytic cells, these complexes can accumulate in capillary beds, such as those found in the skin, the lung, and especially the kidney. Such complexes are able to activate the complement system, inducing an inflammatory response, inflammation that can be extremely damaging to the surrounding tissues. Antibodies can also cause damage when they bind directly to antigens on the surface of tissue cells. Often, these antibodies are directed to autoantigens, as will be discussed in a subsequent section. The cell may suffer injury through activation of complement or through phagocytosis.

In addition to cooperating with B cells in the production of antibodies, CD4 T cells help in the production of a second population of T cells bearing the CD8 marker. These T cells recognize their corresponding, or cognate, antigen presented by MHC class I products. MHC class I is expressed by all nucleated cells, and proteins generated from within the cell are co-expressed with MHC class I on tissue cell surfaces. If CD8 T cells find their cognate antigen on such tissue cells in conjunction with MHC class I, they are capable of destroying the tissue cell. Such cytotoxic reactions are particularly important in controlling infections that reside within cells — for example, infections induced by viruses and other intracellular pathogens. Cancer cells and transplanted tissue cells can also be destroyed by CD8 T cells with the appropriate specificity. If CD8 T cells are capable of recognizing an autologous antigen, autoimmune damage can result, as will be discussed subsequently.

In addition to their direct effects, CD8 T cells, as well as CD4 T cells, produce a number of cytokines when they are activated. Some of them are important in amplifying the immune response itself — for example, by influencing the class of antibody produced. Other cytokines engender inflammatory reactions. Although useful in limiting infection, inflammation may have adverse effects. To protect itself, the body also produces anti-inflammatory cytokines.

Sometimes, materials are presented by tissue cells in conjunction with MHC class I. Under these circumstances, CD8 T cells may recognize these antigens and initiate a local inflammatory reaction. Since these reactions depend upon the migration of cells to the site of the response or local cell proliferation, they appear relatively slowly (requiring two to four days) and are referred to as delayed hypersensitivity reactions. Injection of the offending antigen (or allergen) into the skin to induce a localized inflammatory reaction is called a delayed-hypersensitivity skin test. It is defined as an immune reaction occurring in the absence of antibody.

3.3.3 *Ageing*

The immune response develops, matures, and then declines over the lifespan. Most newborn mammals are unable to produce an effective immune response and depend for protection upon antibody transferred from the mother during the first few days or weeks of life. Antibody of the IgG class crosses the placenta and temporarily protects the newborn. In addition, colostrum can provide IgM and IgG antibody, followed by IgA in the milk. Later, the more mature infant produces its own IgM and then IgG antibody, as well as cell-mediated immunity.

At the other end of the age spectrum, the elderly are often more susceptible to infection because of a general decline in immune function. Although total immunoglobulin levels and the number of T and B cells in the blood do not change perceptively with age, several T cell responses are significantly lower. The reason may be that the thymus, which plays a key role in T cell maturation and proliferation, gradually involutes after puberty. Antibody responses to a number of test antigens also decline in older individuals. In contrast, there is often an increase in restricted, monoclonal immunoglobulins and in autoantibodies (Lambré & Alaoui-Silimani, 1986).

3.4 Mechanisms of self-tolerance

To carry out its function of recognizing the universe of possible molecules, the immune system generates a great diversity of receptors. Inevitably, some of these receptors will react with antigens present in the body of the host itself. Recognition of autoantigens may result in harm to the host, referred to as autoimmune disease. It is important for survival that these self-directed reactions be avoided or limited so that harm does not follow, the phenomenon called self-tolerance.

The mechanisms involved in self-tolerance can be divided into central and peripheral. During the generation of T cells in the thymus, a process of negative selection takes place. Antigens presented to immature T cells during their education by thymic stromal cells result in programmed cell death or apoptosis of those T cells. Many autoantigens are presented in the thymus in this manner, resulting in deletion of the precursors of self-reactive clones. The great majority of T cells die during their sojourn in the thymus, suggesting that many of them are precommitted to autoantigens. B cells undergo a similar process of negative selection in the bone marrow or in lymph nodes. In addition to deletion of self-reactive clones directed to the most critical autologous antigens, B cells may undergo a unique process of clonal editing, which allows them to reformulate the B cell receptor on their surface by reactivating the immunoglobulin recombination process.

Even under the best circumstances, however, clonal deletion must be regarded as incomplete, because many self-reactive B cells and T cells escape to peripheral sites. Self-reactive B cells are evident from their low-affinity IgM products, which form a network of natural autoantibodies found in all normal sera. The presence of self-reactive T cells in the periphery can now be shown directly by the use of peptide tetramers.

The presence of self-reactive T and B cells in the periphery presents a constant risk for the development of autoimmune disease. A number of mechanisms are in place to maintain self-tolerance and avoid the harmful effects of autoimmunity that are responsible for disease. We now know that T cells and B cells require two signals from an antigen-presenting cell in order to proliferate: an antigen-specific stimulus and a nonspecific second signal. Anergy is a state of unresponsiveness of T cells or B cells due to the absence of a required co-stimulatory (second) signal in the presence of the antigen-specific stimulus. Anergy can be overcome by administering the second signal, often in the presence of one of the inflammatory cytokines. Another mechanism of self-tolerance in the periphery is ignorance. The discovery of immunological ignorance resulted from studies in which autoantigen was expressed in tissue, but ignored by the corresponding T cells. An active viral infection can break such ignorance. The destructive power of the immune system requires that control measures be in place to prevent an overexuberant response. Many of these regulatory mechanisms may also play a role in avoiding harmful immunological reactions. A great deal of attention, for example, is now focused on populations of regulatory T cells that are capable of dampening or preventing immune responses. The $CD4^+CD25^+$ regulatory T cells have become a central concept in the immunology lexicon. Although their mechanism of action is still not fully understood, it is thought that these cells can control autoimmunity by preventing T cell activation, expansion, and differentiation during lymph node priming, by controlling T cell trafficking to tissues as well as their activation and effector function development (Bluestone & Tang, 2005). Other cells, including macrophages, double-negative T cells (lacking both CD4 and CD8 on their surface), and NK T cells (which have markers of both NK and T cells), have also been shown to suppress autoimmune reactions.

3.5 Immunopathogenesis of autoimmune disease

Autoimmune diseases can affect any site and any organ system in the body. Therefore, their clinical manifestations vary greatly. Some general principles, however, underlie the immunopathogenesis of all of the autoimmune diseases. Most autoimmune diseases are currently considered to depend upon the activation of self-reactive CD4 helper T cells.

3.5.1 *Mechanisms of induction*

There is compelling evidence, described above, that central tolerance induced by negative selection is incomplete and that self-reactive B cells and T cells find their way to peripheral sites. These cells are normally quiescent due to the mechanisms of anergy, ignorance, or suppression. The induction of autoimmunity begins by overcoming one of these peripheral mechanisms. Self-reactive B cells are rather easily activated, as shown by the common presence of natural autoantibodies in normal sera. The critical step, in most cases, is the triggering of self-reactive CD4 T cells. Historically, the earliest mechanism proposed was based on the premise that certain autologous antigens are anatomically sequestered from the immune apparatus. Indeed, there are barriers that normally impede the easy entrance of immunologically competent cells into the lens of the eye, the sperm in the testes, and, to some extent, the brain. More modern research has suggested that the barriers are more physiological than anatomical and may depend upon the local expression of signals that initiate apoptosis of activated T lymphocytes. Moreover, the general notion of sequestration has re-emerged as the doctrine of cryptic epitopes. Immune responses may be induced to antigens that were masked or cryptic, but revealed due to foreign agents (Sercarz et al., 1993). This concept suggests that certain epitopes of autologous proteins are unlikely to be expressed by the tolerance-inducing, antigen-presenting stromal cells in the thymus. Therefore, T cells reactive with these cryptic determinants are most likely to escape central tolerance and, if they are encountered in the periphery, are the ones most likely to initiate autoimmune responses.

A second possible mechanism to initiate an autoimmune response is based on the concept of molecular mimicry. It is well known that microorganisms often bear epitopes closely resembling epitopes of autoantigens. An encounter with a cross-reacting antigen from an invading microorganism may initiate a response that affects the similar autoantigen. In fact, rising titres of autoantibodies are frequently found following infection by many different microorganisms. There are, however, few, if any, clear examples of molecular mimicry actually causing human disease. Although it is well documented that streptococcal pharyngitis may precipitate rheumatic fever in susceptible individuals, we are only beginning to define the antigen(s) of the streptococcus that can reproduce the typical pathogenetic manifestations of the disease (see also chapter 9).

Another possible mechanism to explain the origin of autoimmunity is based on the premise that foreign agents, including infectious organisms, environmental chemicals, and radiation, may alter an autoantigen in a manner that makes it antigenic and/or immunogenic. The immune response to the altered "self" may then extend to the unaltered autologous antigen. While there are many experiments demonstrating the production of antibody to altered autoantigens, there are, as yet, no good examples of situations where they are clearly responsible for an autoimmune disease.

The infectious process affects changes in the body of the host that favour the induction of autoimmunity. Many microorganisms produce superantigens that activate an entire family of T cells. Superantigens are toxins that bind to MHC class II molecules, forming a complex; the complex is subsequently recognized by T cells bearing the appropriate variable β chain elements, resulting in the stimulation of large numbers of T cells. Some members of the T cell family may be committed to responding to autoantigens and could thereby initiate an autoimmune response. In the past, we have often compared the effects of infection with the actions of complete Freund's adjuvant, a mixture of mineral oil and bacterial bodies that is known to combine with antigen, to enhance immune responses, and to favour the transition from harmless to pathogenetic autoimmunity. The infectious process itself can act like an adjuvant: it can drive B cells to differentiate into antibody-producing cells that produce the natural autoantibodies so often seen following infection. There are instances, moreover, where class switching results in IgG antibodies, indicating that helper T cells may also be activated, perhaps through the infectious process. Inadequate affinity maturation of adaptive responses can be harmful, as the host responds not only to the infectious agent, but also to closely related autoantigens.

Affinity maturation may lead to the production of high-affinity autoantibodies with pathogenetic potential. Moreover, self-reactive effector T cells may also be generated and induce autoimmune disease. These effects may even be apparent in dealing with memory T cells, suggesting that an infection occurring long after the initial sensitization of the host to autoantigen can cause an enhanced autoimmune response.

The mechanisms described above are likely to be involved in the induction of organ-localized autoimmune diseases, where damage is largely confined to a single organ or cell target, such as seen in diabetes mellitus type 1, chronic lymphocytic thyroiditis, or multiple sclerosis. An alternative mechanism by which autoimmunity may arise is a defect in negative selection in the thymus and a failure of clonal deletion to rid the periphery of self-reactive T cells. Such a defect in clonal deletion is most likely to give rise to multiple autoimmune responses, such as seen in the generalized or systemic autoimmune diseases (e.g. systemic lupus erythematosus). The MLr/lpr/lpr mouse is an example of an animal carrying a genetic defect in the expression of Fas, a receptor involved in the induction of extrinsic apoptosis pathways, leading to impaired intrathymic apoptosis and faulty negative selection. These animals characteristically produce a large spectrum of autoantibodies similar to those seen in human cases of lupus.

As stated previously, the critical event in the progression from a harmless autoimmune response to autoimmune disease is activation of self-reactive, $CD4^+$ helper T cells. This event requires presentation of the appropriate autoantigen on an MHC-compatible antigen-presenting cell, such as a macrophage, dendritic cell, or B cell. Once activated, the T cells amplify the immune response to the point where the body's natural homeostatic mechanisms are no longer able to contain the dangerous reaction. The amplification mechanisms include epitope spread, which involves the recruitment of additional antigenic determinants on the self-reactive antigen molecule. We distinguish this intramolecular epitope spreading from immune escalation, which describes the extension of the autoimmune response to other antigenic molecules in the same target organ. It is characteristic of almost all of the autoimmune diseases that multiple autoantibodies are produced after the disease is under way, probably reflecting an adjuvant effect. For these reasons — epitope spread and immune escalation — it is difficult to define the original

Introduction to the Immune System

autoantigenic determinant responsible for initiation of an autoimmune disease in human cases. Thus, the use of animal models, where the disease can be induced under controlled conditions, can provide important insights into this process. In addition, prospective epidemiological studies that examine the development, persistence, and progression of autoantibodies before the clinical expression of disease can also advance our understanding of the etiology of autoimmune diseases in humans. Several studies of this type are now being conducted in diabetes mellitus type 1 research (Parks et al., 2004b).

3.5.2 Effector mechanisms

The mechanisms used by the immune system to respond to invading microorganisms are presumably the same ones that are involved in response to autoantigens. The important factors determining the cytotoxic mechanisms involved in any situation include the accessibility of the antigen to the immune effectors as well as the quality and quantity of the immune response itself. There is some heuristic value in distinguishing Th1 responses from Th2 responses, although this dichotomy is rarely clear-cut or complete. This dichotomy is largely based on mouse studies that may not entirely apply to human beings or all animal species. In general, Th1 responses are characterized by production of IFN-γ, resulting in a robust CD8 cytotoxic T cell production, and, in the mouse, antibodies in the IgG2a subclass. Th2 responses are primarily associated with IL-4 production and with the appearance of IgG1 and IgE antibody in the mouse. Thus, broadly speaking, Th1 responses are thought of as cell-mediated, whereas Th2 responses are associated with antibody-mediated effector mechanisms.

Among the autoimmune diseases, a direct demonstration of pathogenetic mechanisms has been possible until now only with antibody-mediated disorders. Antibodies in general can act upon antigens available at the cell surface. Antibodies to blood cells are responsible for the haemolytic anaemias and thrombocytopenias, either through enhanced phagocytosis by reticuloendothelial cells or by complement-mediated lysis. Antibodies to receptors on the surface of a tissue cell may block or stimulate the receptors and produce functional effects, such as the muscle weakness of myasthenia gravis, where the acetylcholine receptor is blocked, or Graves disease, where the thyrotropin receptor is stimulated to produce hyperthyroidism. Pemphigus vulgaris and bullous pemphigoid are due to antibodies that destroy intercellular substances that hold together cells of the skin, inducing blister or bullous formation. In lupus, multiple autoantibodies to cellular antigens are produced. The most important antibodies from a clinical point of view are directed to components of the cell nucleus. When these nuclear antigens are released into the bloodstream, they combine with autoantibody to produce immune complexes that can deposit in capillary beds in the brain, skin, kidneys, and other organs, where they induce a pathogenetic inflammatory response.

Autoimmune diseases affecting solid organs are believed to be caused mainly by T cell-mediated Th1 mechanisms. This has been proved as far as diabetes mellitus type 1 is concerned; however, it is not certain whether this also applies to any other autoimmune diseases, such as thyroiditis or hepatitis (Atkinson & Eisenbarth, 2001). Because T cells have greater access to tissue sites than do antibodies, self-reactive T cells will localize and proliferate in the targeted organ. They produce inflammatory cytokines, suggesting that most of the T cells present in tissue-localized sites are attracted by relatively non-antigen-specific inflammatory signals. Once present, the T cells can induce a number of damaging effector mechanisms. Cytotoxic CD8 T cells can act directly on targets in an antigen-specific manner and perhaps are predominant mediators of cell injury in such diseases as multiple sclerosis and diabetes mellitus type 1, as suggested by studies of animal models. Indirect injury may occur through T cell products, such as lymphotoxin or tumour necrosis factor. If B cells are also present, local production of antibody may occur and is often suggested by the presence of germinal centres in the affected organ. Finally, T cells activate macrophages, which produce a long list of injurious products, including reactive oxygen and nitrogen intermediates.

3.6 Summary

Although the autoimmune diseases are quite disparate clinically, they are united by common pathobiological mechanisms. Their signature is an immune response directed to an antigen present in the body of the host, shown by the presence of circulating autoantibodies, even if tissue damage may be due to T cells. This immune response can be initiated by a foreign or an autologous antigen and follows the rules of all adaptive immune responses. Its onset and subsequent course are determined in some measure by the initial innate immune response, which directs the subsequent adaptive immune reaction. Because of the amplification that accompanies the immune response, autoimmunity is a common event following any antigen stimulus. There are homeostatic mechanisms that tend to control autoimmune responses and to limit their pathological effects. These mechanisms include both central tolerance, which aborts the production of T and B cells, and peripheral mechanisms, which hold self-reactive T cells and B cells in check. When these mechanisms fail due to a combination of inborn genetic traits and/or environmental factors, autoimmune responses can result. Once the autoimmune response has reached a threshold level and the appropriate effector mechanism is mobilized, autoimmune disease is the consequence.

4. INTRINSIC FACTORS IN AUTOIMMUNITY

4.1 Genetic factors involved in the induction of or susceptibility for autoimmune diseases

The etiologies and pathological mechanisms involved in the development of autoimmune diseases are incompletely understood. Genetic as well as environmental factors are responsible for the induction, development, and progression of most autoimmune diseases. The familial clustering and the higher rate of concordance for autoimmune disease in monozygotic compared with dizygotic twins indicate that genetic factors are important determinants of susceptibility to autoimmune disease. The highest rates of monozygotic twin concordance, 25–35%, have been reported in systemic lupus erythematosus (Cooper et al., 1999), whereas the concordance rate is much lower (5%) in systemic sclerosis and is similar to that seen in dizygotic twins (Feghali-Bostwick et al., 2003). Thus, the relative contribution of environmental influences may vary among the autoimmune diseases; even in systemic lupus erythematosus, however, it is clear that genetics alone cannot explain the etiology of the disease.

Only a few autoimmune syndromes are probably due to mutations in a single gene (Table 1). In the majority of autoimmune diseases, a multigenic process with multiple susceptibility genes working in concert is suggested. In theory, all genes coding for products that are involved in the induction and maintenance of self-tolerance and in regulating immune effector functions as well as organ-specific functions may be involved in the mosaic of pathogenesis. The research on monogenic autoimmune syndromes has shown the importance of mutations in defined proteins acting in the Fas-mediated T cell apoptosis, thymic negative selection, and the development and activation of regulatory T cells.

4.1.1 *Probable monogenic autoimmune syndromes*

Human autoimmune syndromes in which one gene seems to be responsible for the development of the disease have been rarely described so far (Bennett et al., 1995; Fisher et al., 1995; Rieux-Laucat et al., 1995; Drappa et al., 1996; Vogel et al., 2002).

Table 1. Gene defects in human monogenic autoimmune syndromes

Gene defect	Mechanism	Syndrome
Mutations in the AIRE-1 gene coding for the autoimmune regulator protein	Impaired self-tolerance by failure in the induction to thymic negative selection	Autoimmune polyendocrinopathy with candidiasis and ectodermal dysplasia (APECED) or autoimmune polyglandular syndrome type 1 (APGS 1)
Mutations in the FOXP3 gene	Impaired development and functional activity of regulatory $CD4^+CD25^+$ T cells	Immunodysregulation, polyendocrinopathy, enteropathy, X-linked syndrome (IPEX)
Mutations in the FAS gene	Impaired self-tolerance by preventing the elimination of activated peripheral T cells	Autoimmune lymphoproliferative syndrome (ALPS) type Ia
Mutations in the FAS-L gene		ALPS-Ib
Mutations in the CASP10 gene		ALPS-II
Probably mutations hitting the FAS signalling pathway downstream from FAS		ALPS-III, Dianzani autoimmune lymphoproliferative disease (DALD)

Mutations in genes coding for transcription factors that are critically involved in tolerance induction (e.g. AIRE, FOXP3) seem to be the major cause of autoimmune syndromes associated with immunodeficiency and immune dysregulation. The autoimmune polyendocrinopathy with candidiasis and ectodermal dysplasia syndrome (APECED), also known as autoimmune polyglandular syndrome type 1 (APGS 1), is characterized by the loss of self-tolerance to multiple organs caused by defective negative selection in the thymus due to mutations in the AIRE (autoimmune regulator) gene (Vogel et al., 2002; Park et al., 2003). Immunodysregulation, polyendocrinopathy, enteropathy, X-linked syndrome (IPEX), another syndrome with multiple organ-specific (endocrine) autoimmune manifestations, is caused by mutations in FOXP3, a master control gene for the development and function of $CD4^+CD25^+$ T cells (Bennett et al., 2001; Owen et al., 2003). This regulatory T cell population is involved in the maintenance of peripheral self-tolerance by actively suppressing the activation and expansion of self-reactive T cells (Shevach, 2000).

Deficiencies in the Fas apoptosis pathway may cause a variety of autoimmune lymphoproliferative syndromes (Fisher et al., 1995; Rieux-Laucat et al., 1995; Drappa et al., 1996; Dianzani et al., 1997; Wang et al., 1999). The autoimmune lymphoproliferative syndrome (ALPS) or Canale-Smith syndrome, characterized by lymphadenopathy/splenomegaly, autoimmune cytopenias, and expanded populations of double-negative ($CD3^+CD4^-CD8^-$) T cells, is caused by mutations in the Fas, the Fas ligand, or caspase 10 gene (Fisher et al., 1995; Rieux-Laucat et al., 1995; Drappa et al., 1996; Wang et al., 1999). Other variants of autoimmune lymphoproliferative syndromes (e.g. ALPS-III or Dianzani autoimmune lymphoproliferative disease, DALD) may be due to mutations hitting the Fas signalling pathway downstream from Fas (Dianzani et al., 1997). In mice, mutations in the Fas receptor (lpr) or its ligand (gld) are associated with lymphadenopathy and lupus-like autoimmunity (Nagata & Suda, 1995).

Although in most cases the described syndromes are inherited, it cannot be excluded that environmental as well as additional genetic factors may interact, which may explain the wide spectrum of disease signs and symptoms, the possibility of manifestations in adulthood, and the healthy state of parents carrying mutations (Rieux-Laucat et al., 1999; Deutsch et al., 2004). In this sense, these syndromes are not truly monogenic. The development of autoimmune lymphoproliferative syndromes seems to require accumulations of several genetic defects involved in apoptosis (Ramenghi et al., 2000).

4.1.2 Multigenic autoimmune diseases

Compared with the autoimmune polyglandular and autoimmune lymphoproliferative syndromes described above, all other known autoimmune diseases and syndromes may not be inherited; nonetheless, genes are responsible for differences in the susceptibility for disease development. Multiple genes, acting in concert with various environmental factors, seem to be involved in the autoimmune pathogenesis of most autoimmune diseases (see chapter 9).

4.1.2.1 Immune deficiencies

Many primary immunodeficiency syndromes in which genetic defects are known or suggested are associated with a variety of autoimmune manifestations. A selection of immunodeficiencies together with their associated autoimmune manifestations is shown in Table 2. Immune dysregulation, persistent antigen stimulation, recurrent tissue damage, and defective clearance of immune complexes are pathogenetic factors that may lead to autoimmunity in immunodeficient individuals (Etzioni, 2003).

Table 2. Association of immunodeficiency with autoimmune diseases in humans

Immunodeficiency	Gene defect(s)	Autoimmune disease
X-linked agammaglobulinaemia (XLA): lack of mature immunoglobulin-producing B cells	Mutations in Bruton's tyrosine kinase (BTK)	Arthritis, dermatomyositis, autoimmune haemolytic anaemia (AIHA), scleroderma
Common variable immunodeficiency (CVID): not a single disease, various degrees of defective antibody production	Unknown; susceptibility locus termed IGAD1 in the HLA-DQ/DR region	Cytopenias, intestinal diseases, arthritis, hepatitis, Guillain-Barré syndrome (GBS)
Selective IgA deficiency (SIgAD)	Unknown; susceptibility locus termed IGAD1 in the HLA-DQ/DR region	Systemic lupus erythematosus (SLE), rheumatoid arthritis (RA), coeliac disease, and many other autoimmune manifestations
Hyper IgM syndrome (HIGM)	Mutations in the CD40L	Neutropenia, other cytopenia, arthritis, sclerosing cholangitis
Complement deficiencies (C1q, C2, C3, C4)	Deletions, insertions, and point mutations in the complement factor encoding genes	SLE
Defensin deficiency	Mutation in NOD2	Crohn disease

1) Selective IgA and common variable immunodeficiency

The most common primary immunodeficiency syndromes are selective IgA deficiency (SIgAD) and common variable immunodeficiency (CVID), characterized by defect(s) in the terminal stage of lymphocyte differentiation leading to impaired production of one or more immunoglobulin isotypes. In both diseases, autoimmunity is very common and occurs in 10–36%. Autoimmune response, which is not necessarily pathogenetic, may be the first presentation prior to the diagnosis of immunodeficiency. It has been suggested that both primary immunodeficiency syndromes may be a part of a spectrum of disease caused by common genetic factor(s) (Hammarstrom et al., 2000). Recently, it has been shown that HLA-DQ/DR is the major susceptibility locus. Furthermore, immunogenic, immunological, and clinical features strongly suggest that (at least a part of) SIgAD/CVID is not inherited but autoimmune in nature (Kralovicova et al., 2003). Thus, SIgAD/CVID may provide a helpful model for the study of the pathogenesis of autoimmune disease.

2) Complement deficiencies

Deficiencies of early components of the classical complement pathway (e.g. C1q, C1r/C1s, C2, C3, C4) are associated with the development of systemic lupus erythematosus. The prevalence of systemic lupus erythematosus in homozygous C1q, C4, or C2 deficiency is approximately 90%, 75%, and 10–30%, respectively. The strongest susceptibility genes for the development of systemic lupus erythematosus in humans are null mutants of C1q. Several findings are compatible with the hypothesis that complement deficiency causes systemic lupus erythematosus by the failure to clear immune complexes and apoptotic cells (Botto, 2001). In consequence, uncleared apoptotic bodies may provide the source of the autoantigens that drive the autoimmune response of systemic lupus erythematosus.

3) Defensin deficiency

Clinical observations, immunological and genetic studies, as well as animal models and therapeutic approaches suggest that the initial event in the development of Crohn disease, even if not necessarily causative, might not be characterized by a loss of self-tolerance but rather resembles an immunodeficiency (Folwaczny et al., 2003). Decreased α-defensin expression and impaired induction of human β-defensins 2 and 3 have been found in patients with Crohn disease, especially if associated with NOD2 mutations

(Fellermann et al., 2003). The deficient induction of β-defensins may be due to mutations of the intracellular peptidoglycan receptor NOD2 and to changes in the intracellular transcription by NFκB. The resulting deficient mucosal barrier function may lead to a permanent but slow bacterial invasion, triggering the inflammatory process and probably autoimmunity.

4.1.2.2 Defects and dysregulation in apoptosis pathways and cell cycle regulation

A breakdown in the balance between survival and apoptosis (programmed cell death) has been implicated in a number of autoimmune diseases by different mechanisms (Vaishnaw et al., 1997; Pittoni & Valesini, 2002). For example, (i) defects in apoptotic pathways may promote the survival of potentially autoreactive cells, (ii) failure to eliminate activated cells can result in prolonged effector cell function, (iii) accelerated apoptosis may account for autoantigen selection, and (iv) impaired clearance of apoptotic cells may modify the balance between tolerance induction and activation of T cells. Thus, genetic defects of molecules regulating apoptosis may be involved in autoimmune disease development (Table 3). In mouse models of lupus-like autoimmunity with lymphadenopathy, mutations in Fas or its ligand (FasL) have been described (e.g. Chu et al., 1993; Nagata & Suda, 1995). In humans, mutations of Fas, FasL, and other proteins of the Fas signalling pathway are associated with a variety of autoimmune lymphoproliferative syndromes (see section 4.1.1, Table 1). In patients with systemic lupus erythematosus, however, such mutations seem to be vary rare (Vaishnaw et al., 1997). On the other hand, Fas expression in lymphocytes of patients with systemic lupus erythematosus and other systemic autoimmune diseases is often increased, and Fas gene or Fas promotor gene polymorphisms associated with the development of systemic lupus erythematosus have been described (Horiuchi et al., 1999; Kanemitsu et al., 2002).

Many regulators of the cell cycle are also involved in regulation of apoptosis. There is growing evidence that some of these genes are also dysregulated in autoimmune animal models as well as in patients with autoimmune disease (for examples, see Table 3). In particular, the cell cycle blockade at the G_0/G_1-phase could be a major factor in the apoptosis resistance and accumulation of activated/memory T cells in systemic autoimmunity. The expression of the cell cycle inhibitor p21 is upregulated in lupus patients and autoimmune-prone mice (Lawson et al., 2004). Moreover, p53 is upregulated in T cells of lupus patients, and this upregulation correlates with disease activity (Liu et al., 2000).

Table 3. Proteins involved in different pathways of apoptosis and genetic defects or polymorphisms that may be involved in the pathogenesis of autoimmune diseases

Mechanism	Involved proteins	Genetic defects or polymorphisms in animal models (a) or human autoimmune disease (b)
Apoptosis inducers (ligands)	FasL TNF-α TRAIL	FasL gene mutations: (a) lupus-prone mice; (b) ALPS (see Table 1), SLE (vary rare)
Apoptosis receptors (death receptors)	Fas TNFRI, TNFRII	Fas gene mutations: (a) lupus-prone mice; b) ALPS (see Table 1), SLE (very rare)
		Fas gene and promotor gene polymorphism: (b) SLE
Signal transducers and intracellular regulators	Caspases Serin proteases Bcl-2 family	Bcl-2 knockout mice: (a) development of lymphomas or SLE-like features
		CASP10 gene mutation: (b) ALPS (see Table 1)
Apoptotic cell clearance factors	Collectins (e.g. C1q)	(a) Mer receptor: Mer^{kd} mouse (Scott et al., 2001)
	Scavenger receptors (e.g. Mer)	(b) Homozygous C1q deficiency: SLE (see section 4.1.2.1)
Apoptosis regulators at cell cycle checkpoint	p53 p21$^{WAF1/Cip1}$ Mdm2 Survivin	p53 mutations: (b) RA synoviocytes (Firestein et al., 1997; Han et al., 1999)
		p21 deletion: (a) inhibition of spontaneous autoimmunity (Lawson et al., 2004)
Apoptosis protectors	LMP2/NF-κB	LPM2 promoter mutation: (a) NOD mice (model for diabetes mellitus type 1) (Kühtreiber et al., 2003)
Immunoregulatory signals (Rosenblum et al., 2004)	CD200 (OX-2)	CD200 knockout: (a) mice prone to induction of autoimmune disease (Hoek et al., 2000)

In summary, inherited or acquired mutations in genes encoding regulators of the cell cycle and/or apoptosis may not only increase the risk of cancer development but also predispose to autoimmunity. Furthermore, environmental factors influencing the expression of such genes may be of importance for autoimmune disease development.

4.1.2.3 Associations with MHC alleles or haplotypes

Genetic susceptibility to most, if not all, autoimmune diseases is predominantly associated with genes of the MHC. The MHC consists of a large number of highly polymorphic genes, most of which are essential to the immune system, including genes encoding human leukocyte antigen (HLA). Certain MHC haplotypes or alleles are associated with susceptibility or resistance to specific autoimmune diseases (Table 4). It is important to note that those associations can be different in different ethnic groups and are (in most cases) not caused by mutant alleles that are exclusively found in patients. Positive associations may be interpreted as either a direct involvement of a given allele in disease pathogenesis or the involvement of genes that are in linkage disequilibrium with the test allele. HLA alleles/haplotypes may contribute to autoimmune disease susceptibility by presentation of triggering peptide epitopes in the periphery and/or by ineffective presentation of autoantigens in the thymus, which leads to more aggressive T cells or fewer numbers of regulatory T cells. Besides "epitope selection" (Gregersen et al., 1987), other mechanisms, such as the differential expression of HLA class II genes, may also account for disease susceptibility and progression (Heldt et al., 2003).

1) MHC class I genes

Only some autoimmune diseases are almost exclusively associated with MHC class I alleles of the HLA-A, HLA-B, or HLA-C locus. One of the strongest MHC disease associations is between HLA-B27 and the spondyloarthropathies, especially ankylosing spondylitis and reactive arthritis. B27 molecules seem to play a direct role in disease pathogenesis (David, 1997). Although the exact mechanism is unknown, it has been shown that HLA-B27 is capable of presenting potentially "arthritogenic" peptides to cytotoxic T cells (Bowness, 2002).

Table 4. Examples of some important associations between MHC region genes and autoimmune-like diseases

Disease	MHC allele/haplotype association(s)
Behcet disease	Complete absence of the TAP1C allele.[a] Linkage disequilibrium between HLA-DQB1*0501 and TAP2B (González-Escribano et al., 1995).
Coeliac disease (gluten-sensitive enteropathy)	Nearly all cases are associated with HLA-DQ2 (DQA1*05/DQB1*02) or HLA-DQ8 (DQA1*0301/DQB1*0302) (Sollid & Thorsby, 1993). HLA-DQ2 is expressed in up to 95%. The expression of these HLA-DQ2 or HLA-DQ8 molecules is necessary, but not sufficient, to develop the disease. Gluten-reactive T cells recognize peptides from gluten in the context of HLA-DQ2 or HLA-DQ8 (Lundin et al., 1993).
Multiple sclerosis	In the European population, susceptibility to multiple sclerosis is associated with HLA-DR2 (DRB1*1501) and HLA-DQ6 (DQB1*0602) (Dyment et al., 2004).
Psoriatic arthritis	HLA-Cw*0602 and MICA-A9[b] appear to be the strongest genetic susceptibility factors for psoriatic arthritis (González et al., 2002).
Rheumatoid arthritis (RA)	In most Caucasian populations, susceptibility to (or severity of) RA is due to a closely related set of polymorphic sequences (the "shared epitope") on several different HLA-DRB1 alleles, especially certain subtypes of the DR4 and DR1 allelic families (Gregersen et al., 1987; Nepom, 1998). Some genetically distant populations exhibit a different association (e.g. HLA-DR9 in Native Americans, HLA-DR3 in RA patients from Finland) (Hakala et al., 1997). Ferucci et al. (2005) found genetic susceptibility to the development of RA in the American Indian/Alaskan Native populations at least partially associated with different HLA alleles, such as HLA-DRB1*1402, among other possible genetic factors yet elucidated.
Spondyloarthropathies	HLA-B27 is a very strong disease susceptibility marker. The relative risk for ankylosing spondylitis is up to 150. Under the influence of environmental and other inherited factors (e.g. MHC class II alleles), HLA-B27 seems to be directly involved in the development of spondyloarthropathies (Westman et al., 1996; David, 1997; Khan, 2000; Bowness, 2002). The HLA-linked LMP2 gene is involved in the expression of ankylosing spondylitis (Maksymowych et al., 1995).
Systemic lupus erythematosus (SLE)	Three class II-containing risk haplotypes have been identified: DRB1*1501 (DR2)/DQB1*0602, DRB1*0801 (DR3)/DQB1*0402, and DRB1*0301 (DR3)/DQB1*0201 (Graham et al., 2002).

Table 4 (Contd)

Disease	MHC allele/haplotype association(s)
Diabetes mellitus type 1 (T1D)	In Caucasians, T1D is strongly associated with HLA-DR3 and HLA-DR4 alleles. Diabetes risk is particularly high for individuals with DR3/4 and DR4/4 genotypes, which contain DQB1 alleles carrying non-Asp at residue 57 (Ronningen et al., 1992). In contrast, certain MHC haplotypes (e.g. HLA-DRB1*1501/DQB1*0602) provide significant protection, with protection dominant over susceptibility (Nepom, 1993).

[a] TAP: transporters associated with antigen processing, genes map in MHC class II region.
[b] MICA: MHC class I chain related gene A.

Besides classical MHC class I genes, other polymorphic genes of the MHC I region may also be susceptibility markers, such as the MHC class I chain related gene A (MICA). MICA-A9 has been described as a strong genetic susceptibility marker for psoriatic arthritis (González et al., 2002).

2) *Classical MHC class II genes*

Most autoimmune diseases are primarily associated with MHC class II polymorphism within the HLA-DR, HLA-DQ, and HLA-DP loci — e.g. HLA-DR2 with systemic lupus erythematosus, multiple sclerosis, Addison disease, Graves disease, and myasthenia gravis; HLA-DR4 with rheumatoid arthritis; and HLA-DR3/DR4 with diabetes mellitus type 1. Most of the MHC class II associations can be accounted for by sequence polymorphisms in the hypervariable regions of the HLA-DQB1, HLA-DRB1, and/or HLA-DPB1 genes. Through high-resolution typing of class II alleles by either polymerase chain reaction-based oligotyping or nucleotide sequencing, specific disease-associated alleles or sequences have been identified. To show the complexity of MHC/disease associations, we will focus on rheumatoid arthritis. Other examples are shown in Table 4.

In most Caucasian populations with rheumatoid arthritis, genetic susceptibility is conferred by HLA-DRB1 alleles that share a common amino acid sequence ("shared epitope") in the third hypervariable region of the HLA-DRB1 chain (amino acids 70–74: QRRAA, QKRAA, RRRAA) (Gregersen et al., 1987; Nepom,

1998). The shared epitope may serve as the binding site for an arthritogenic peptide or may itself be the autoantigen that activates T cells. Homozygosity for the rheumatoid arthritis-associated HLA-DRB1 alleles has been associated with a more severe course of the disease. In a population-based study, only weak associations between rheumatoid arthritis and specific shared epitope alleles, with the exception of the clearly distinct influence of HLA-DRB*0404, have been shown (Thomson et al., 1999). In another study, no important allelic differences between patients with mild disease and controls could be observed (Khani-Hanjani et al., 2002). Ferucci et al. (2005) found genetic susceptibility to the development of rheumatoid arthritis in the American Indian/Alaskan Native populations at least partially associated with different HLA alleles, such as HLA-DRB1*1402, among other possible genetic factors yet to be elucidated.

In conclusion, there is a variable strength of positive association of high-risk alleles and a preferential expression in patients with severe disease. HLA-DRB1 alleles encoding an aspartic acid at position 70 protect against development of rheumatoid arthritis even in individuals carrying one shared epitope positive allele (Mattey et al., 2001). Interestingly, a striking gene–environment interaction between smoking and shared epitope alleles was seen for rheumatoid factor positive rheumatoid arthritis (Padyukov et al., 2004). The molecular mechanisms for this interaction are not yet known. Substances in the smoke may induce modifications of the potential autoantigen or deliver neoantigens that might be bound to shared epitope-containing alleles or might act as adjuvants. Furthermore, the gene involved in the gene–environment interaction may be not the shared epitope-carrying allele but a gene in linkage disequilibrium with the shared epitope allele.

3) *Non-classical MHC class II genes*

Besides polymorphisms in classical MHC class II genes, other genes of the MHC II region, such as HLA-DMA and HLA-DMB, as well as genes involved in the HLA class I- and class II-associated antigen processing pathways (e.g. LMP2, LML7, TAP1, TAP2), may influence autoimmune disease susceptibility (González-Escribano et al., 1995; Maksymowych et al., 1995; Yen et al., 1999).

4) MHC class III genes

The MHC class III region maps between the MHC class I and class II gene clusters and contains genes for tumour necrosis factor, heat shock protein 70, and some components of the complement system (for review, see Arnett & Moulds, 1991). Many proteins coded by MHC class III genes may be involved in the development of autoimmunity. The importance of deficiencies in complement factors has been described in subsection 2) of section 4.1.2.1. The role of tumour necrosis factor gene polymorphisms is shown in section 4.1.2.2.

4.1.2.4 *Polymorphisms in genes coding for regulatory and effector molecules of the immune system*

Theoretically, polymorphisms in all genes that code for molecules involved in regulatory or effector pathways of the immune system may be associated with autoimmune disease development. In the following, we will focus on some important examples.

1) Polymorphisms in receptors of the immune system

Receptors of antigen recognition and presentation: The T cell repertoire is shaped by negative and positive selection based on T cell interaction with antigen-presenting cells. Genotype-specific differences in this process could be the basis for associations between HLA genes and autoimmune diseases (see section 4.1.2.3). The involvement of the trimolecular complex of T cell receptor (TCR)–peptide–HLA suggests that an autoimmune susceptibility allele of TCR might confer susceptibility only in individuals with a specific HLA allele. Germline polymorphisms in the variable regions of the T cell receptor β (TCRB) gene complex have been found associated with rheumatoid arthritis among individuals possessing HLA-DR4 allele(s) and pauciarticular-onset juvenile idiopathic arthritis among patients with HLA-DQA1*0101 (Charmley et al., 1994; Mu et al., 1996).

Receptors of the Fc portion of IgG: Receptors of the Fc portion of IgG (FcγR) play a role in handling immune complexes as well as in clearance of apoptotic cells. Functionally polymorphic genes encoding FcγRIIA, FcγRIIIA, and FcγRIIIB have been implicated as genetic factors in determining the pathogenesis and course of many autoimmune diseases (van der Pol & van de Winkel, 1998). Associations have been reported for systemic lupus erythematosus, rheumatoid arthritis, Wegener granulomatosis, myasthenia gravis, multiple sclerosis, and Guillain-Barré syndrome. In patients with systemic lupus erythematosus, polymorphisms in Fcγ RIIA, FcγRIIIA, and FcγRIIIB have been shown to be associated with clinical manifestations and disease course (Manger et al., 2002). Another study provided genetic evidence supporting a role for a physiologically relevant single nucleotide polymorphism of the FcγIIIA gene in the pathophysiology of systemic lupus erythematosus (Edberg et al., 2002). Furthermore, it has been observed that low-affinity FcγR alleles (FcγRIIA-R131 and FcγRIIIA-F176) were inherited independently and were present at higher frequency in patients with systemic lupus erythematosus. FcγRIIA is implicated as a possible disease-modifying gene in rheumatoid arthritis (Brun et al., 2002). Patients homozygous for the FcγRIIA-R allele have less efficient binding of the IgG2 subclasses than patients homozygous for the H allele. Thus, a genetically defined modulation of processing of circulating immune complexes may contribute to disease severity in rheumatoid arthritis.

CD28 family of receptors: The CD28 family of structurally related proteins expressed on T cells and activated B cells, of which CD28 is a member, also includes cytotoxic T lymphocyte antigen-4 (CTLA-4). These receptors are important in regulating antigen responsiveness by controlling the production of cytokines. Polymorphisms in regulatory regions of genes coding for the immunoinhibitory receptors programmed cell death 1 (PD-1) and CTLA-4 are important for autoimmune disease susceptibility. Both receptors have a critical role in downregulating T cell activation, which has a profound impact on inflammation and autoimmunity (Salomon & Bluestone, 2001). The gene encoding human CTLA-4 contains multiple polymorphisms, certain of which affect the expression and function of the protein. Also, regulatory polymorphisms in the PD-1 coding gene PDCD1 exist that may influence T cell regulation, affecting susceptibility for autoimmune diseases.

Cytokine and chemokine receptors: An association between systemic sclerosis and polymorphisms in the CXCR-2 gene has been reported (Renzoni et al., 2000).

2) Polymorphisms of mediators of the immune system

Gene polymorphisms that affect the function or the level of expression of regulatory or effector molecules of inflammation, fibrosing, or other pathological processes involved in autoimmune disease development have been observed, for example, in systemic sclerosis (transforming growth factors TGFβ1, TGFβ2, TGFβ3), juvenile idiopathic arthritis (IL-1β), rheumatoid arthritis (IL-4), systemic lupus erythematosus (IL-10), Sjögren syndrome (IL-10), juvenile idiopathic inflammatory myopathies (IL-1RA), and Wegener granulomatosis (IL-10) (McDowell et al., 1995; Cantagrel et al., 1999; D'Alfonso et al., 2000; Rider et al., 2000; Susol et al., 2000; Anaya et al., 2002; Crilly et al., 2002; Zhou et al., 2002). In many autoimmune diseases (e.g. systemic lupus erythematosus, rheumatoid arthritis, Behcet disease, coeliac disease, inflammatory bowel diseases, and diabetes mellitus type 1), various TNF-α promoter or microsatellite polymorphisms have been found. The tumour necrosis factor polymorphism may be part of a disease-associated MHC haplotype (due to linkage disequilibrium) and represents a haplotype-dependent association (Hajeer et al., 1996; Sturfelt et al., 1996). Nevertheless, tumour necrosis factor polymorphisms as independent susceptibility factors for rheumatoid arthritis and systemic lupus erythematosus have been described in some populations (Martinez et al., 2000; Rood et al., 2000; Parks et al., 2004b). Such polymorphisms may be directly involved in pathogenesis, because TNF-α is known to be the strongest inflammatory factor and a major candidate for long-lasting immune response modifications, and associations of in vitro TNF-α production with tumour necrosis factor microsatellite polymorphisms have been reported (Pociot et al., 1993).

4.1.2.5 Hormones and genes

Immunomodulating influences of estrogens, androgens, and gonadotropins seem to be important for the disproportionate number of women with autoimmune diseases, especially with systemic lupus erythematosus and rheumatoid arthritis (see section 4.2). An altered sex hormone metabolism (e.g. peripheral estrogen hydroxylation, increased aromatase activity) may predispose to or modify autoimmune disease development (Cutolo et al., 2004). The hormone metabolism as well as effects of sex hormones on the immune system (cell growth, differentiation and activation, apoptosis) could be genetically influenced at different levels (e.g. at the level of hormonal structure, metabolizing enzymes, hormonal receptor alleles). In contrast, hormones may be involved in the regulation of the expression of a number of genes that are important for mediating immune responses. It has been hypothesized that prolactin modulates the biological activities of immune cells through the activation of the transcription factor gene, interferon regulatory factor-1 (IRF-1) (Yu-Lee et al., 1998). The prolactin gene is in close proximity to the HLA complex, and genotype aberrations could be genetically linked to disease predisposition in some subsets of patients with systemic lupus erythematosus. A functionally significant polymorphism that alters prolactin promoter activity and mRNA levels in lymphocytes has been demonstrated (Stevens et al., 2001a). Furthermore, a linkage disequilibrium between HLA-DRB1 susceptibility alleles and microsatellite marker alleles close to the prolactin gene among women with rheumatoid arthritis and systemic lupus erythematosus has been described (Brennan et al., 1997). Another example of hormonal involvement in inflammatory processes is corticotropin-releasing hormone (CRH), a key regulator of anti-inflammatory glucocorticoid release. Genetic variation at the CRH locus is linked to and associated with rheumatoid arthritis (Fife et al., 2000). Further studies are necessary to understand the genetic background of hormonal influences on the immune system.

4.1.2.6 Genetic polymorphisms of xenobiotic-metabolizing enzymes

Genetic polymorphisms of xenobiotic-metabolizing enzymes may result in expression of inactive enzymes or enzymes with a reduced or increased metabolic activity (Daly, 1995). For example, the incidence of hydralazine- and procainamide-induced lupus is higher or the disease starts earlier in individuals with the slow acetylator phenotype caused by mutant NAT-2 alleles than in individuals exhibiting the fast-acetylator phenotype (Woosley et al., 1978; von Schmiedeberg et al., 1999).

The generation of protein adducts and neoantigens is another mechanism of drug-induced autoimmunity that is modulated by the polymorphism of metabolizing enzymes. Patients with dihydralazine-induced hepatitis are more often of the slow-acetylator phenotype (Siegmund et al., 1985). They produce autoantibodies against cytochrome P4501A2 (CYP1A2) due to a higher risk of adduct formation, because slow-acetylators can use only the pathway mediated by CYP1A2 for detoxification of dihydralazine. Polymorphisms of genes encoding *S*-mephenytoin 4-hydroxylases (CYP2C19) or organic solvent-metabolizing enzymes (CYP2E1) are associated with systemic sclerosis. The CYP2E1*3 allele seems to be involved in increased susceptibility to scleroderma among individuals who have been exposed to organic solvents (Povey et al., 2001). These findings need to be confirmed.

In conclusion, associations with genetic polymorphisms of xenobiotic-metabolizing enzymes would indirectly point to xenobiotics as etiological agents of immune-mediated diseases and may provide information as to the type of chemical compound to be searched for (Griem et al., 1998). It is important to note that the research on polymorphisms of metabolizing enzymes in relation to xenobiotics may reveal novel insights into gene–environment associations. For example, a 3-fold increased risk of systemic lupus erythematosus associated with 24 or more months of occupational sun exposure with GSTM1 null genotype was observed, although the authors did not find any association of glutathione-*S*-transferase with an increased risk of lupus, nor did they find any association of occupational sun exposure with an increased risk of lupus (Fraser et al., 2003).

4.1.2.7 *Genes coding for autoantigens*

Germline and acquired mutations as well as polymorphisms of genes that code for autoantigens may be susceptibility factors or even involved in the development of autoimmune disease.

1) Mutations

The expression of mutated autoantigens may be one mechanism of the break of immune tolerance against self. For example, a mutant La mRNA was isolated from an La/SS-B antibody-positive patient with systemic lupus erythematosus (Bachmann et al., 1996). The expression of mutant La in experimental mice results in systemic autoimmunity (Bachmann, 2004), most likely by an impaired regulation of the cell cycle inhibitor p21 (see also section 4.1.2.2).

2) *Polymorphisms*

The thyroglobulin gene is both linked and associated with autoimmune thyroid diseases and therefore is likely a susceptibility gene for these diseases (Tomer et al., 2002). An important susceptibility locus for diabetes mellitus type 1 (called IDDM2) maps upstream of the human proinsulin gene to a variable number of tandem repeats (VNTR) (Bennett et al., 1995). Homozygosity at the INS VNTR class I allele is associated with up to 5 times increased risk for diabetes mellitus type 1, whereas the class III alleles are dominantly protective (Bennett et al., 1995). Because insulin expression in the thymus is modulated by INS VNTR alleles at the IDDM2 locus (the class I allele is associated with lower and the class III VNTR allele with higher levels of proinsulin mRNA expression in the thymus), effects in terms of central tolerance appear to influence the risk of developing diabetes mellitus type 1 (Pugliese et al., 1997, 2001). An intron 3 polymorphism of the Ro52 gene (coding for a Sjögren syndrome and systemic lupus erythematosus autoantigen) is strongly associated with the presence of Ro52 autoantibodies in patients with Sjögren syndrome (Nakken et al., 2001).

4.1.2.8 *Genes coding for enzymes involved in post-translational modification of autoantigens*

Post-translational modifications that generate neo-epitopes from self-proteins can be involved in the induction of autoimmunity (Anderton, 2004). Such modifications may be influenced by exogenous and genetic factors. The only genetic association so far has been described for rheumatoid arthritis: a case–control linkage disequilibrium study identified a haplotype associated with susceptibility in peptidylarginine deiminase type 4 (PADI4) but not in neighbouring PADI genes (Suzuki et al., 2003). PADI4 is one of five known PADI genes that code enzymes to change arginine into citrulline, which is important in generating rheumatoid arthritis-specific autoimmunity. The rheumatoid arthritis susceptibility haplotype in PADI4 produces a more stable transcript and is associated with higher levels of autoantibody to citrullinated peptides.

4.1.2.9 DNA methylation

Altered gene expression due to changes in DNA methylation is implicated in the pathogenesis of autoimmunity (Richardson, 2003). Endogenous as well as exogenous (e.g. ultraviolet radiation, drugs, diet) factors can alter DNA methylation patterns. Two lupus-like disease-inducing drugs (procainamide, hydralazine) have been reported to inhibit DNA methylation, cause overexpression of the adhesion molecule LFA-1, and induce autoreactivity in human and murine T cells (Yung et al., 1995). Furthermore, age-dependent changes in T cell DNA methylation may contribute to the development of some forms of autoimmunity in the elderly (reviewed in Richardson, 2002).

4.1.3 Problems and perspectives

In the etiologically complex autoimmune diseases, multiple genes and environmental factors may interact in different ways to initiate or modify disease development. This makes it very difficult to search for disease-specific initiating or modifying factors. With regard to genetic factors, there may be incomplete penetrance (i.e. not all susceptible individuals are affected), several disease susceptibility loci, interaction between these loci, and heterogeneity (i.e. different alleles may cause disease in different groups). Therefore, it is difficult to localize disease genes, ascertain the number and relation of disease loci involved, understand modes of inheritance and interaction effects, and understand the mechanisms by which these genetic changes give rise to disease (Lander & Schork, 1994).

The heterogeneity of most of the systemic but also organ-specific autoimmune diseases is an additional important factor that complicates genetic analyses. Careful disease classification is necessary, and differentiation of subgroups according to clinical presentation, autoantibody production, ethnic background, as well as environmental exposures may be helpful. The risk associated with one genetic risk factor for an autoimmune disease may be strongly influenced by the presence of an environmental factor, as has been shown for smoking and shared epitope alleles or sun exposure and GSTM1 allele (Fraser et al., 2003; Padyukov et al., 2004). Therefore, genes/alleles with no or weak disease association may also be involved in gene–environment interactions. For better understanding of the complex nature of autoimmune diseases, it is very important to search for the involved genetic and xenobiotic factors and their interactions.

4.2 Hormonal influence on autoimmunity

4.2.1 Pregnancy

4.2.1.1 Suppression of autoimmunity

While the mechanisms of protection against rejection of the fetus are not well understood, the immune status in pregnant women is generally characterized as having localized immunosuppression or tolerance and elevated systemic immune responses. Fetal cytokines may downregulate the production of proinflammatory cytokines in the mother, shifting the balance of the maternal immune environment towards Th2 dominance. Other factors, including corticosteroids, maternal cytokines, estrogens, prostaglandins, and pregnancy-associated proteins, may affect the Th1/Th2 balance. Pregnancy has been associated with an amelioration of Th1-mediated autoimmune diseases, including multiple sclerosis, psoriasis, rheumatoid arthritis, thyroiditis, and uveitis. Graves disease frequently becomes quiescent during pregnancy, with a corresponding decrease in antithyroid microsomal, antithyroglobulin, and thyroid-stimulating antibody levels (Amino et al., 2003; Shah et al., 2003). Similar reductions in circulating autoantibodies have been reported in patients with subclinical autoimmune hepatitis (Izumi et al., 2003). For some diseases, particularly multiple sclerosis and Graves disease, the exacerbation rate is increased in the first several months following delivery (Tamaki et al., 1993; Confavreux et al., 1998). However, it has been suggested that, at least for multiple sclerosis, past history of relapse is the best indicator of clinical course during gestation and postpartum (Dwosh et al., 2003). Postpartum thyroiditis has been estimated to occur with a prevalence rate of 7.2% in women who were asymptomatic prior to pregnancy; while the majority of women become euthyroid within the first year, approximately 25%

will develop permanent hypothyroidism (Stagnaro-Green, 2002). The risk of developing new-onset rheumatoid arthritis is significantly decreased during pregnancy; however, it is markedly increased in the postpartum period (Silman et al., 1992).

4.2.1.2 Stimulation of autoimmunity

In contrast to the putative protective effects of pregnancy on Th1-mediated diseases, there have been reports of a worsening of symptoms in autoimmune diseases with strong Th2 components, such as systemic lupus erythematosus (Petri et al., 1991; Ruiz-Irastorza et al., 1996; Huizinga et al., 1999). However, there is still considerable debate as to whether patients with lupus have flares of the disease (Khamashta et al., 1997). Physiological changes that commonly occur during pregnancy, such as tiredness, mild proteinuria, elevated complement levels, and thrombocytopenia, mimic lupus activity and have made the diagnosis of pregnancy-associated flares fairly complicated (Boumpas et al., 1995; Ruiz-Irastorza et al., 2004). An accurate definition of lupus flare in pregnancy is of significant clinical relevance, as lupus-associated renal disease may mask life-threatening conditions, such as pre-eclampsia. Recently developed and validated diagnostic tools may provide a more accurate platform to clarify the risk of increased disease onset and/or exacerbation during pregnancy (Ruiz-Irastorza et al., 2004).

A number of mediators have been suggested to be responsible for the shift from Th1 to Th2 immunity during pregnancy and the corresponding protective effects for autoimmune diseases with Th1-mediated pathogenesis. These include early pregnancy factor, estriol, human chorionic gonadotropin, prolactin, gender-related hormones such as estrogen and progesterone, and vitamin D derivatives. In laboratory rodents, early pregnancy factor has been shown to suppress clinical signs of experimental autoimmune encephalomyelitis and reduce the proliferation of antigen-specific T cell clones in response to myelin basic protein (Harness & McCombe, 2001; Harness et al., 2003). Studies of other hormones that increase during pregnancy and decrease during the early postpartum period have shown similar effects. Using murine T cells, Miyaura & Iwata (2002) demonstrated that progesterone and glucocorticoids might interact to induce a shift to the Th2 phenotype during pregnancy. The production of IL-12, a critical factor in the proliferation and differentiation of Th1 effector cells, is inhibited in human macrophages following treatment with cortisol or 1,25-dihydroxyvitamin D3 (Lemire et al., 1995; Elenkov et al., 1996). Moreover, monocytes taken from women in the third trimester of pregnancy showed a reduced capacity to produce IL-12 and TNF-α, and the alterations in cytokine production paralleled significant increases in urinary cortisol, 1,25-dihydroxyvitamin D3, estrogen, and progesterone (Elenkov et al., 2001). Similarly, Soldan et al. (2003) reported decreased production of TNF-α and increased production of the Th2-promoting cytokines IL-5 and IL-10 in multiple sclerosis patients receiving estriol treatment. In a pilot study, these authors reported an inverse association between increased estriol levels and relapsing/remitting multiple sclerosis, where the changes in cytokine profiles correlated with decreases in enhancing lesion volume and number compared with pretreatment baseline values (Soldan et al., 2003). It is clear that multiple factors may be involved in the protective effect of these factors during pregnancy. Oral estrogen treatment alone, either through the use of oral contraceptives or as hormone replacement therapy, does not appear to be protective for progression of either rheumatoid arthritis or multiple sclerosis (Hall et al., 1994; Hernán et al., 2000; Drossaers-Bakker et al., 2002).

Although the hormone prolactin is most commonly recognized for its role in the promotion and support of lactation, there is increasing evidence that it functions as a cytokine in immune tissues (Pellegrini et al., 1992; Sabharwal et al., 1992). Prolactin is structurally related to growth-promoting cytokines such as erythropoietin and granulocyte–monocyte colony stimulation factor (GM-CSF; Horseman & Yu-Lee, 1994), and prolactin receptors are members of the cytokine receptor superfamily. Elevated serum prolactin levels have been associated with disease flares that occur during pregnancy and the postpartum period in individuals with systemic lupus erythematosus, rheumatoid arthritis, and multiple sclerosis (Neidhart, 1998). The genes encoding prolactin and its receptor map to regions with linkage to autoimmune disease, and several studies have suggested the prolactin and prolactin receptor genes as candidates for susceptibility genes. Brennan et al. (1997) studied DNA from a cohort of European women with systemic lupus erythematosus or rheumatoid arthritis and found excess frequency of specific marker alleles close to the prolactin gene, suggesting that there may be linkage disequilibrium between the

HLA-DRB1*0301 and HLA-DRB1*0401 alleles and the prolactin gene. Stevens et al. (2001b) characterized the T→G^{-1149} polymorphism in the lymphocytic promoter in the human prolactin gene. In a cohort study of 143 patients with systemic lupus erythematosus from the United Kingdom, there was a significant association with the −1149 extrapituitary promoter polymorphism genotype in the patient group compared with a group of control subjects ($P = 0.047$ for comparison of genotypes). These authors suggest that the polymorphism increases prolactin production in T cells, contributing to B cell activation and antibody production (Stevens et al., 2001b). Mellai et al. (2003) screened 19 prolactin and prolactin receptor single gene polymorphisms in DNA from Italian patients with systemic lupus erythematosus or multiple sclerosis. In a subset of 147 patients with systemic lupus erythematosus and 98 controls, these authors examined the T→G^{-1149} prolactin gene polymorphism that had been found previously to be associated with systemic lupus erythematosus. In contrast to the findings of Stevens et al. (2001b), these studies found no differences in the expression of the allele between the patients and controls. Discrepancies in the two studies may be explained by variations in the HLA distribution in the two study populations (Mellai et al., 2003).

Laboratory studies also support the association between elevated prolactin levels and autoimmune disease. Lupus-prone NZB×NZW mice receiving syngeneic pituitary transplants to simulate prolactin concentrations expected during pregnancy demonstrated elevated IgG levels, increased frequency of autoantibodies, and accelerated renal disease compared with sham-operated controls (McMurray et al., 1991). Treatment with the dopaminergic antagonist bromocriptine, which suppresses prolactin release or suppresses the release of other compounds that modulate serum prolactin levels, has been shown to ameliorate disease progression in rodent models of antiphospholipid syndrome, systemic lupus erythematosus, and multiple sclerosis (McMurray et al., 1991; Riskind et al., 1991; Tomita et al., 1993; Blank et al., 1995; Neidhart, 1997). Clinical studies in relatively small numbers of patients have evaluated the efficacy of bromocriptine treatment in patients with systemic lupus erythematosus (McMurray et al., 1995; Alvarez-Nemegyei et al., 1998).

4.2.2 Psychological stress

There is also evidence to suggest that a number of autoimmune diseases such as diabetes mellitus type 1 and multiple sclerosis may be exacerbated by factors such as psychological stress. This is not surprising, given the degree of reciprocal interactions between the immune system and the central nervous system. Stress activates the hypothalamic–pituitary–adrenocortical (HPA) axis to ultimately release glucocorticoids and catecholamines, which modulate immune function. Deficient corticosteroid production has been suggested as a factor in the progression and pathogenesis of rheumatoid arthritis, as there appears to be a blunting of the HPA axis in patients with rheumatoid arthritis (Masi & Chrousos, 1996). Alterations in the HPA axis have also been observed in patients with Sjögren syndrome and systemic lupus erythematosus (Gutierrez et al., 1998; Johnson et al., 1998). Although the linkage between psychological stress and disease was recognized in the early 19th century, the study of actual risk has been challenging due to differences in definition of stressors, limited follow-up, and generally small sample sizes (J. Li et al., 2004). A meta-analysis of 14 studies showed a significant increase in risk of exacerbation of multiple sclerosis following stressful life events (Mohr et al., 2004). However, a number of other studies have shown equivocal results or improvement of multiple sclerosis, suggesting that different stressors may influence disease outcomes in different ways (Nisipeanu & Korczyn, 1993; Goodin, 2004).

The interactions between the immune and nervous systems and the potential mechanisms by which psychological stress can influence autoimmune diseases are still poorly understood; however, laboratory studies are providing some mechanistic insights. Transgenic mice with a dysfunctional glucocorticoid receptor had reduced susceptibility to experimental allergic encephalomyelitis (EAE), the experimental model for multiple sclerosis (Marchetti et al., 2001). Changes in disease susceptibility were associated with decreased T cell proliferation and increased macrophage activity. The secretion of glucocorticoids and catecholamines has been shown to be increased in mice subjected to restraint stress, and in vivo administration of these factors augmented Fas ligand-mediated cytotoxicity of self-reactive NK T cells (Oya et al., 2000).

5. CLINICAL EXPRESSION OF HUMAN AUTOIMMUNE DISEASES

5.1 Introduction

To date, more than 60 diseases have a proven or suspected autoimmune etiology. Table 5 lists the most important systemic autoimmune diseases that are, in general, clinically manifest in multiple organs; Table 6 categorizes most of the organ-specific autoimmune diseases based on the organ system that is involved. It remains a matter of debate how to prove that a given disease is indeed an autoimmune disease. For some autoantibody-mediated autoimmune diseases (e.g. pemphigus and myasthenia gravis), there is clear agreement that the adaptive immune response to an autoantigen causes the observed pathology. Other diseases, such as coeliac disease and inflammatory bowel diseases, have an autoimmune component, but the role of autoimmunity in their pathogenesis is not clear.

Table 5. Systemic autoimmune diseases

Systemic autoimmune disease	Section
ANCA-associated vasculitis	5.3
Churg-Strauss syndrome	5.3
Microscopic polyangiitis	5.3
Wegener granulomatosis	5.3
Antiphospholipid syndrome	5.4
CREST syndrome	5.23
Dermatomyositis	5.15
Henoch-Schönlein purpura	ND
Juvenile rheumatoid arthritis	ND
Polymyositis	5.15
Rheumatoid arthritis	5.22
Sjögren syndrome	5.24
Systemic lupus erythematosus	5.25
Systemic sclerosis	5.23

ND, Not discussed in the current chapter

Table 6. Organ-specific autoimmune diseases (established or suspected)

Organ	Autoimmune disease	Section
Ears	Autoimmune sensorineural hearing loss	ND
	Meniere disease	ND
Endocrine system	Addison disease	5.2
	Autoimmune polyglandular syndrome type 1 (APECED), type 2 (Schmidt syndrome), and type 3	5.19
	Diabetes mellitus type 1 (IDDM)	5.6
	Graves disease	5.27.1
	Hashimoto thyroiditis	5.27.2
	Idiopathic hypoparathyroidism	ND
Eyes	Sympathetic ophthalmitis	ND
	Uveitis	ND
	Vogt-Koyanagi-Harada disease	ND
Gastrointestinal tract	Autoimmune gastritis	5.18
	Coeliac disease	5.5
	Crohn disease	5.11.1
	Ulcerative colitis	5.11.2
Heart	Congenital heart block	ND
	Myocarditis (dilated cardiomyopathy)	5.14
	Dressler syndrome	ND
Haematological diseases	Autoimmune neutropenia	ND
	Haemolytic anaemia	5.9
	Immune (idiopathic) thrombocytopenic purpura	5.26.1
	Pernicious anaemia	5.18
	Thrombotic thrombocytopenic purpura	5.26.2
Kidney	Anti-TBM (tubular basement membrane) nephritis	ND
	Goodpasture disease/anti-GBM (glomerular basement membrane) nephritis	5.7
	IgA-nephropathy	ND
	Interstitial nephritis	ND
	Membranoproliferative glomerulonephritis types I and II	ND

Table 6 (Contd)

Organ	Autoimmune disease	Section
Kidney (contd)	Necrotizing crescentic glomerulonephritis	5.3
Liver	Autoimmune hepatitis types I and II	5.10
	Primary biliary cirrhosis	5.20
	Primary sclerosing cholangitis	5.10
Lung	Goodpasture disease	5.7
	Primary pulmonary hypertension	5.23
Neuromuscular system	Guillain-Barré syndrome	5.8
	Lambert-Eaton syndrome	5.13
	Miller-Fisher syndrome	5.8
	Multiple sclerosis	5.12
	Myasthenia gravis	5.13
	Paraneoplastic neurological syndromes	5.16
	Rasmussen's encephalitis	ND
	Stiff-person syndrome	ND
Skin	Bullous pemphigoid	5.17.2
	Dermatitis herpetiformis (Morbus Duhring)	ND
	Epidermolysis bullosa aquisita	ND
	Herpes gestations	ND
	Linear IgA bullous dermatosis	ND
	Paraneoplastic pemphigus	ND
	Pemphigus foliaceus	5.17.1
	Pemphigus vulgaris	5.17.1
	Psoriasis	5.21
	Vitiligo	ND

ND, Not discussed in the current chapter

The focus of this chapter is on those diseases that are generally accepted to be autoimmune diseases, but descriptive information about some of the other common, potential autoimmune diseases is also included. Diseases that are only recently postulated to be autoimmune (e.g. atherosclerosis) will be mentioned only briefly at the end of this chapter. The respective autoimmune diseases will be discussed in alphabetical order. The topics discussed include epidemiology, clinical features, diagnostic criteria, pathogenesis, evident genetic associations, and possible links with xenobiotics, such as drugs and environmental risk factors.

Even though a number of diseases have been suspected to have autoimmune etiology, available evidence is insufficient to establish a close relationship in many instances.

This book addresses chemical risk, but other relevant environmental risk factors possibly able to cause autoimmune disorders, such as ultraviolet radiation, will be briefly taken into account in a specific section (section 8.8 of chapter 8).

Epidemiological patterns are discussed in more detail in chapter 6.

5.2 Addison disease

Idiopathic Addison disease is the most common form of adrenal insufficiency and is caused by autoimmune destruction of the steroid-producing cells in the adrenal glands — i.e. primary adrenocortical insufficiency — whereas secondary forms may occur as a result of pituitary or hypothalamic diseases (Betterle et al., 2002). Primary Addison disease is relatively rare, with a prevalence of 5–15 per 100 000 in Europe and the United States (Jacobson et al., 1997; Lovas & Husebye, 2002). This disease is usually slowly progressive, and patients generally present with such manifestations as malaise, anorexia, hyperpigmentation, hypotension, and salt wasting. The laboratory diagnosis primarily rests on the lack of a cortisol response to adrenocorticotropic hormone stimulation. The diagnosis may be supported by radiological procedures, revealing small, non-calcified adrenal glands, or by detection of autoantibodies to adrenal cortical cells. These autoantibodies are directed to enzymes involved in steroid synthesis, such as 21-hydroxylase. Antibody deposition and complement fixation to adrenal cortical cells is apparent upon microscopic examination. The involvement of T cells is postulated due to a major association with HLA-B8 and HLA-DR3. Nevertheless, the exact role of autoantibodies and/or T cells in the pathogenesis of Addison disease remains elusive. Addison disease can present as an isolated entity or in combination with other autoimmune diseases: the distinct autoimmune polyglandular syndromes (APGS) 1 and 2 and insulin-dependent diabetes mellitus (IDDM) or diabetes mellitus type 1. The latter is probably the result of the shared risk genotype HLA-DR3/4, HLA-DQ2/8.

5.3 ANCA-associated vasculitis

Primary vasculitis is a condition characterized by inflammation of blood vessels, resulting in thrombosis and rupture of these vessels and subsequent ischaemic tissue damage. The clinical presentation may vary greatly depending on the type and size of vessels involved. A categorization of primary vasculitides, according to the 1993 Chapel Hill Consensus Conference definitions, distinguishes large-vessel, medium-sized vessel, and small-vessel vasculitides. The antineutrophil cytoplasmic antibody (ANCA)-associated vasculitides are a subgroup of the small-vessel vasculitides and include Wegener granulomatosis, Churg-Strauss syndrome, microscopic polyangiitis, and the renal limited form of those diseases, which is idiopathic necrotizing crescentic glomerulonephritis (Rutgers et al., 2003). Altogether, the ANCA-associated vasculitides have a prevalence of approximately 15 per 100 000 (Watts et al., 2000). In contrast to many other autoimmune diseases, ANCA-associated vasculitides occur more often in men than in women; 60% of patients are male (Watts et al., 2000). Patients generally present with malaise, weight loss, fever, and arthralgias. In the case of Wegener granulomatosis, presentation often includes signs of chronic inflammation of the upper and/or lower respiratory tract and, in particular, bloody nasal discharge. Patients with Churg-Strauss syndrome usually have manifestations such as nasal obstruction due to polyposis nasi, asthma, diarrhoea, and eosinophilia. The diagnosis is based on clinical findings and on detection of antineutrophil cytoplasmic autoantibodies in the circulation. The antineutrophil cytoplasmic autoantibodies encountered in vasculitis patients are mostly directed against the neutrophil azurophilic granule proteins proteinase 3 (PR3) and myeloperoxidase (MPO) (Savige et al., 2000). The final diagnosis depends on biopsy evidence of vasculitis in the affected organs, in particular the kidney, nose, skin, lungs, nerve, and/or muscle. Levels of PR3-ANCA are considered especially relevant for monitoring disease activity, as well as for predicting renal outcome. Although a pathogenetic role of MPO-ANCA has recently been established in animal models, the pathogenetic mechanism still remains obscure. ANCA-associated vasculitides may also be caused by several drugs

(Merkel, 2001). The clinical manifestations of this type of drug-induced vasculitides range from single organ involvement, most commonly the skin, to life-threatening systemic disease. Most drug-induced ANCA vasculitis is associated with antithyroid drugs, such as propylthiouracil. In these cases, antineutrophil cytoplasmic autoantibodies are often directed to multiple specificities, including MPO, PR3, and elastase. There is no strong association with HLA genes, although HLA-DR6 seems to be protective. However, a number of non-HLA loci have been identified as contributing to disease severity.

5.4 Antiphospholipid syndrome

Antiphospholipid syndrome (APS) is now widely accepted as a systemic autoimmune disease characterized by a thrombophilic state and by obstetrical complications (Levine et al., 2002). The condition is primary if associated autoimmune disease (especially systemic lupus erythematosus) has been excluded. Up to 15% of patients with systemic lupus erythematosus will have antiphospholipid syndrome, and about 50% of patients with antiphospholipid syndrome have systemic lupus erythematosus. The female to male ratio is 2:1. The clinical features of antiphospholipid syndrome result from thromboembolism of large vessels, thrombotic microangiopathy, or both. Obviously, these may affect many different organs and tissues. By far the most common manifestation is deep venous thrombosis of the legs, with or without pulmonary emboli. Arterial thrombosis mostly results in strokes and transient ischaemic attacks in the brain or in myocardial infarction. In the case of adverse pregnancy outcomes in women with antiphospholipid syndrome, thrombotic events in the placenta may cause poor placental perfusion. However, antiphospholipid antibodies may also impair trophoblastic invasion. While most patients with antiphospholipid syndrome present with a single thrombotic event, a minority present with multiple simultaneous vascular occlusions throughout the body, often resulting in death. This syndrome is termed the "catastrophic antiphospholipid syndrome". For diagnosis of antiphospholipid syndrome, the Sapporo classification criteria can be used (Wilson et al., 1999a). A definite antiphospholipid syndrome is considered to be present if at least one clinical criterion and one laboratory criterion are met. The clinical criteria include vascular thrombosis, arterial, venous, or small-vessel thrombosis, and complications of pregnancy, such as unexplained death after the 10th week of gestation, premature birth before the

34th week of gestation, or at least three unexplained consecutive spontaneous abortions before the 10th week of gestation. The laboratory criteria include repeated detection of β_2-glycoprotein-I-dependent IgG and/or IgM anticardiolipin antibodies at least six weeks apart or repeated detection of lupus anticoagulant antibodies at least six weeks apart. How antiphospholipid antibodies promote thrombosis is unknown. Activation of endothelial cells or platelets, oxidant-mediated injury of the vascular endothelium, interference with the function of phospholipid-binding proteins involved in the regulation of coagulation, or events similar to those in heparin-induced thrombocytopenia have been proposed as pathogenetic mechanisms, and supporting in vitro evidence has been suggested for each possibility. The mere presence of antiphospholipid antibodies is considered insufficient to generate thrombosis; a second event may be required. Such events may include vascular injury, medication, atherosclerotic disease, or infections.

5.5 Coeliac disease

Coeliac disease is characterized by hypersensitivity to gluten, a cereal grain storage protein (Farrell & Kelly, 2002). The prevalence of clinically diagnosed coeliac disease is estimated to be 1:1000; however, screening trials suggest a prevalence of up to 1:100. The gluten-sensitive enteropathy results in weight loss, diarrhoea, symptoms due to nutritional deficiencies, such as anaemia and fatigue, and growth failure. These symptoms are the result of the mucosal lesions that develop and eventually result in villous atrophy. Coeliac disease may also present as extraintestinal manifestation, such as dermatitis herpetiformis, or may remain clinically silent. Diagnostic criteria of coeliac disease are well established. Firstly, there is the appearance of flat small intestinal mucosa with the histological features of hyperplastic villous atrophy while the patient is still eating adequate amounts of gluten. Secondly, there should be unequivocal and full clinical remission after withdrawal of gluten from the diet. The clinical response to a gluten challenge is not essential for diagnosis. Detection of antibodies to gliadin, the ethanol-extractable fraction of gluten, and in particular of auto-antibodies to the endomysial autoantigen tissue transglutaminase (tTG), supports the diagnosis. T cells from the mucosal lesions recognize deamidated epitopes of gliadin in the context of HLA-DQ2 or HLA-DQ8. Autoreactive T cells recognizing tTG have not been described. The presence of anti-tTG autoantibodies is considered to be secondary to the selective lack of T cell tolerance for deamidated gliadin, combined with the inherent characteristics of tTG to catalyse post-translational modification (deamidation) of gliadin and thereby enable the formation of gliadin–tTG complexes. In the presence of these complexes, tTG-specific B cells can be supported by gliadin-specific T helper cells and eventually produce the anti-tTG autoantibodies. Altogether, coeliac disease is a typical example of an environmental factor — in this case gluten — triggering an autoimmune antibody response, although this autoimmune response is not maintained in the absence of the environmental trigger. Prolonged exposure to gluten may eventually result in small bowel lymphoma.

5.6 Diabetes mellitus

Insulin-dependent diabetes mellitus (IDDM) or diabetes mellitus type 1 is a disorder in which the insulin-producing β-cells of the islets of Langerhans in the pancreas are attacked by the immune system, eventually resulting in insulin deficiency and hyperglycaemia (Atkinson & Eisenbarth, 2001). Diabetes mellitus type 1 is one of the most common of the autoimmune diseases, with a prevalence of about 200 per 100 000 (Betterle et al., 2002). Onset of disease is typically during childhood or adolescence and peaks between 10 and 14 years. The clinical features of insulin-dependent diabetes mellitus result from derangement of insulin function and include polyuria, polydipsia, polyphagia, and ketoacidosis. Longstanding diabetes is associated with renal insufficiency, blindness due to retinopathy, neuropathy, and atherosclerotic events such as myocardial infarction, cerebrovascular accidents, and gangrene of an extremity. The diagnosis of diabetes is made on the basis of hyperglycaemia (>7.0 mmol/l). Autoantibodies reactive with islet-associated antigens, such as islet cell antibodies (ICA), insulin autoantibodies (IAA), glutamic acid decarboxylase (GAD) antibodies, and insulinoma antigen 2 (IA2) antibodies, may further support the diagnosis. Indeed, about 90% of Caucasian children will have at least one of these antibodies at the time of diagnosis. However, these antibodies are most valuable as tools to identify those at risk of developing insulin-dependent diabetes mellitus. Pancreatic lesions show evidence of lymphocytic infiltration in the islets in early diabetes. The infiltrate consists of macrophages and both CD4 and CD8 T cells causing cell-mediated destruction of islet β-cells by induction of apoptosis. Whether any of the autoantibodies are involved in the pathogenesis of disease remains unclear. It is well recognized that HLA class II genes are important genetic factors that determine susceptibility to insulin-dependent diabetes mellitus: HLA-DR3/DQ2 and HLA-DR4/DQ8 are susceptibility haplotypes, whereas HLA-DQ6 is a protective haplotype. Besides these, about 20 non-HLA loci have been identified as contributing to disease susceptibility. There is a clear association of insulin-dependent diabetes mellitus with coeliac disease, possibly due to linkage with similar HLA-DQ alleles.

Environmental factors have been suggested as triggers for the autoimmune response. These suggested factors include viral infections, infant feeding practices, toxins such as N-nitroso derivates, vaccinations, and arsenic exposure, but for the most part evidence supporting these links is lacking.

5.7 Goodpasture disease

Goodpasture disease, also referred to as anti-glomerular basement membrane (anti-GBM) disease, is characterized by rapidly progressive glomerulonephritis and/or pulmonary haemorrhage (Ball & Young, 1998). Anti-GBM disease is very rare, with an incidence of approximately 1 case per 100 000 per year (F.K. Li et al., 2004). It affects primarily white males. Patients present with respiratory insufficiency due to alveolar haemorrhage, rapidly progressive renal insufficiency, or both. Kidney biopsy may reveal necrotizing crescentic glomerulonephritis with a typical linear deposition of anti-GBM antibodies. Early diagnosis is mandatory in order to prevent end-stage renal disease or death. Detection of circulating anti-GBM antibodies and/or the in situ presence of anti-GBM antibodies in kidney biopsies are diagnostic for anti-GBM disease. Anti-GBM antibodies are directed to the non-collagenous domain of the alpha 3 chain of type IV collagen. The pathogenicity of these autoantibodies is well established: they cause damage to the basement membrane in the lung and kidneys via a type II hypersensitivity reaction. A genetic association has been made between anti-GBM disease and HLA-DR15. This HLA type appears to have the unique capacity to bind many peptide sequences within the non-collagenous domain of type IV collagen. Environmental factors that play a role in disease triggering or severity include penicillamine, hydrocarbon exposure, and smoking.

5.8 Guillain-Barré syndrome

Guillain-Barré syndrome (GBS) is the most common cause of acute flaccid paralysis and is one of the best examples of a post-infectious autoimmune disease (Winer, 2001). The incidence is 1–2 cases per 100 000 per year, with higher rates in males and at older ages (Bogliun & Beghi, 2004; Cuadrado et al., 2004; Kuwabara, 2004). In North America and Europe, the most frequent pattern of Guillain-Barré syndrome is an acute inflammatory demyelinating polyneuropathy (AIDP). Patients present with rapidly progressive tingling, numbness, muscle weakness, and sometimes pain. The acute motor (and sensory) axonal neuropathy (AMAN) pattern of Guillain-Barré syndrome, in which primary axonal degeneration occurs with little or no demyelination, is more common in China and Japan, especially in areas where *Campylobacter jejuni* infections are frequent. About one to three weeks after infection, patients exhibit a progressive paralysis for up to four weeks that reaches a plateau phase. In most patients, recovery is complete or near complete within a period of several months. Diagnostic criteria include progressive weakness of more than two limbs, areflexia, and progression for no more than four weeks. Neurophysiological testing may further confirm the presence of a peripheral neuropathy. Immunopathological examination has revealed that in AIDP, both cellular (T cells and macrophages) and humoral mechanisms are involved in the pathogenesis, while in AMAN, complement-fixing antibodies directed to gangliosides are held responsible for the tissue damage. This is also consistent with the rate of recovery being accelerated by plasma exchange or intravenous immunoglobulin. Immunological studies suggest that at least one third of Guillain-Barré syndrome patients, in particular with the AMAN variant, have in the acute phase of the disease antibodies against nerve gangliosides, such as GD1a and GM1 (Willison & Yuki, 2002). Cross-reactivity with constituents of the lipopolysaccharide of *C. jejuni* sets up the autoimmune responses. The best support for a pathogenetic role of antiganglioside antibodies comes from Miller Fisher syndrome (MFS), a variant of Guillain-Barré syndrome that is clinically characterized by acute onset of ophthalmoplegia, ataxia, and areflexia. The annual incidence has been estimated at 0.9 cases per million population, and, like Guillain-Barré syndrome, Miller

Fisher syndrome has been associated with previous *C. jejuni* infection. In Miller Fisher syndrome, antibodies to the ganglioside GQ1b have been shown to produce neuromuscular block and may in part explain the clinical signs of that disorder (Willison & Yuki, 2002).

The antidepressant drug zimeldine was also transiently withdrawn because of an association with Guillain-Barré syndrome (see section 8.11.5).

5.9 Autoimmune haemolytic anaemia

Autoimmune haemolytic anaemia (AIHA) is caused by antibody production by the body against its own red cells (Gehrs & Friedberg, 2002). Autoimmune haemolytic anaemia is a rare disorder; the estimated incidence, based on studies conducted in the 1960s, is 1–3 cases per 100 000 per year (Gehrs & Friedberg, 2002). Two criteria must be met to diagnose autoimmune haemolytic anaemia: serological evidence of an autoantibody, and clinical or laboratory evidence of haemolysis. These diseases are characterized by a positive direct antiglobulin (Coombs') test and divided into warm and cold autoimmune haemolytic anaemias according to whether the antibody reacts more strongly with red cells at 37 °C or at 4 °C. Furthermore, several drugs may cause so-called drug-induced autoimmune haemolytic anaemia. Distinction of these three mechanisms can be made on the basis of serological reactions of the serum and the eluate.

5.9.1 Warm autoimmune haemolytic anaemia

Warm autoimmune haemolytic anaemia may be either idiopathic or secondary to chronic lymphocytic leukaemia, lymphomas, systemic lupus erythematosus, or other autoimmune disorders or infections. Warm autoantibodies are responsible for 48–70% of autoimmune haemolytic anaemia cases and may occur at any age; due to the secondary causes, however, the incidence increases starting around 40 years of age. There is an approximate 2:1 female predilection, possibly due to the association with other autoimmune diseases. Warm autoimmune haemolytic anaemia presents as a haemolytic anaemia of varying severity. The symptoms are those of anaemia (i.e. weakness, dizziness, fatigue, pallor, oedema, and dyspnoea on exertion) and haemolysis (i.e. jaundice, dark urine, and splenomegaly). The laboratory evaluation shows a reduced haemoglobin and haematocrit and a mean corpuscular volume that is elevated due to reticulocytosis. Red cells are typically coated with IgG and/or complement, as detected in the direct antiglobulin test, and eliminated by cells of the reticuloendothelial system. Furthermore, red cells may become spherical and are ultimately destroyed in the spleen. Infants born to mothers with autoimmune haemolytic anaemia may also suffer transient haemolysis due to passively acquired maternal autoantibodies. The symptoms of autoimmune haemolytic anaemia may precede the recognition of the underlying illness in the case of secondary autoimmune haemolytic anaemia. When associated with idiopathic thrombocytopenic purpura (ITP), which is a similar condition affecting platelets (see below), it is known as Evans syndrome.

5.9.2 Cold autoimmune haemolytic anaemia

As in warm autoimmune haemolytic anaemia, cold autoimmune haemolytic anaemia may be idiopathic or secondary to lymphoproliferative disorders or infections, in particular infectious mononucleosis or *Mycoplasma* pneumonia. Cold autoimmune haemolytic anaemia represents about 16–32% of autoimmune haemolytic anaemia cases. Primary cold autoimmune haemolytic anaemia affects primarily older adults, with a slight female preponderance. Patients with primary disease or disease secondary to a lymphoproliferative disorder commonly have a mild, chronic haemolytic anaemia, resulting in pallor and fatigue. Obviously, a cold environment may exacerbate the condition; especially in the extremities, acrocyanosis due to agglutination of red cells may be observed in the small vessels. Symptoms due to autoimmune haemolytic anaemia secondary to infection are similar, but transient, and appear two to three weeks after the infection starts. Red cells are typically coated with IgM and/or complement, as detected in the direct antiglobulin test. The cold autoantibodies in idiopathic autoimmune haemolytic anaemia and secondary to a lymphoproliferative disorder are IgM monoclonal antibodies mostly directed against the I-antigen of the *Ii* blood group system, while antibodies in autoimmune haemolytic anaemia secondary to infections are polyclonal IgM, directed to the I-antigen in the case of *Mycoplasma pneumoniae* and to the i-antigen in the case of infectious mononucleosis. IgM-sensitized red blood cells are generally associated with a combination of intra- and extravascular haemolysis, the latter being more common. Intravascular haemolysis occurs because IgM antibodies readily activate the classical complement pathway. Kupffer cells in the liver are the principal effectors of IgM-associated extravascular haemolysis.

5.9.3 Drug-induced autoimmune haemolytic anaemia

Drug-induced immune haemolytic anaemia may occur when the drug (e.g. methyldopa or fludarabine) induces autoantibodies directed to red blood cells. Drug-induced immune haemolytic anaemia secondary to neoantigen formation or drug absorption has a positive direct antiglobulin test and can be serologically distinguished from true autoimmune haemolytic anaemia because of the requirement for an exogenous drug to detect the antibody. The incidence of all these types of drug-induced immune haemolytic anaemia clearly varies with changes in drug usage in clinical practice. Typically, the haemolytic anaemia gradually disappears when the drug is discontinued, but with true autoimmune haemolytic anaemia, the autoantibodies may persist for several months.

5.10 Autoimmune hepatitis

Autoimmune hepatitis (AIH) is a chronic liver disease that frequently progresses to cirrhosis. It is divided into three types, according to the autoantibody profile, but only two types have mutually exclusive autoantibodies and different clinical profiles (Ben-Ari & Czaja, 2001). Type 1 autoimmune hepatitis is associated with the presence of antinuclear antibodies and/or anti-smooth muscle antibodies, while in type 2 autoimmune hepatitis, antibodies to liver/kidney microsome type 1, in particular to CYP2D6, can be detected. Anti-soluble liver antigen antibodies were originally considered typical for type 3 autoimmune hepatitis. Since clinical and laboratory features of patients with anti-soluble liver antigen antibodies are indistinguishable from those of patients with type 1 autoimmune hepatitis, the presence of these antibodies is probably not a hallmark of a separate entity. There are limited data concerning disease rates, but a recent study from Norway estimated an incidence of autoimmune hepatitis of approximately 2 cases per 100 000 per year and a prevalence of 15 per 100 000 (Boberg et al., 1998). Both forms of autoimmune hepatitis typically affect women. Typical symptoms of disease result from liver dysfunction and include fatigue, jaundice, dark urine, anorexia, and abdominal discomfort. Extrahepatic symptoms include arthralgias and Raynaud phenomenon. Diagnostic criteria for autoimmune hepatitis have been established. The clinical features should be dominated by raised transaminases without significant cholestasis, presence of autoantibodies as described above, liver biopsy findings showing necrosis of hepatocytes in the periportal region, and disruption of the limiting plate of the portal tract with infiltrating lymphoid cells, in particular plasma cells and CD4 T cells. A *definite* diagnosis requires exclusion of viral, drug-induced, alcoholic, and hereditary liver disease. If not all criteria are met, a *probable* diagnosis can be made. The mechanism by which hepatocytes are destroyed in autoimmune hepatitis has not been unravelled, but both T cell-mediated and antibody-dependent cellular cytotoxicity mechanisms have been postulated (Vergani & Mieli-Vergani, 2003). The susceptibility to autoimmune hepatitis is associated with human leukocyte antigens: DR3 (DRB1*0301) and DR4 (DRB1*0401) in Caucasians with type 1 autoimmune hepatitis and, to a lesser extent, DR7 (DRB1*0701) with type 2 autoimmune hepatitis. Finally, autoimmune hepatitis-like disease in association with anti-liver–kidney microsome type 1 (anti-LKM1) has also been described in 15% of patients with autoimmune polyglandular syndrome (APGS) type 1. This syndrome is the result of mutations in the AIRE gene. However, this type of autoimmune hepatitis is a distinct clinical entity, different from idiopathic autoimmune hepatitis. Although by definition autoimmune hepatitis is a non-viral disease, there is a clear association between viral infection and the autoimmune response. In particular, autoantibodies associated with autoimmune hepatitis commonly occur in chronic hepatitis B and C infection.

Several drugs and chemicals or their metabolites have been shown to induce hepatitis with autoimmune involvement. Halothane is a general anaesthetic agent that has been associated with hepatitis (Neuberger, 1998). Hepatitis is the result of toxic metabolites that are generated by cytochrome P450-mediated drug metabolism and bind covalently to liver components. Additionally, covalent binding of toxic metabolites to cytochrome P450 can lead to the formation of neoantigens and subsequently of anticytochrome P450 antibodies, resulting in immune-mediated hepatitis associated with dihydralazine, tienilic acid, and iproniazid.

In addition to autoimmune hepatitis, other liver autoimmune diseases include primary biliary cirrhosis (PBC) and primary sclerosing cholangitis (PSC). He et al. (2001) reviewed these autoimmune liver diseases and indicated that these relatively uncommon diseases are most likely initiated by the combination of environmental factors, such as xenobiotics, and a susceptible genetic predisposition.

5.11 Inflammatory bowel disease

The inflammatory bowel diseases (IBD) are chronic non-infectious inflammations manifest in the gastrointestinal tract, due to dysregulated immune responses to antigenic compounds in the intestinal lumen. Since the antigens are ill defined in terms of being endogenous or exogenous antigens, it remains questionable whether the inflammatory bowel diseases are bona fide autoimmune disorders. However, the occurrence of autoantibodies in these diseases warrants further description of the two most common, but distinct, forms of inflammatory bowel disease: Crohn disease and ulcerative colitis.

5.11.1 Crohn disease

Crohn disease usually presents with diarrhoea, abdominal pain, and/or weight loss. The illness characteristically waxes and wanes and eventually may lead to serious intestinal complications, such as strictures, perforation, and fistulae (Podolsky, 2002). Its incidence is estimated as 2–10 cases per 100 000 per year (Timmer, 2003). The onset typically occurs in teenagers and young adults. The sex ratio is nearly equal to one. The clinical manifestations of Crohn disease are the results of transmural inflammation of the bowel wall. Any part of the alimentary tract may be involved, although most typically the terminal ileum, colon, and small intestine are affected. The disease is associated with arthritis, uveitis, and sclerosing cholangitis, as well as features of malabsorption. Histopathology reveals granulomatous lesions, associated with crypt abscesses, fissures, and aphthous ulcers with submucosal extensions. The infiltrates consist of lymphocytes (T and B cells), plasma cells, and macrophages, and these are associated with increased production of Th1 cytokines, such as IL-12 and IFN-γ. The diagnosis of Crohn disease is based on the finding of typical clinical and pathological features and absence of evidence of other mimicking conditions. Gastrointestinal endoscopy with biopsy and imaging studies, such as computed tomography and barium contrast studies, are most specific for diagnostic purposes. The presence of anti-*Saccharomyces cerevisiae* antibodies, in the absence of perinuclear antineutrophil cytoplasmic antibody (pANCA), may be helpful in distinguishing Crohn disease from ulcerative colitis. Factors involved in the pathogenesis of Crohn disease include genes, the mucosal immune system, and the microbial environment in the gut. Genetic linkage studies have identified the NOD2/CARD15 gene on chromosome 16, which is mutated in as many as 50% of the patients (Bouma & Strober, 2003). The gene product is involved in signal transduction upon binding of bacterial lipopolysaccharide. The defect may eventually result in an imbalanced immune system due to insufficient immune suppression by regulatory T cells and regulatory cytokines such as IL-10. The effectiveness of anti-TNF-α therapy suggests that TNF-α, a product of activated macrophages, plays a pivotal role in the pathogenesis of Crohn disease. Although HLA antigens have been studied extensively, the resulting associations with Crohn disease have been variably reproducible. Smoking is the only recognized environmental risk factor for Crohn disease.

5.11.2 Ulcerative colitis

Ulcerative colitis is an idiopathic, chronic, relapsing, and remitting inflammatory condition of the colon (Ghosh et al., 2000). Ulcerative colitis, in contrast to Crohn disease, is limited to the colon and involves mainly the superficial layers of the bowel. Its incidence is approximately 5–20 cases per 100 000 per year (Timmer, 2003). Men and women are equally affected. Patients typically present with diarrhoea, tenesmus, relapsing rectal bleeding, and lower abdominal cramps and pain with defecation. Ulcerative colitis may present in a very severe form, with transmural damage to the colon, which has a high risk of perforation and death. Extraintestinal manifestations include arthritis, uveitis, pyoderma gangrenosum, erythema nodosum, and sclerosing cholangitis. The superficial mucosal inflammation and ulceration of the rectal and colonic mucosa occur in a continuous pattern, typically decreasing in severity in more proximal areas of the colon. The mucosa has intense infiltration of the colonic crypts with polymorphonuclear cells and surrounding accumulations of lymphocytes and plasma cells. Cytokine analysis of infiltrating cells shows increased expression of the Th2 cytokines IL-5 and IL-13, but not IL-4. The diagnosis of ulcerative colitis is based on exclusion of infections and subsequent visualization of the rectal and colonic mucosa by flexible sigmoidoscopy and biopsy and either total colonoscopy or double-contrast barium enema examination. The presence of pANCA in the absence of anti-*S. cerevisiae* antibodies may be helpful in distinguishing ulcerative colitis from Crohn disease. Antigen specificities revealing the pANCA pattern have been only partially elucidated. Environmental factors, in particular factors that trigger detrimental mucosal immune responses to enteric bacteria, are considered more important than genetic factors in the pathogenesis of ulcerative colitis (Farrell & Peppercorn, 2002). Indeed, no clear-cut HLA association has been described so far. Of all environmental factors, the protective effect of cigarette smoking remains the most consistent. Nicotine is probably the main active ingredient in this association, but the mechanisms remain unknown. In patients with long-standing disease, there is an increased risk of colonic dysplasia and adenocarcinoma.

5.12 Multiple sclerosis

Multiple sclerosis (MS) is an inflammatory, demyelinating autoimmune disorder of the central nervous system, affecting most commonly young adults between the ages of 20 and 40 years. The prevalence of the disease is approximately 60 cases per 100 000, and the incidence is 3 cases per 100 000 per year (Jacobson et al., 1997), but these vary considerably between countries. The most apparent clinical presentation of multiple sclerosis includes chronic or relapsing paralysis and problems of vision, sensation, strength, and coordination. Several disease patterns can be distinguished: relapsing-remitting (60–70%), primary progressive (10–20%), and secondary progressive multiple sclerosis (15–25%), all resulting in the accumulation of significant neurological disability (Compston & Coles, 2002). Multiple sclerosis is diagnosed based on the objective demonstration of dissemination of lesions in both time and space, and diagnosis incorporates evidence from magnetic resonance imaging (McDonald et al., 2001). Berger et al. (2003) showed that the presence of serum antibodies directed to myelin oligodendrocyte glycoprotein (MOG), with or without antibodies against major basic protein (MBP), in patients with an initial event suggestive of central nervous system demyelination and evidence of multifocal lesions on magnetic resonance imaging studies of the brain is highly predictive of subsequent clinical events that establish the diagnosis of clinically definite multiple sclerosis (Berger et al., 2003). The pathology of multiple sclerosis lesions is characterized by the presence of large multifocal sclerotic plaques with reactive glial scar formation. Active lesions show inflammation and active myelin degradation and phagocytosis. Further analysis of the demyelinating lesions may reveal, besides a T cell- and macrophage-dominated immune response, immunoglobulin and complement deposition, myelin protein loss, and distinct patterns of oligodendrocyte degeneration. On the basis of these findings, four patterns of demyelination have been identified, suggesting that there exist distinct pathogenetic mechanisms (Kornek & Lassmann, 2003). The primary injury is directed at the myelin itself or its cell of origin, the oligodendrocyte, being responsible for synthesis and maintenance of the myelin sheath of nerve axons. The main concept holds activated autoreactive T cells responsible for driving chronic inflammation and macrophage/microglia activation in the lesions. The importance of T helper cells is further supported by the consistent association of multiple sclerosis in European populations and the HLA class II alleles DR2 (DRB1*1501) and DQ6 (DQB2*0302). However, CD8 T cells are considered to be even more directly involved in tissue destruction. The presence of antibodies against myelin proteins may add to the immunopathogenetic mechanism. Although the genetic involvement in multiple sclerosis is well defined, no certain susceptibility genes outside the HLA gene complex have been unequivocally identified, possibly as the result of disease heterogeneity (Compston & Coles, 2002).

5.13 Myasthenia gravis

Myasthenia gravis (MG) is a disorder of transmission at the neuromuscular junction characterized by muscle weakness (Vincent et al., 2001). The estimated prevalence of disease varies between 5 and 15 cases per 100 000 (Jacobson et al., 1997; Kalb et al., 2002). There are two peak disease incidences with different male/female ratios: before age 40, women are 3 times more commonly affected, whereas in the older age group, males predominate. The prominent clinical feature of myasthenia gravis is painless, fatigable weakness of selected muscle groups. The disease frequently presents with ptosis and diplopia. Limb and neck flexor weakness typically occurs later in the disease. Anti-acetylcholine receptor antibodies are present in about 85–90% of patients and, when identified in the appropriate clinical setting, are diagnostic for myasthenia gravis. The presence of anti-muscle-specific kinase (MuSK) antibodies in patients lacking anti-acetylcholine receptor antibodies may identify a subgroup of myasthenia gravis patients. Furthermore, a similar syndrome, Lambert-Eaton syndrome, is associated with antibodies against the presynaptic, voltage-gated calcium channels. Reversibility of clinical symptoms with anticholinesterase inhibitors in myasthenia gravis is another hallmark of diagnosis. Once a diagnosis has been made, computed tomography or magnetic resonance imaging of the chest should be done to exclude an associated thymoma, which is apparent in about 10% of the patients. Myasthenia gravis is a prototypic autoimmune disease, since its antibody-mediated pathogenesis is exclusively directed to the postsynaptic membrane of the neuromuscular junction. The muscular nicotinic acetylcholine receptor is the major autoantigen. Antibodies directed to the acetylcholine receptor lower the number of functional receptors, leading to an impaired neuromuscular signal transduction, resulting in the characteristic fatigable skeletal muscle weakness. Indeed, in muscle biopsy specimens from myasthenia gravis patients, antibodies are attached to the postsynaptic membrane, receptors are lost, and postsynaptic folds are sparse and shallow. The immunopathogenetic role of the autoantibodies is further established by the occurrence of neonatal myasthenia gravis in babies born to women with the disease. In these cases, spontaneous resolution usually occurs within a few weeks due to disappearance of maternal antibodies. The HLA-DR3 B8 A1 extended ancestral haplotype has been reproducibly associated with the most frequent form of myasthenia gravis, which presents with thymus hyperplasia. This haplotype has also been involved in other human autoimmune diseases, including systemic lupus erythematosus, coeliac disease, insulin-dependent diabetes mellitus, and autoimmune thyroiditis, suggesting that the respective genes could determine non-antigen-specific immune dysregulation rather than specify a particular "self" target to the immune system (Garchon, 2003). For instance, a gene within the HLA gene complex and close to the tumour necrosis factor gene has been implicated in increased antibody production. This may also explain why myasthenia gravis is often associated with other autoimmune diseases, such as insulin-dependent diabetes mellitus and autoimmune thyroiditis. Nevertheless, several other HLA associations have been identified, which are partly correlated to the phenotypic heterogeneity of myasthenia gravis. Although some drugs, such as quinoline derivatives, may induce, aggravate, or expose myasthenia gravis by directly interfering with neuromuscular transmission to alter both presynaptic and postsynaptic components, D-penicillamine therapy has been reported to be the drug most frequently associated with autoimmune myasthenia gravis. Disease manifestations disappear upon withdrawal of this drug (Delamere et al., 1983).

5.14 Myocarditis

Myocarditis is an inflammatory disease of the myocardium; it may be idiopathic, infectious, or autoimmune and may heal or lead to dilated cardiomyopathy (DCM) (Fairweather et al., 2001; Mason, 2003). The prevalence of dilated cardiomyopathy is estimated to be 0.1 per 100 000 in adults and 4.1 per 100 000 in children (Jacobson et al., 1997). Clinical features of the disease are unexplained congestive heart failure, chest pain mimicking myocardial infarction, arrhythmias, syncope, and sudden death. Early and definite diagnosis of myocarditis depends on the detection of inflammatory infiltrates in endomyocardial biopsy specimens according to the Dallas criteria. Histopathology reveals lymphocytic infiltrates, interstitial oedema, myocardial necrosis, and fibrosis. Additionally, circulating cardiac autoantibodies may be detected. These antibodies are directed against a multitude of autoantigens, such as the β_1-adrenoreceptor and α-myosin, and have only limited sensitivity (Caforio et al., 2002). For some of these autoantibodies, there is in vitro evidence for a functional role. On the whole, myocarditis is considered a progressive disease with three distinct, chronologically successive stages. The initial insult to the myocardium is believed to be a viral infection. Depending on the genetic makeup of the patient, this initiating infection may go unnoticed or may trigger an autoimmune reaction that causes further myocardial injury, eventually resulting in the typical picture of dilated cardiomyopathy (Mason, 2003). The genes involved in this dichotomous outcome remain to be identified.

5.15 Autoimmune myositis

Inflammatory muscle diseases include dermatomyositis (DM) and polymyositis (PM) (Dalakas & Hohlfeld, 2003). These diseases affect skeletal muscle and/or skin, leading to profound tissue modification. The prevalence of these diseases is approximately 5 cases per 100 000 (Jacobson et al., 1997). Dermatomyositis, affecting both children and adults, is more common than polymyositis, which strongly predominates in adults. Women are affected twice as commonly as men. Both dermatomyositis and polymyositis present with insidious onset of symmetrical muscle weakness. The proximal muscles of the extremities are most often affected, usually progressing from the lower to the upper limbs. Later on, lung disease may complicate the clinical picture. In the case of dermatomyositis, a characteristic erythematous rash over bony prominences of the extremities is observed. The clinical diagnosis of dermatomyositis and polymyositis is confirmed by elevation of muscle enzymes in the serum, electromyographic findings of myopathy, and biopsy evidence of myositis. In dermatomyositis, the inflammation consists of CD4 T cells and B cells and is predominantly perivascular or in the interfascicular septa. The muscle fibres undergo phagocytosis and necrosis, eventually resulting in perifascicular atrophy. These effects are possibly the result of vascular damage mediated by antibodies and complement. Dermatomyositis is associated with autoantibodies directed to the nuclear antigen Mi-2, but these antibodies are of low sensitivity. In contrast to dermatomyositis, in polymyositis, the cellular infiltrate is primarily characterized by CD8 T cells focused on the muscle fibres, especially in the endomysial areas. Destruction of myocytes is evidently T cell-mediated in polymyositis. Autoantibodies to the histidyl-tRNA synthetase (Jo-1) are associated with polymyositis, but are considered to be not pathogenic. As for several other organ-specific autoimmune diseases, the strongest genetic risk factor for myositis is the ancestral HLA-DR3 B8 A1 haplotype. Associations of environmental factors with myositis onset have been identified — for instance, intake of drugs such as penicillamine, tiopronine, and pyritinol and the old anticonvulsant trimethadione. Also, the ingestion of contaminated L-tryptophan preparations may be implicated in the development of myositis.

5.16 Paraneoplastic neurological syndromes

The paraneoplastic syndromes of the nervous system arise in association with a cancer (Darnell & Posner, 2003). However, the neurological symptoms are characteristic of certain types of cancer and often precede the identification of the underlying malignancy. Therefore, proper identification of the neurological disorder will be of help in finding the cancer that causes the neurological disability. Most of these disorders are immune-mediated and characterized by the presence of autoantibodies. Sensory neuropathy and limbic encephalomyelitis, characterized by memory impairment, psychiatric changes, and seizures, are associated with anti-Hu antibodies that cross-react with the nuclei of all neurons. The presence of these antibodies warrants a search for small-cell lung cancer, neuroblastoma, and prostate cancer. In paraneoplastic cerebellar degeneration, patients present with slurred speech, gait instability, and tremor. Anti-Yo antibodies, reacting with a cytoplasmic component of Purkinje cells, may be found, and these antibodies are indicative of the presence of ovarian, breast, or lung cancer. Other antibodies associated with cerebellar degeneration, such as anti-Tr and anti-mGluR1 antibodies, are a sign of Hodgkin lymphoma. Ataxia with or without opsoclonus-myoclonus syndrome is related to anti-Ri antibodies, which recognize neuronal nuclei, and these antibodies have been associated with breast, gynaecological, lung, and bladder cancers. Finally, the Lambert-Eaton myasthenic syndrome is caused by antibodies to voltage-gated calcium channels, which are indicative of a small-cell lung cancer. Overall, the paraneoplastic neurological syndromes are rare, affecting perhaps only 0.01% of patients with cancer. The pathogenetic mechanism is based on the ectopic expression of a nervous system-specific antigen by a tumour. Antigen expression outside the immunologically privileged site results in an immune response that may control the growth of the tumour, but also causes the neurological disease when immune cells are enabled to cross the blood–brain barrier. However, the site of damage and the exact mechanism may vary from syndrome to syndrome.

5.17 Pemphigus/pemphigoid

Pemphigus and pemphigoid are cutaneous, antibody-mediated autoimmune diseases characterized by loss of cell–cell or cell–matrix adhesion, resulting in blister formation. The disease affects the skin and mucous membranes. Differences in type of disease depend on the antigen to which the autoantibodies are directed. Here we will describe the major subtypes of pemphigus — i.e. pemphigus vulgaris (PV) and pemphigus foliaceus (PF) — and bullous pemphigoid.

5.17.1 Pemphigus

Pemphigus vulgaris and pemphigus foliaceus are two rare blistering skin diseases that will be fatal if unrecognized or untreated (Blauvelt et al., 2003). Pemphigus may occur at all ages, but most people are middle-aged at the time of presentation. While pemphigus vulgaris is the most common form of pemphigus, it is still a rare disease, with an incidence of less than 1 per 100 000 per year (Jacobson et al., 1997). Pemphigus vulgaris, but not pemphigus foliaceus, is most prevalent in people of Jewish or Mediterranean heritage. Persistent painful oral erosions are an almost invariant feature of pemphigus vulgaris. Skin lesions are flaccid and fragile bullae without surrounding erythema. Pemphigus foliaceus presents with more superficial blistering without mucosal involvement. Diagnosis is based on the presence of the typical epidermal lesions and appropriate immunofluorescence studies. Direct immunofluorescence reveals the deposition of IgG and complement components on the epidermal cell surface, forming the characteristic chickenwire appearance. The diagnosis may be further supported by the detection of circulating antibodies reacting with the desmosomal cadherins desmoglein 1 (Dsg1) and Dsg3. It is now well established that these antidesmosomal antibodies are pathogenic via a type 2 hypersensitivity reaction (Martel & Joly, 2001). Indeed, neonates from women with an active disease at delivery may also present with pemphigus. Curiously, most cases of neonatal pemphigus have been reported in women with pemphigus vulgaris and not with pemphigus foliaceus. Pemphigus vulgaris is associated with HLA-A10 and HLA-DR4/DQw3 or HLA-DRw6/DQw1; for pemphigus foliaceus, no associations have been described yet. Studies in Brazil on the endemic form of pemphigus foliaceus (fogo selvagem) suggest that pemphigus foliaceus may be triggered by an infectious agent, perhaps transmitted by an insect vector.

Pemphigus may also be induced by drugs, such as penicillamine and captopril. Because several drugs containing a thiol group, including penicillamine and capropril, have been associated with autoimmune reactions, a role of sulfhydryl groups present in most proteins in inducing autoimmune reactions has been suspected, but has failed to be clearly demonstrated.

Here a distinction is made between drug-induced pemphigus, which may regress spontaneously when the drug is discontinued, and drug-triggered pemphigus, which does not improve upon drug withdrawal.

5.17.2 Pemphigoid

Bullous pemphigoid, the most common pemphigoid disease, is an autoimmune subepidermal blistering disease. There is no sex or race predominance in this disease, and it is primarily a disease of individuals above the age of 60. Bullous pemphigoid is characterized by large, tense blisters that are often pruritic; the blisters are distributed over the extremities and trunk. Diagnosis requires these characteristic skin lesions, due to detachment of basal keratinocytes from the underlying dermis at the level of the lamina lucida, in combination with linear deposits of IgG and complement components at the epidermal basement membrane zone. The autoantibodies in bullous pemphigoid recognize two distinct keratinocyte hemidesmosomal proteins: the cytoplasmic BP 230 and the transmembrane BP 180. The diagnosis may be supported by detection of circulating autoantibodies that bind to the basement membrane of skin tissue in indirect immunofluorescence. In particular, the autoantibodies reactive with BP 180 are considered pathogenic (Liu, 2002). Bullous pemphigoid is usually a self-limited disease with a benign, but sometimes prolonged, course. There are no known patterns of inheritance or HLA associations.

5.18 Pernicious anaemia

Pernicious anaemia, or autoimmune (type A) gastritis, is a disorder characterized by vitamin B_{12} deficiency caused by autoimmune attack on the gastric mucosa (Toh et al., 1997). More females than males are affected (1.6:1), with a peak occurrence at 60 years of age. A population survey revealed that even 1.9% of persons at the age of 60 or more have undiagnosed pernicious anaemia, but not all have an autoimmune pathogenesis. The disease is found worldwide, but is most common in northern Europe. Clinical findings are megaloblastic anaemia and irreversible neurological complications, due to the vitamin B_{12} deficiency, and achlorhydria. Pernicious anaemia may be associated with autoimmune endocrinopathies and antireceptor autoimmune diseases. Furthermore, patients with pernicious anaemia have increased risks of gastric carcinoma and carcinoid tumours. Diagnosis is based on the histological picture revealing a plasma cell and lymphoid infiltrate of the lamina propria of the gastric mucosa. The infiltrate is accompanied by loss of parietal and zymogen cells, leading to atrophy of the stomach, in particular the fundus and body, but not the antrum. The diagnosis is confirmed by the presence of an abnormal Schilling's test for the detection of vitamin B_{12} malabsorption. This test consists of the administration of radiolabelled vitamin B_{12} by mouth, followed by measurement of the uptake of the label and its appearance in the stool. Reduced uptake due to decreased production of intrinsic factor and/or to antibodies that block intrinsic factor function indicates the presence of pernicious anaemia. Detection of circulating autoantibodies to gastric parietal cells and to intrinsic factor may further add to the diagnosis. Destruction of the gastric parietal cells, with concomitant loss of intrinsic factor production, is considered to be mediated by CD4 T cells that are specific for the β subunit of gastric H^+/K^+-ATPase. Additionally, the B cells are responsible for production of anti-intrinsic factor antibodies, which interfere with uptake of vitamin B_{12}. Chronic immune stimulation predisposes patients to gastric carcinoma. Pernicious anaemia is associated with HLA-B8, HLA-B12, and HLA-B15; environmental factors have not been identified.

5.19 Autoimmune polyglandular syndromes

Autoimmune polyglandular syndromes (APGS) are groupings of multiple endocrine dysfunctions of autoimmune origin in a genetically susceptible individual. On the whole, component autoimmune diseases present similarly to the individual diseases. The syndromes are organized and classified in three main types, as described below (Betterle et al., 2002). The fourth type is a rare syndrome characterized by the association of autoimmune combinations not falling into the other three categories, and this type will not be discussed.

5.19.1 APGS type 1

The first type of autoimmune polyglandular syndrome, also referred to as APECED, is characterized by the presence of three major component diseases: chronic candidiasis, hypoparathyroidism, and autoimmune Addison disease. It has primarily been seen, to date, among the Iranian Jewish community, in Finland, and in Sardinia. The syndrome occurs in childhood, with a female to male ratio varying between 0.8 and 2.4. APGS type 1 is inherited in an autosomal recessive fashion. The gene responsible for this condition has been identified as AIRE (autoimmune regulator). The AIRE protein is considered to be primarily involved in intrathymic tolerance induction.

5.19.2 APGS type 2

APGS type 2, also referred to as Schmidt syndrome, is characterized by Addison disease in association with autoimmune thyroid diseases and/or diabetes mellitus type 1. APGS type 2 may occur at any age and in both sexes (the female to male ratio is 2:1), but it is most common in middle-aged females and very rare in childhood. Several studies have revealed an association of this syndrome with various alleles within the HLA-DR3-carrying haplotype.

5.19.3 APGS type 3

The least well characterized autoimmune polyglandular syndrome is the type 3 syndrome. This syndrome is defined by the presence of autoimmune thyroid disease with another autoimmune disease, such as diabetes mellitus type 1, autoimmune gastritis, or myasthenia gravis, but in the absence of Addison disease. APGS type 3 primarily involves females (the female to male ratio is 7:1) who have HLA-DR3-associated autoimmune disease and is probably the most common of the autoimmune polyglandular syndrome disorders. Since different and multiple clinical combinations can be found, the classification of this type of autoimmune polyglandular syndrome is probably more complicated than originally anticipated.

5.20 Primary biliary cirrhosis

Primary biliary cirrhosis (PBC) is an idiopathic autoimmune liver disease characterized by chronic inflammation and destruction of intrahepatic bile ducts (Talwalkar & Lindor, 2003). The disease typically affects middle-aged women (the female to male ratio is 9:1). The prevalence of the disease, which is found worldwide, has been estimated to be 4 cases per 100 000 (Feld & Heathcote, 2003). With advances in diagnosis, a growing proportion of patients are being identified with asymptomatic early-stage disease. Clinical presentation includes pruritus, fatigue, increased skin pigmentation, arthralgias, and dryness of the mouth and eyes. Due to necrosis of the intrahepatic bile ducts, there is chronic cholestasis, hepatic fibrosis, cirrhosis, and eventually liver failure. The occurrence of hepatocellular carcinoma is amplified, which is usually recognizable in late-stage disease. The diagnosis of primary biliary cirrhosis is based on rises in serum alkaline phosphatase and typical histological abnormalities on liver biopsy: chronic inflammation leading to destruction and disappearance of intrahepatic bile ducts and progressive portal fibrosis, which ultimately leads to cirrhosis. Furthermore, high-titre antimitochondrial antibodies are considered a hallmark feature of this disease; the antibodies are probably not pathogenic. These antibodies are predominantly directed to the E2 subunit of the pyruvate dehydrogenase complex. It has been suggested that the induction of these autoantibodies and the subsequent development of autoimmune disease are the result of exposure to xenobiotics. Halogenated compounds, in particular, may bind to the autoantigen, break tolerance, and lead to an intense mucosal immune response (Long et al., 2002). Although the genetic basis of primary biliary cirrhosis is only poorly understood, linkage with HLA-DRB1*08 has been described.

5.21 Psoriasis

Psoriasis is a relatively common chronic skin disease (Blauvelt et al., 2003; Lebwohl, 2003). Estimates of its prevalence vary from 0.5% to 4.6%, with rates varying between countries and races. Prevalence is almost equal in men and women, whereas Caucasians are affected twice as often as blacks or Asians. The most common form of psoriasis is chronic plaque disease. This presents as well defined red scaly plaques typically distributed over the scalp, lower back, and extensor aspects of the limbs. Clinical variants include guttate psoriasis, sebopsoriasis, and pustular forms of psoriasis. Between 5% and 42% of patients have psoriatic arthritis, a destructive and occasionally disabling joint disease. Diagnosis of psoriasis relies almost entirely on characteristic clinical features — i.e. the presence of sharply demarcated, erythematous, scaling plaques — and rarely requires histological confirmation. Histologically, psoriasis is characterized by marked keratinocyte hyperproliferation, a dense inflammatory infiltrate consisting of CD4 T cells and neutrophils, and activation of the cutaneous vasculature.

Psoriasis is considered as a primary T cell-mediated inflammatory disease driven by proinflammatory and type 1 cytokines, such as IFN-γ. A possible autoantigen has not yet been identified. Alternatively, a growing body of evidence implicates streptococcal and staphylococcal superantigens in the development of psoriasis. Superantigens have a proven ability to induce high levels of inflammatory cytokines and/or initiate autoimmune responses that contribute to the development of skin disorders. Psoriasis is genetically a complex trait, but there is general agreement that one of the psoriasis genes (PSORS1) is located in the short arm of chromosome 6 (6p21.3), whereas other susceptibility genes are scattered throughout the genome.

Exacerbation of psoriasis can be seen after drug treatment, with, for example, beta-blockers and recombinant IFN-α (Abel, 1992).

5.22 Rheumatoid arthritis

Rheumatoid arthritis (RA) is considered a systemic autoimmune disease featured by joint inflammation that results in joint damage and loss of function. It affects approximately 1% of the population (Jacobson et al., 1997), with a female to male ratio of 3:1. The typical clinical presentation of rheumatoid arthritis is a symmetrical arthritis affecting many joints, often in association with constitutional symptoms such as fever and malaise. The disease begins in the small joints of the hands and feet and progresses in a centripetal and symmetric fashion, eventually resulting in severe deformities. Extra-articular manifestations include vasculitis, atrophy of skin and muscle, lymphadenopathy, splenomegaly, and leukopenia. The diagnosis of rheumatoid arthritis depends primarily on clinical manifestations of the disease. Seven criteria (revised) have been formulated by the American Rheumatology Association; rheumatoid arthritis is diagnosed when at least four criteria are present (Arnett et al., 1988). The presence of rheumatoid factor, an autoantibody directed to the Fc portion of immunoglobulin, is one of these criteria, but this autoantibody is not very specific for rheumatoid arthritis. More recently, antibodies reactive with citrullinated peptides have been described that share high sensitivity and specificity for rheumatoid arthritis (Schellekens et al., 2000). The pathology of rheumatoid arthritis lesions reveals a prominent CD4 T cell synovial infiltrate in close apposition to macrophages, resulting in high production of pro-inflammatory cytokines, such as TNF-α and IL-1, and proteolytic enzymes (Firestein, 2003). In addition, antibody-producing B cells are abundantly present in the synovium. Local autoantibody production, such as rheumatoid factor or anti-cyclic citrullinated antibodies, may be pathogenic by formation and deposition of immune complexes in the lesions. Although the immune complex theory could explain many of the acute inflammatory features of rheumatoid arthritis, the prominent T cell infiltrate, combined with the association with several HLA-DR genes, including HLA-DR4 and HLA-DR1, suggests a key role for T cells. A multitude of potential autoantigens have been suggested to be implicated in T cell activation. The important role of TNF-α and IL-1 is well established, since neutralization of these antibodies results in amelioration of disease. Importantly, however, anti-TNF-α treatment induces humoral autoimmunity, possibly by inhibition of cytotoxic T lymphocyte responses that normally suppress autoreactive B cells (Via et al., 2001). This may result in the induction of antibodies to double-stranded DNA (dsDNA).

Ferucci et al. (2005) described a relationship of genetic factors and prevalence of rheumatoid arthritis and presented evidence for the increased prevalence of a severe, early-onset rheumatoid arthritis in some populations of American Indians (including Alaskan Natives) that is associated with a high frequency of some HLA alleles, such as HLA-DRB1*1402. However, evidence suggests that other genetic factors or components, possibly non-HLA-associated genes, play contributing roles in rheumatoid arthritis risk.

There is considerable evidence that tobacco smoking is associated with an increased risk of rheumatoid arthritis and with an increased prevalence of rheumatoid factor among people without clinical disease. The role of occupational exposure to silica dust in rheumatoid arthritis is also an active area of research (see chapter 8).

5.23 Scleroderma (systemic sclerosis)

Scleroderma (systemic sclerosis) is a disease of unknown etiology characterized by abnormally increased collagen deposition in the skin and visceral organs, alterations in the microvasculature, and numerous cellular and humoral immune abnormalities. A recent study in the United States estimated the disease prevalence to be approximately 25 per 100 000 (Mayes et al., 2003). Besides a racial predisposition in African Americans, these patients present with more pronounced systemic involvement and a higher frequency of pulmonary fibrosis, as compared with Caucasian patients. Scleroderma can be subdivided based on the nature and extent of end-organ involvement: diffuse systemic sclerosis (dSSc) is characterized by diffuse skin involvement and severe fibrosis of multiple internal organs, and limited systemic sclerosis (lSSc) shows limited skin sclerosis (sclerodactyly or acrosclerosis) with minimal signs of fibrosis in internal organs. The CREST syndrome, defined by the presence of soft-tissue calcinosis, Raynaud phenomenon, oesophageal dysmotility, and telangiectasias, is the major form of limited scleroderma. Primary pulmonary hypertension is one of the most severe manifestations of the CREST syndrome. The diagnosis of scleroderma is based primarily on clinical symptoms. The diagnosis may be hampered when the visceral complaints (predominantly in lungs, heart, and kidney) are not associated with classic skin changes and Raynaud phenomenon. The diagnosis may be supported by detection of anticentromere antibodies (80–96%), common in patients with limited systemic sclerosis, or anti-topoisomerase 1 (Scl-70) antibodies, typically seen in patients with diffuse systemic sclerosis (30–40%). The pathological changes in skin biopsies of systemic sclerosis patients reveal thinning of the epidermis with flattening of the rete pegs, atrophy of the dermal appendages, hyalinization and fibrosis of arterioles, and massive accumulation of dense collagen in the reticular dermis. Also in the visceral organs, the triad of fibrosis, narrowing of blood vessels, and perivascular inflammation is observed, eventually resulting in end-stage atrophy of the affected organs. In particular, the T cell population in affected systemic sclerosis tissues is believed to release cytokines, which initiate and/or perpetuate the fibrotic process as well as the endothelial and vascular alterations (Derk & Jimenez, 2003). Owing to the potent profibrotic and immunomodulatory activities of TGFβ, this cytokine has been considered one of the dominant molecules in the pathogenesis of systemic sclerosis. Initially, this cytokine may be produced by infiltrated leukocytes, and production may be further enhanced by sensitized fibroblasts. Altogether, because of the progressive fibrosis and organ failure, diffuse systemic sclerosis in particular is associated with a high mortality rate, with an estimated five-year survival of approximately 40%. New therapeutic options for treatment of pulmonary hypertension in the CREST syndrome, such as endothelin receptor antagonists, prostacyclin derivatives, or phosphodiesterase inhibitors, may improve this outcome in the near future.

A fairly strong and consistent association between exposure, primarily in occupational settings, to solvents (e.g. trichloroethylene) and scleroderma has been reported in numerous epidemiological studies (see chapter 8). Scleroderma-like diseases can also be induced by other chemical compounds, such as drugs (D'Cruz, 2000) and silica ("Erasmus syndrome"). Workers exposed to vinyl chloride monomers exhibit clinical features that resemble systemic sclerosis, such as fibrotic skin lesions, pulmonary fibrosis, and skin capillary abnormalities. However, vinyl chloride disease also harbours several features that are clearly distinct from systemic sclerosis. After exposure is discontinued, skin lesions, capillary abnormalities, and acroosteolytic lesions revert to nearly normal (Haustein & Ziegler, 1985).

Scleroderma-like manifestation is a typical clinical feature of the toxic oil syndrome (see chapter 7).

Some data also suggest an increased risk of systemic sclerosis in workers exposed to hand-transmitted vibration due to the use of vibrating tools (Bovenzi et al., 2001).

5.24 Sjögren syndrome

Sjögren syndrome is an autoimmune exocrinopathy characterized by both organ-specific autoimmunity, preferentially affecting the salivary and/or lacrimal glands, and systemic manifestations (Jonsson et al., 2000). The diminished gland secretion results in keratoconjunctivitis sicca and xerostomia. Primary Sjögren syndrome is diagnosed if no other autoimmune disease is present; secondary Sjögren syndrome is associated with rheumatoid arthritis or other connective tissue disorders. Prevalence of Sjögren syndrome is estimated to be 15 per 100 000. Like many other connective tissue diseases, there is a female preponderance, with a female to male ratio of 9:1. Patients typically present with dry eyes and mouth, but other mucosal sites may also be affected. Furthermore, a majority may present with systemic complaints, such as arthralgias, fibromyalgia, or chronic fatigue. The gold standard for diagnosis is a minor labial salivary gland biopsy, showing focal lymphocytic infiltrates consisting predominantly of CD4 T cells. Quantitative immunohistological criteria based on percentages of IgA- and IgG-containing plasma cells are, however, more sensitive and specific for the diagnosis of Sjögren syndrome (Bodeutsch et al., 1992). Additionally, decreased salivary flow and tearing can be demonstrated. The presence of anti-SSA/Ro and/or anti-SSB-La antibodies and polyclonal hypergammaglobulinaemia may further support the diagnosis of Sjögren syndrome. Although the pathogenesis of this disease is still ill defined, it has been suggested that infiltrating lymphocytes induce destruction of the mucosal glands, eventually resulting in the dryness of these mucosal sites. Alternatively, autoantibodies to the M3 muscarinic acetylcholine receptors may be the causative agents (Yamamoto, 2003). Circulating immune complexes, in contrast, are held responsible for the systemic manifestations. So far, no definite genetic markers have been identified for predisposition to Sjögren syndrome. In the long term, patients with Sjögren syndrome are at risk of developing mucosa-associated B cell lymphomas, probably due to chronic stimulation of the humoral immune system.

5.25 Systemic lupus erythematosus and lupus syndrome

Systemic lupus erythematosus (SLE) is considered the prototype systemic autoimmune disease, and its clinical manifestations are extremely diverse and variable (Hochberg & Petri, 1993).

Drug-induced lupus (lupus syndrome) is a different disease with more or less similar clinical manifestations.

5.25.1 *Systemic lupus erythematosus*

The prevalence of systemic lupus erythematosus in the general population is 40–50 cases per 100 000 persons. Systemic lupus erythematosus has a clear female preponderance (female to male ratio is 9:1). Furthermore, systemic lupus erythematosus is more prevalent in African Americans and Asians than in Caucasians. In addition to constitutional symptoms, such as fever, weight loss, and malaise, nearly every organ system can be involved (e.g. glomerulonephritis, dermatitis, thrombosis, vasculitis, seizures, and non-erosive arthritis). Owing to marked interindividual variability in the clinical expression of the disease, a list of 11 clinical criteria has been proposed, of which 4 must be satisfied for the diagnosis.

Systemic lupus erythematosus is an autoimmune disease characterized by a multitude of autoantibodies, in particular directed against nuclear components. For diagnostic purposes, antibodies to double-stranded DNA and the Sm antigen are most useful. Since antiphospholipid syndrome is frequently encountered in patients with systemic lupus erythematosus, antiphospholipid syndrome-associated autoantibody detection is relevant for recognition of this syndrome. Furthermore, systemic lupus erythematosus follows a course of exacerbations and remissions. In particular, increases in the level of anti-dsDNA antibodies can predict relapses. Autoantibodies appear to play a key role in the pathogenesis of systemic lupus erythematosus. All antinuclear autoantibodies are probably the result of inappropriate removal of apoptotic material in systemic lupus erythematosus, eventually resulting in an immune response to these normally sequestered autoantigens. Next, the tissue deposition of antibodies and immune complexes could cause inflammation and injury of multiple organs. The pathogenicity of autoantibodies is probably the best proven by the occurrence of neonatal lupus and congenital complete heart block. Since systemic lupus erythematosus is primarily an immune complex-mediated disease, it is evident that deficiencies and/or polymorphisms in genes of the complement system and the Fcγ receptors are associated with systemic lupus erythematosus (Tsao, 2003). Furthermore, HLA associations with the HLA-DR2 and HAL-DR3 genes have been consistently described for the Caucasian population. There are rare instances where systemic lupus erythematosus can be more prevalent in exposed human subjects. More recently, induction of autoantibodies to double-stranded DNA have been described in relation to treatment with anti-TNF-α therapy for rheumatoid arthritis or inflammatory bowel disease. However, systemic lupus erythematosus is only infrequently observed in these patients (De Rycke et al., 2003; Vermeire et al., 2003).

5.25.2 Lupus syndrome

Certain drugs, such as hydralazine, procainamide, isoniazid, chlorpromazine, and minocycline, can provoke lupus-like manifestations (D'Cruz, 2000). Clear differences between systemic lupus erythematosus and lupus syndrome can be identified — hence the recommended different terminology. Typical clinical features of the drug-induced lupus syndrome include arthralgias, arthritis, rash, and fever. Involvement of the kidney or the central nervous system hardly ever occurs, whereas pleural and pericardial effusions are far more frequent in lupus syndrome than in systemic lupus erythematosus. Circulating antibodies are often directed to histones in lupus syndrome instead of the classical antinuclear antibodies associated with systemic lupus erythematosus. Importantly, discontinuation of the drug typically results in resolution of the clinical findings in patients with lupus syndrome. It should be emphasized that a number of early reports of so-called drug-induced systemic lupus erythematosus were in fact more likely to be drug hypersensitivity syndromes (DRESS), which underlines the involvement of overlapping mechanisms and clinical similarities, often resulting in misleading statements, if not erroneous diagnosis.

5.26 Autoimmune thrombocytopenia

Greinacher et al. (2001) and Aster (2000) reviewed drug-induced autoimmune thrombocytopenias. Abnormal bleeding associated with thrombocytopenia is characterized by spontaneous skin purpura, mucosal haemorrhage, and prolonged bleeding after trauma. Thrombocytopenia may be due to many different causes; here, we discuss only the immune-mediated diseases that are not secondary to systemic lupus erythematosus, malignancy, or infection. These include immune (idiopathic) thrombocytopenic purpura (ITP), thrombotic thrombocytopenic purpura (TTP), and drug-induced thrombocytopenia (McCrae et al., 2001).

5.26.1 Immune thrombocytopenic purpura

Immune thrombocytopenic purpura is an autoimmune disorder having an incidence of about 100 cases per million persons per year, and about half of these cases occur in young children. Childhood onset is often sudden and follows a viral infection. Boys and girls are equally affected. Adult onset is often insidious and is followed by a chronic course of disease. Adult immune (idiopathic) thrombocytopenic purpura has a female to male ratio of 2:1. Physical examination generally reveals only evidence of platelet-type bleeding. The major cause of fatal bleeding, especially in people over 60 years of age, is intracranial haemorrhage. In both children and adults, the IgG autoantibodies are directed against a number of glycoprotein antigens on the platelet surface, in particular against the GPIIb/GPIIIa and Ib/IX complex. The involvement of these antibodies in the pathogenesis is well established, since transient thrombocytopenia occurs in neonates born to affected women. IgG-sensitized platelets are prematurely removed from the circulation by macrophages, especially in the spleen, reducing the lifespan of a platelet to only a few hours. Additionally, the IgG-sensitized platelets may be destroyed via complement-mediated lysis. Diagnosis is based on low platelet counts ($10–50 \times 10^9$ per litre), but normal white cell counts and haemoglobin concentration. The bone marrow shows normal or increased numbers of megakaryocytes, and IgG autoantibodies may be demonstrated on the platelet surface or in the serum. Obviously, exclusion of other causes is imperative (Cines & Blanchette, 2002).

5.26.2 Thrombotic thrombocytopenic purpura

Thrombotic thrombocytopenic purpura is a rare, potentially fulminant and life-threatening disorder characterized by platelet microthrombi in small vessels. The clinical syndrome is manifested by thrombocytopenia, microangiopathic haemolytic anaemia, fever, renal dysfunction, and neurological abnormalities. The pathological platelet aggregation is the result of deficient activity of the von Willebrand factor cleaving protease ADAMTS13, which breaks down high molecular weight multimers of von Willebrand factor that are normally produced by endothelial cells (Tsai, 2003). The deficiency may be due to genetic mutations (familial thrombotic thrombocytopenic purpura) or autoimmune inhibitors (acquired thrombotic thrombocytopenic purpura). Obviously, only the latter has an autoimmune etiology. Detection of an inhibitor, which has been identified as IgG, can distinguish familial from acquired thrombotic thrombocytopenic purpura (Tsai & Lian, 1998).

5.26.3 Drug-induced thrombocytopenia

The drug most commonly used in clinical practice that can produce immune thrombocytopenic purpura is heparin. Other examples are sulfonamides, thiazide diuretics, chlorpropamide, quinidine, and gold. These types of immune thrombocytopenic purpura are reversed when the drug is withdrawn. Molecular mechanisms for the formation of specific drug-dependent antibodies appear to be very similar. The glycoproteins on the platelet surface interact with the drugs to form neo-epitopes. Subsequent sensitization of platelets with antibodies results in removal of platelets from the circulation and in clinical presentation, as observed in autoimmune thrombocytopenic purpura. Diagnosis includes the effect of drug withdrawal on platelet count. Typically, in the case of heparin-induced thrombocytopenia (HIT), the most common antibody-mediated, drug-induced thrombocytopenic disorder, the molecular mechanism and clinical presentation are different. The antibodies bind to a complex of heparin and platelet factor 4 (PF4). It is likely that this interaction occurs predominantly on the surface of activated platelets, endothelial cells, and macrophages. FcRγIIA cross-linking may further activate the platelets, causing aggregation, whereas endothelial cells and macrophages may produce tissue factor, all contributing to a pro-thrombotic tendency. The clinical presentation of heparin-induced thrombocytopenia, therefore, is moderate thrombocytopenia and new thromboembolic complications. Diagnosis of heparin-induced thrombocytopenia includes laboratory testing for the presence of antibodies against heparin/PF4 complexes or the ability of antibodies to activate platelets in a heparin-dependent manner (McCrae et al., 2001).

5.27 Autoimmune thyroid diseases

The autoimmune thyroid diseases, including Graves disease and Hashimoto thyroiditis, are some of the most common human autoimmune diseases (Pearce et al., 2003). These diseases are characterized by immune responses to thyroid antigen, resulting in infiltration of the thyroid by T cells and production of thyroid antibodies. However, the manifestations of these two entities are clearly different, and the two diseases are discussed separately. Furthermore, the effect of iodine supplementation on thyroiditis is discussed briefly.

The role of certain recombinant cytokines (rIL-2 and IFN-α) has been clearly shown in the induction of antithyroid antibodies and of autoimmune thyroiditis.

5.27.1 Graves disease

Graves disease is defined as a form of hyperthyroidism associated with a diffuse hyperplastic goitre. The prevalence is approximately 1% of the general population (Jacobson et al., 1997). The disease is more prevalent in females than in males (female to male ratio is 7:1). Graves disease usually presents with thyrotoxicosis, due to the release of preformed thyroid hormones from the damaged tissue, and a diffusely enlarged thyroid. Disease is often accompanied by exophthalmos. Patients with Graves disease have diffuse lymphocytic infiltration of the thyroid gland, resulting in thyroid destruction, and produce antibodies to a multitude of antigens, such as thyroid peroxidase (low titre), thyroid-stimulating hormone receptor (TSHR), and thyroglobulin. The diagnosis of Graves disease is based on clinical and biochemical manifestations of hyperthyroidism. The hyperthyroidism is due to continuous stimulation of the thyroid-stimulating hormone receptor by autoantibodies. As a consequence, high levels of thyroid hormones, in particular triiodothyronine (T3), are found in the absence of high levels of plasma thyroid-stimulating hormone (TSH). Alternatively, the anti-thyroid-stimulating hormone receptor autoantibodies may be inhibitory instead of stimulating; the presence of these antibodies is associated with hypothyroidism. The anti-thyroid-stimulating hormone receptor autoantibodies are considered to be responsible for transient neonatal hyperthyroidism. Graves disease has been found to be associated with HLA-DR3, and this may partially explain the association with other autoimmune diseases, such as myasthenia gravis and pernicious anaemia (Tomer, 2002). Treatment is generally with either radioiodine therapy or antithyroid medication. Importantly, drugs that are used to treat hyperthyroidism may induce antineutrophil cytoplasmic autoantibodies and occasionally ANCA-associated vasculitis.

5.27.2 Hashimoto thyroiditis

Chronic progressive autoimmune thyroiditis, known as Hashimoto disease, is an inflammatory disorder that results in progressive destruction of the thyroid gland. The prevalence of Hashimoto disease is 0.5–1.0% (Wang & Crapo, 1997; Lind et al., 1998), but subclinical hypothyroidism is much more common, affecting 4% of the general population, with higher rates among women and with increasing age (Hollowell et al., 2002). This disease is found most commonly in the middle-aged and elderly, but it also occurs in children. Females make up the vast majority of patients (female to male ratio is 8:1). The clinical disease is marked by initial thyrotoxicosis, which is invariably followed by progressive hypothyroidism and myxoedema. The clinical diagnosis of Hashimoto disease is based on the presence of a firm, rubbery, painless goitre with initially euthyroidism, but later clinical signs of hypothyroidism are often apparent in combination with the presence of high titres of antithyroid peroxidase and/or antithyroglobulin antibodies. The former autoantibodies are closely associated with overt thyroid dysfunction, and their presence tends to correlate with thyroidal damage and lymphocytic inflammation. Although these antibodies may be cytotoxic to thyrocytes, formal proof of their pathogenicity has not yet been obtained. Histopathology reveals infiltrates of T cells and plasma cells, often containing germinal centres, and eventual fibrosis. T cells are considered to play a critical role in thyroid destruction by interacting with the follicular cells as well as the extracellular matrix. T cells may destroy thyroid tissue by direct cytotoxicity or indirectly by cytokine secretion. Data on association of HLA haplotypes with Hashimoto thyroiditis are somewhat controversial. HLA-DR3, HLA-DR4, and HLA-DR5 have all been reported to be associated with this disease (Tomer, 2002).

5.27.3 *Iodine and thyroid disease*

Bournaud & Orgiazzi (2003) addressed the evidence for a relationship between levels of iodine exposure and Graves disease and Hashimoto thyroiditis. Excess iodine ingestion has been implicated in the induction and exacerbation of autoimmune thyroiditis in human populations. Iodine is a requisite substrate for the synthesis of the thyroid hormones, but in many countries the levels of iodine ingested in the food are far beyond the recommended level of 150 g/day. The administration of pharmacological quantities of iodine, such as iodides for the treatment of pulmonary disease, organic iodine present in medications, and X-ray contrast dyes, and the ingestion of iodine-rich natural foods may result in goitre, hypothyroidism, or hyperthyroidism, especially in patients with underlying thyroid disease (Vagenakis & Braverman, 1975). An autoregulatory mechanism within the thyroid serves as the first line of defence against fluctuations in the supply of iodine. This mechanism also prevents induction of the Wolff-Chaikoff effect, which is associated with inhibition of thyroid stimulating hormone synthesis that can result from exposure to a very large quantity of iodine. The pathological consequences of iodine excess, such as seen with the Wolff-Chaikoff effect, ensue only when thyroid autoregulation is defective or when autoregulation is absent (Woeber, 1991). When the source of iodine has been dissipated, the pathological consequences of iodine excess will resolve.

The issue is further discussed in chapter 8.

5.28 Diseases with autoimmune components

Several diseases that have not been mentioned so far in this chapter have recently been more and more considered to be autoimmune in nature. However, because the autoimmune component has not been identified or other pathogenetic mechanisms dominate disease progression, these diseases have not yet been accepted as true autoimmune diseases. Here, we only briefly discuss some apparent examples, with emphasis on the contribution of the autoimmune response to these conditions.

Sarcoidosis is a multisystem granulomatous disease of unknown origin that occurs most commonly in young adults. Pulmonary manifestations occur in more than 90% of patients. Accumulation of CD4 T cells that proliferate in situ spontaneously produces inflammatory cytokines and causes a lymphocytic alveolitis and granulomatous lesions. The disease is characterized by autoantibodies on erythrocytes (Pilatte et al., 1990), but deregulation of the immune response, in particular the cytokine response, is an alternative explanation to an autoimmune pathogenesis.

Hepatitis C patients treated with IFN-α seem to be at a greater risk of developing sarcoidosis.

A sarcoidosis-like pulmonary disease has been clearly associated with beryllium exposure.

Alzheimer disease is a very heterogeneous disorder that is characterized by dementia due to plaque formation, with a central amyloid core, in frontal and temporal lobes. Although small mononuclear infiltrates have been described, they are not held responsible for the initiation of Alzheimer disease. Nevertheless, secondary immune responses to, for instance, amyloid-β peptides may contribute to the pathogenesis of the disease, but this has not been validated.

Atherosclerosis is a chronic inflammation of the arterial vessel wall resulting in plaque formation that eventually may cause cardiovascular events, such as myocardial infarction or cerebral vascular accidents. The presence of autoimmune components in atherosclerosis is well established. Autoantibodies to heat-shock proteins and oxidized low-density lipoproteins (oxLDL) are prevalent in the circulation of patients with atherosclerosis, but the role of these autoantibodies is debated. While anti-oxLDL IgG antibodies may facilitate uptake of oxLDL by foam cells in the lesions, natural IgM antibodies directed to oxLDL may even protect from atherosclerosis. Atherosclerotic plaques also contain some T cells that are considered to be autoreactive, although the respective autoantigens have not yet been identified. These T cells are probably not involved in the plaque formation as such, but they may cause plaque instability, rupture, and subsequent clinical events.

6. EPIDEMIOLOGY

6.1 Descriptive epidemiology

Descriptive epidemiology is the study of the distribution and burden of disease within a population. The incidence of a disease is the number of new diagnoses that occur in a population in a given time period. The prevalence is the number of people who have the disease and so is determined by the incidence and duration of the illness. The criteria used to define a disease, methods used to identify people with a specific condition, study area, as well as secular changes in rates can contribute to the variability in rates for a specific disease that may be seen among studies.

A recent review of epidemiological studies covering 24 specific autoimmune diseases estimated that approximately 3% of the population in the United States suffers from an autoimmune disease (Jacobson et al., 1997). This estimate is likely to be low, as for many diseases our knowledge of basic epidemiology is quite limited or based on studies conducted 30 or more years ago, and some diseases (e.g. psoriasis) were not included in this summary. A revised estimate of the prevalence of autoimmune diseases presented in a recent report of the United States National Institutes of Health (2000) is 5–8%. Comparable figures for other countries are not available.

Many specific autoimmune diseases are relatively rare, with an estimated incidence of less than 5 per 100 000 persons per year or an estimated prevalence of less than 20 per 100 000 (Table 7). Other diseases (e.g. rheumatoid arthritis, Graves disease, thyroiditis) are quite common, affecting 1% or more of the population (Cotch et al., 1996; Boberg et al., 1998; Cooper et al., 1998; Marie et al., 1999; Boisseau-Garsaud et al., 2000; Watts et al., 2000; Pillemer et al., 2001; Doran et al., 2002; Kalb et al., 2002; Lovas & Husebye, 2002; Feld & Heathcote, 2003; Gonzalez-Gay et al., 2003; Mayes et al., 2003; Bogliun & Beghi, 2004; Cuadrado et al., 2004).

Table 7. Estimated incidence and prevalence rates and demographic distributions of selected autoimmune diseases[a]

Disease	Incidence per 100 000 person-years	Prevalence per 100 000	% female	Usual age at diagnosis	Primary reference(s)
Systemic diseases					
ANCA-associated vasculitis	2	15	40	50–75	Watts et al. (2000); Gonzalez-Gay et al. (2003)
Dermatomyositis and polymyositis	2	5	70	45–60	Jacobson et al. (1997); Marie et al. (1999)
Rheumatoid arthritis (adults)	25	860	75	40–70	Jacobson et al. (1997); Doran et al. (2002)
Sjögren syndrome	4	15	95	40–75	Jacobson et al. (1997); Pillemer et al. (2001)
Systemic lupus erythematosus	2–8	20–60	90	30–50	Jacobson et al. (1997); Cooper et al. (1998)
Systemic sclerosis (scleroderma)	2	25	90	35–65	Jacobson et al. (1997); Mayes et al. (2003)
Organ-specific diseases					
Addison disease	0.6	5–15	93	15–45	Jacobson et al. (1997); Lovas & Husebye (2002)
Diabetes (type 1)	12	200	45	8–15	Jacobson et al. (1997)
Guillain-Barré syndrome	1–2	No data	40	40–70	Bogliun & Beghi (2004); Cuadrado et al. (2004)
Hyperthyroidism (Graves disease)	14	1200	88	40–55	Jacobson et al. (1997)

Epidemiology

Table 7 (Contd)

Disease	Incidence per 100 000 person-years	Prevalence per 100 000	% female	Usual age at diagnosis	Primary reference(s)
Hypothyroidism (Hashimoto thyroiditis)	No data	500–1000	85	45–75	Jacobson et al. (1997); Wang & Crapo (1997); Lind et al. (1998)
Autoimmune hepatitis	2	15	90	biomodal? 0–30; 50–70	Boberg et al. (1998); Feld & Heathcote (2003)
Primary biliary cirrhosis	1	4	90	40–65	Jacobson et al. (1997); Boberg et al. (1998); Feld & Heathcote (2003)
Primary sclerosing cholangitis	1	10	30	20–40	Boberg et al. (1998); Feld & Heathcote (2003)
Multiple sclerosis	3	60	65	25–45	Jacobson et al. (1997)
Myasthenia gravis	0.4	15	75	20–50	Jacobson et al. (1997); Kalb et al. (2002)
Vitiligo	No data	100–500	52	15–30	Jacobson et al. (1997); Boisseau-Garsaud et al. (2000)

[a] Selected on the basis of availability of published data (two or more studies) and incidence of at least 1.0 per 100 000 per year. Diabetes mellitus type 1 rates are for children and adolescents (age <20 years); all other rates are for adult populations.

6.1.1 Demographic patterns

There are differences among the diseases in terms of usual age at onset. Two autoimmune diseases, diabetes mellitus type 1 and myocarditis, are most commonly seen in children and adolescents. Most other autoimmune diseases are much less common in children than in adults. For example, the incidence or prevalence rates of dermatomyositis (Mendez et al., 2003), hypothyroidism (Brownlie & Wells, 1990; Hunter et al., 2000), multiple sclerosis (Gadoth, 2003), myasthenia gravis (Poulas et al., 2001; Kalb et al., 2002), and uveitis (Paivonsalo-Hietanen et al., 2000) are approximately one tenth the rates in adults. Addison disease, multiple sclerosis, and vitiligo occur most often in young adults (and teenagers, in the case of vitiligo) (Table 7). The autoimmune thyroid diseases, lupus, systemic sclerosis, and rheumatoid arthritis usually occur in late-reproductive and early-postmenopausal years, while some other diseases (e.g. systemic vasculitis, Sjögren disease) generally have an older onset.

Almost all autoimmune diseases that occur in adults disproportionately affect women. However, there is considerable variability in the extent of female predominance and no clear relation between degree of female predominance and type of disease or age at onset (Table 7). More than 85% of patients with Sjögren syndrome, systemic lupus erythematosus, systemic sclerosis, the autoimmune thyroid diseases, and primary biliary cirrhosis are female, compared with 65–75% of patients with rheumatoid arthritis and multiple sclerosis. Some diseases (e.g. diabetes mellitus type 1, ANCA-associated vasculitis, primary sclerosing cholangitis) occur more often in males than in females.

The extent to which ethnic, racial, or geographic variability in disease incidence or severity occurs has been well characterized for only the few autoimmune diseases that have been the subject of numerous epidemiological studies. Incidence and/or prevalence rates of diabetes mellitus type 1 (Karvonen et al., 2000), juvenile rheumatoid arthritis (Oen, 2000), and multiple sclerosis (Rosati, 2001) tend to be higher in northern European countries than in southern European countries; rates in Asian countries are also low. In diabetes mellitus type 1, multiple sclerosis, and hyperthyroidism, rates are higher among whites than among minority groups (Kurtzke et al., 1979; Lorenzi et al., 1985; Hollowell et al., 2002). African Americans and other minority groups in the United States, Canada, and the United Kingdom are at higher risk of systemic lupus erythematosus compared with whites (Hopkinson et al., 1993; Johnson et al., 1995; McCarty et al., 1995) and of scleroderma compared with whites (Mayes et al., 2003). Severity of these diseases is worse in these groups, too, with increased disease activity, increased organ

Epidemiology

damage (particularly renal involvement), and higher mortality risks (Laing et al., 1997; Alarcon et al., 1998; Sutcliffe et al., 1999; Peschken & Esdaile, 2000).

6.1.2 Co-morbidity of autoimmune diseases

Co-morbidity of the autoimmune disorders (i.e. the co-occurrence of different autoimmune disorders) is of particular interest, since it may indicate a common genetic susceptibility or common environmental etiological factors. Thus, it may permit the detection of genes or environmental factors that can inform preventive action. Co-morbidity can be observed at a number of levels, including the individual, the household, the family (genetically related), and population levels.

Animal models suggest that both genetic and environmental factors are important in co-morbidity, and of particular interest is the way in which environmental factors can modify genetic susceptibility. Thus, non-obese diabetic (NOD) mice develop thyroiditis and sialo-adenitis in addition to autoimmune diabetes (Skarstein et al., 1995). This expression of autoimmune disorders is modified by the degree of microbial contamination of the environment (Rossini et al., 1995) and by early life exposure to filarial worms (Imai et al., 2001). In both cases, early immune stimulation leads to lower incidence of diabetes, showing how genetic susceptibility to multiple autoimmune disorders may be disguised by environmental factors.

Data pertaining to co-morbidity of autoimmune diseases in humans are surprisingly sparse. Few studies are population-based, and few are of sufficient size to address potentially important biological associations, given the relative rarity of many diseases (Scofield, 1996). A recent unpublished review of co-morbidity of rheumatoid arthritis, diabetes mellitus type 1, multiple sclerosis, Crohn disease, and autoimmune thyroid disease found evidence of an increased incidence of autoimmune thyroid disease in patients with rheumatoid arthritis and in autoimmune diabetes (E. Somers, unpublished data).

Familial association studies have reported an increased risk of several autoimmune diseases (including lupus, rheumatoid arthritis, and thyroid diseases) among relatives of patients with a systemic autoimmune disease (Cooper et al., 1999). Studies in this area are also few and most of a small size, which makes control of confounding difficult. One study of the household showed that those living with subjects suffering from systemic lupus erythematosus were more likely to have related autoantibodies (DeHoratius et al., 1975). The study was not able to fully distinguish between a genetic and environmental relationship, but it raises many intriguing questions.

6.2 Epidemiology of autoantibodies

6.2.1 Prevalence of autoantibodies in the general population

Studies of autoantibodies in the general population allow us to determine the prevalence of specific autoantibodies among people who do not have a clinically evident autoimmune disease, whether the prevalence of autoantibodies reflects the demographic variation in disease risk and whether specific environmental exposures are related to the expression of specific autoantibodies. These studies are most feasible for the autoantibodies associated with the most common autoimmune diseases: diabetes mellitus type 1, autoimmune thyroid disease, and rheumatoid arthritis. Important issues with respect to interpreting these types of studies include the type of test used and definition of a "positive" result.

Islet cell antibodies (ICA) were first described by Bottazzo et al. (1974), a pivotal point in establishing diabetes mellitus type 1 as an autoimmune disease. Insulin autoantibodies and antibodies directed against specific islet cell proteins, including glutamic acid decarboxylase and a member of the protein tyrosine phosphatase family, islet antigen 2 (IA-2A or ICA512), were subsequently identified (Pozzilli et al., 2001). Approximately 5% of high-risk groups (defined on the basis of family history or genetic susceptibility) have two or more of these antibodies, compared with 0.5% of the general population. The presence of diabetes-related autoantibodies is strongly associated with subsequent risk of developing disease. In the high-risk groups (e.g. family members of patients with diabetes mellitus type 1), approximately 30–60% of people with any specific diabetes-related autoantibody develop diabetes mellitus type 1 over 5–10 years of follow-up, with an increased risk seen as the number of antibodies increases (Bruining et al., 1989; Schatz et al., 1994; Verge et al., 1996; Bingley et al., 1997; Kulmala et al., 1998;

Ziegler et al., 1999; Yu et al., 2000; Kimpimaki et al., 2001; LaGasse et al., 2002).

The prevalence of antithyroglobulin and antithyroid peroxidase antibodies (formerly called antimicrosomal antibodies) increases with age, and the antibodies are more common among women than among men (Hawkins et al., 1980; Prentice et al., 1990; Vanderpump et al., 1995; Hollowell et al., 2002). In the recent population-based sample in the United States, approximately 18% of people ages 12–80 who were not taking thyroid medications and did not report a history of thyroid disease or goitre had one or both of these antibodies. The highest prevalence of these antibodies was seen in whites (Hollowell et al., 2002). In the cross-sectional analysis of the full population (including those with thyroid disease), antithyroid peroxidase antibodies, but not antithyroglobulin antibodies, were highly predictive of hypothyroidism and hyperthyroidism (defined on the basis of thyroid stimulating hormone and thyroxine [T4] levels). The predictive ability of antithyroid peroxidase antibodies for the subsequent development of hypothyroidism was also seen in a longitudinal study in the United Kingdom (Vanderpump et al., 1995).

Rheumatoid factor is seen in 3–10% of people over age 60 (Enzer et al., 2002; Korpilähde et al., 2003). In the Pima Indians, a population with an extremely high incidence of rheumatoid arthritis, the prevalence of rheumatoid factor is higher in females than in males (Enzer et al., 2002), but in other populations there is little difference by sex (Korpilähde et al., 2003). Rheumatoid factor and anti-cyclic citrullinated peptide antibodies have been shown to be predictive of the development of rheumatoid arthritis (del Puente et al., 1988; Rantapaa-Dahlqvist et al., 2003).

Several large studies of antinuclear antibodies in the general population have been conducted using blood donors (Fritzler et al., 1985; Craig et al., 1999), community-based sampling (Rosenberg et al., 1999), or other sampling approaches (Tan et al., 1997). Similar estimates were seen in these studies, with a prevalence of approximately 25–30% at a titre of 1:40 and 3–4% at a titre of 1:320. The prevalence of antinuclear antibodies is lower in children than in adults, but is fairly constant through the reproductive years. Other studies have reported increased antinuclear antibody (ANA) prevalence among the elderly, but this finding may be limited to those with chronic diseases. There are limited, and somewhat conflicting, data comparing prevalence of high-titre antinuclear antibodies by sex (Craig et al., 1999; Rosenberg et al., 1999). None of these studies was able to provide data pertaining to ethnic differences in the prevalence of antinuclear antibodies.

We do not currently have data pertaining to the predictive ability of antinuclear antibodies with respect to development of lupus. However, a study using serum samples from 130 active-duty personnel in the United States military who developed systemic lupus erythematosus documented the presence of antinuclear antibodies, anti-Ro antibodies, anti-La antibodies, antiphospholipid antibodies, and anti-dsDNA antibodies a mean of 1–3 years before the occurrence of symptoms (Arbuckle et al., 2003).

6.2.2 Associations between autoantibodies and environmental exposures

Relatively few studies have examined environmental influences on the development of autoantibodies. A complex relation is seen between dietary iodine and prevalence of antithyroid antibodies, with increased prevalence reported in relation to iodine deficiency and to excess intake. This issue is discussed in greater detail in section 8.10 on iodine.

Smoking history has been associated with the prevalence of rheumatoid factor in several studies (Regius et al., 1988, 1990), including a population-based study in Finland (Heliovaara et al., 2000) and a longitudinal study in Iceland (Jonsson et al., 1998). These studies reported an increased prevalence of rheumatoid factor among smokers. A similar association was also seen between smoking and antinuclear antibodies in one study (Regius et al., 1990). With respect to thyroid antibodies, however, smoking was associated with a decreased prevalence of antithyroid peroxidase antibodies in a study of 759 women in the Netherlands (Strieder et al., 2003).

Some organochlorine chemicals (including some pesticides and industrial by-products, such as polychlorinated biphenyls [PCBs] and hexachlorobenzene) may interfere with the metabolism of thyroid hormones (Brouwer et al., 1999; Sala et al., 2001).

Abnormal levels of thyroid stimulating hormone and thyroxine and an increased prevalence of antithyroid antibodies have been reported among workers in a highly contaminated PCBs manufacturing plant in East Slovakia (Langer et al., 1998). Anti-glutamic acid decarboxylase antibodies were also found at an increased prevalence among these workers (Langer et al., 2002), but additional information regarding parameters related to glucose metabolism and diabetes mellitus type 1 are not available. There is also evidence of thyroid-related effects, including increased thyroid volume, abnormal thyroid stimulating hormone, and antithyroid peroxidase antibodies from environmental, rather than occupational, exposure to PCBs (Langer et al., 2003) and dithiocarbamates, especially ethylenebis-dithiocarbamates (Marinovich et al., 1997).

There are also other studies on pesticide immunotoxicity following exposure to the pesticide mancozeb (Colosio et al., 1996; Corsini et al., 2005). Both of these studies suggest a slight immunostimulatory effect exerted by mancozeb. Little is known about pesticide exposure and autoantibodies. Small studies examining pentachlorophenol (McConnachie & Zahalsky, 1991; Colosio et al., 1993), chlordane (McConnachie & Zahalsky, 1992), and chlorpyrifos (Thrasher et al., 1993) have reported inconsistent associations in relation to antinuclear antibodies, anti-smooth muscle antibodies, and thyroid antibodies. Rosenberg et al. (1999) examined the prevalence of low-titre (1:40) antinuclear antibodies in relation to various farming tasks and pesticide exposure in a population-based study of 322 residents in Saskatchewan, Canada. There was a 2-fold increased prevalence with history of exposure to insecticides and herbicides, but not with exposure to fungicides or algicides. This association was seen with several specific organochlorine pesticides, but was not seen in analyses of higher-titre antinuclear antibodies.

7. MECHANISMS OF CHEMICAL-ASSOCIATED AUTOIMMUNE RESPONSES

7.1 General

When discussing mechanisms of chemical-induced autoimmunity, it should be stressed that autoimmunity is an ill-understood phenomenon. It is also important to realize that normal healthy individuals possess natural autoantibodies as well as autoreactive T and B cells to provide a necessary and protective immunological homeostasis (Avrameas, 1991; Schwartz & Cohen, 2000). At the present time, it is not precisely known why on certain occasions autoimmune responses can lead to pathological conditions (i.e. autoimmune diseases). Another important consideration is that mechanisms of systemic allergy may resemble those of autoimmune reactions, at least to some extent.

Compounds can induce the release of neoantigens (cryptic epitopes) or alter autoantigens so that they appear foreign (Griem et al., 1998). Specificity of an immune response induced by a compound may be initially directed exclusively towards this neoantigen, but after a certain time it spreads to include autoantigen-directed responses. For instance, it has been shown that T cells from mice exposed to mercury(II) chloride for only one week responded to mercury(II) chloride or mercury-modified fibrillarin, whereas after eight weeks of exposure, the T cells responded to native fibrillarin as well (Kubicka-Muranyi et al., 1996). This process, referred to as epitope or determinant spreading (Sercarz et al., 1993), may explain why individuals, after a certain period of exposure, have an autoimmune response. Individual properties of patients may determine whether the immune response is eventually more allergy-like or more autoimmune-like in nature.

The immune system is highly host-specific (for instance, based on MHC haplotypes). Whether exposure to a chemical results in immune-related diseases may depend more on a patient's individual predisposing characteristics and circumstances of exposure than on the characteristics of the chemical itself (Lehmann et al., 1993). The multifactorial nature of the process may explain why only relatively few patients develop adverse clinical responses.

The complexity of chemical-induced systemic allergy and autoimmunity is a major hurdle for the development of models predictive for such adverse effects of chemicals. To illustrate the possible mechanisms of chemical-induced autoimmunity, in particular regarding initiation of processes, it is reasonable to consider results of studies with allergenic drugs as well.

Mechanisms through which chemicals cause sensitization of the immune system are very diverse, but they can mostly be categorized according to the general strategy that is followed by the immune system (Janeway & Medzhitov, 2002; Hoebe et al., 2004) (see Fig. 1). According to this strategy, immunization occurs only when cells of the adaptive immune system (T and B lymphocytes) encounter antigen-specific signals (providing so-called signal 1 to the lymphocyte) from antigen-presenting cells in combination with additional, adjuvant-like costimulatory signals (collectively called signal 2). Once sensitized, T cells may activate various effector mechanisms that in turn may cause protective immunity or, depending on the antigen that is recognized and under certain circumstances, adverse (i.e. allergic or autoimmune) disorders. All steps in this process are strongly regulated by a number of factors, including immune, neuroendocrine, and environmental factors (see Fig. 1). Together, this strategy aims to tailor the immune response so as to effectively get rid of the initiating antigen and at the same time to prevent the immune response from persisting or possibly proceeding to adverse effects.

Drugs may interfere with all phases of this immune strategy. For instance, chemicals may interfere with antigen-specific stimulation (signal 1) by forming neoantigens (section 7.2.1), inducing targets for cross-reactivity (section 7.2.2), releasing non-tolerant epitopes (section 7.2.3), or interfering with central tolerance (section 7.2.4). Chemicals may also elicit adjuvant-like processes, reminiscent of danger signals, leading to increased costimulation, and thus provide signal 2 to lymphocytes (section 7.2.5). And obviously, chemicals may directly (e.g. through modification of immune regulatory processes) or indirectly (e.g. through the neuroendocrine system) (section 7.2.6) affect the functionality of the immune system.

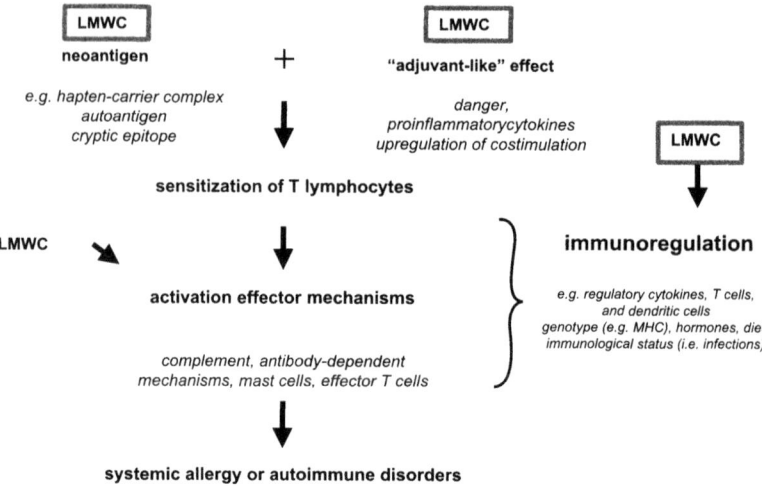

Fig. 1. Schematic view of chemical-induced adverse immune responses. LMWC are low molecular weight compounds.

7.2 Induction of antigen-specific responses

Many chemicals have been suggested to induce antigen-specific immune responses, but it is not always known to which antigenic structure the immune response is directed. Most chemicals are low molecular weight compounds with a molecular weight often less than 500 daltons, which is actually too small to be recognized by a specific T cell that usually recognizes amino acid stretches of about 9–12 amino acids in the groove of MHC molecules.

7.2.1 Formation of neoantigens

Although low molecular weight compounds cannot be recognized directly by T cells, they can be recognized as part of a larger self-protein structure (i.e. a skin protein or antigen on the surface of an erythrocyte). Once a low molecular weight compound has bound to a larger protein, a so-called hapten–carrier complex is formed. This hapten–carrier complex can then be processed by antigen-presenting cells and presented by MHC molecules to, and recognized by, specific T cells. In the case of hapten–carrier complex formation, the binding between the chemical and the carrier protein is supposed to be covalent in nature. This concept is the basis of the "hapten hypothesis" (Griem et al., 1998). In contrast to most chemicals, such as industrial chemicals, sensitizing drugs, however, are usually not chemically reactive, and it is hypothesized that they need to be bioactivated through metabolism to bind covalently to a carrier and become immunogenic.

Chemicals may also directly alter MHC molecules — for instance, on the surface of autoreactive B cells that are normally present in healthy individuals (Klinkhammer et al., 1989). This altered-self hypothesis is in fact an extension of the hapten hypothesis and proposes that specific T cells that recognize altered MHC molecules may provide "help" signals so that the autoreactive B cells carrying these molecules start to produce autoantibodies. In this case, T cell help is called non-cognate help, because T and B cells recognize different antigens. This hypothesis is supported by studies with allergenic chemicals such as trinitrochlorobenzene (Weltzien et al., 1996) and with certain metals (e.g. nickel and gold) (Sinigaglia, 1994).

It has also recently been shown that T cells isolated from patients with a history of drug allergy can respond to the offending drug when it is presented by MHC molecules without the need to bind covalently. Based on these findings, the pharmacological interaction concept has been formulated (Pichler, 2002). According to this concept, metabolic activation of the drug is not required. However, whether drugs are also capable of inducing adverse immune reactions by this mechanism is as yet unknown.

7.2.2 Cross-reactivity

Generation of cross-reactive T cells might be another way by which chemicals can induce hypersensitivity and stimulate autoimmune responses (Pichler, 2002; Depta & Pichler, 2003). Cross-reactivity implies that T cells may recognize not only the best-fitting MHC–peptide complex, but also completely different peptides in the groove of unrelated MHC molecules.

It has been found that certain drug-reactive T cell clones (e.g. allopurinol, carbamazepine, lamotrigine, sulfamethoxazole) were

MHC allele-unrestricted and at the same time highly drug-specific, which means that they did not respond to metabolites with even small chemical alterations. Other drug-induced T cell clones appeared less stringent with respect to the drug structure they recognized, but they were highly MHC allele-restricted. Still other drug-induced T cells responded to MHC–peptide complexes in the absence of the initiating drug and in an MHC allele-unrestricted manner. Thus, the specificity of drug-reactive T cells may range from highly drug-specific and non-MHC-restricted to highly MHC-restricted and non-drug-specific. From these findings, it can be inferred that drug-induced T cells can also react with autoantigens through cross-reactivity.

7.2.3 Release of non-tolerant epitopes

Non-tolerant epitopes can be defined as parts of antigenic self-proteins to which no tolerance has developed and to which an immune response can take place when recognized by T lymphocytes. Examples of non-tolerant epitopes are sequestered epitopes and cryptic epitopes (Sercarz et al., 1993; Moudgil & Sercarz, 1994).

Anatomically sequestered epitopes (as part of an antigen) are part of immunologically privileged sites, such as the eye, brain, and testis, but also intracellular epitopes that normally do not come in contact with lymphocytes. As these antigens do not come in contact with the developing immune system, tolerance does not exist. As a consequence of tissue damage, however, antigens may be released in the system, and naive specific T cells may become activated. As these T cells are then reactive to self-proteins, a destructive autoimmune response may follow. In principle, chemicals, once being reactive and membrane damaging, may induce autoimmune responses in this manner.

Foreign proteins as well as self-proteins contain dominant and cryptic epitopes (Sercarz et al., 1993; Moudgil & Sercarz, 1994). Dominant epitopes of a protein are those epitopes or stretches of peptide that survive enzymatic proteolysis and in addition bind with sufficiently high affinity to MHC molecules to be presented to T cells. Peptide stretches that do not survive antigen processing (e.g. survive enzymatic splicing), that do not bind to MHC molecules, or with too low affinity remain unnoticed and are considered cryptic to

T cells. T cells that recognize dominant epitopes with too high an affinity or avidity have a high chance of being eliminated during the intrathymic selection process, whereas T cells that are specific to cryptic epitopes will usually not encounter their epitope in the thymus. Hence, these T cells will not be eliminated in the thymus and appear in the peripheral system.

It has been shown that certain chemicals (e.g. Au^{III} salts; Griem et al., 1996) and *para*-substituted benzene derivatives (Wulferink et al., 2002) may interfere with the antigen itself or with antigen processing in such a way that cryptic epitopes end up in the peptide binding groove of the MHC molecule in sufficiently high levels to be efficiently presented to T cells. The underlying mechanisms are unknown, but may include (i) changes in antigen processing, (ii) structural alterations of the antigen, (iii) interference with antigen processing (e.g. altered splicing), or (iv) increased expression of MHC molecules (e.g. as a result of cytokines).

7.2.4 Interference with central tolerance

The classical example of a chemical that interferes with the generation of central tolerance is cyclosporin. Under specific circumstances (e.g. perinatal or neonatal T cell development, bone marrow reconstitution after irradiation), the interference with negative thymocyte selection that occurs as a result of cyclosporin treatment results in an autoimmune syngeneic graft versus host disease with scleroderma-like symptoms (Barendrecht et al., 2002; Damoiseaux, 2002). Administration of cyclosporin to newborn mice has been shown to abrogate production of mature thymocytes and cause various organ-specific autoimmune diseases, including thyroiditis, oophoritis, orchitis, insulitis, and adrenalitis (Sakaguchi & Sakaguchi, 1989).

A recently suggested mode of action of the induction of immune responsiveness as a result of drug exposure also involves interference with central tolerance induction in the thymus. It has been demonstrated that intrathymic injection of procainamide-hydroxylamine, a metabolite of procainamide, alters positive selection and results in systemic lupus erythematosus-like changes (appearance of antibodies to a histone [H2A-H2B]–DNA complex) in C57BL/6 mice (Kretz-Rommel et al., 1997; Rubin & Kretz-Rommel, 2001).

This mechanism may be age-dependent, as central tolerance induction may be more or less pronounced at various stages in life.

7.2.5 Signal 2 increasing mechanisms

7.2.5.1 Importance of signal 2

Importantly, in the absence of co-stimulatory help, signal 1 is known to induce a state of immunological tolerance, whereas signal 2 alone will not elicit any response. In other words, signal 2 can be considered to be more decisive than signal 1 for inducing an immune response.

Signal 2 or co-stimulation is provided by non-antigen-specific receptor–ligand interactions and is required for optimal sensitization of both T and B lymphocytes. The most crucial co-stimulatory signals for T cells are mediated through receptor–ligand couples CD40-CD154 and by the CD80/CD86 (B7 molecules)-CD28/CTLA-4 pathway (Salomon & Bluestone, 2001; Carreno & Collins, 2002). Over the past years, more B7 homologues and ligands have been discovered and new pathways have been described that seem to be important in regulating adaptive immune responses, resulting in the recognition of a B7 family (Henry et al., 1999; Carreno & Collins, 2002). Some of these co-stimulatory interactions have stimulatory effects, whereas others have an inhibitory or regulatory effect (in particular, CTLA-4). To better understand the regulation of T cell activation, it has been suggested that all critical signalling molecules (in the vicinity of the TCR complex) constitute a so-called signalosome. The signalosome is directly related to the immunological synapse and organized as a flexible aggregation of lipid rafts at the interface between T cells and antigen-presenting cells. Altogether, it is important to realize that the interaction of antigen-presenting cells and T cells involves a complex set of interacting and modulatory receptor–ligand couples. In addition, a number of cytokines are regarded as inducers and mediators of co-stimulatory help. Among these are, for instance, IL-2, IL-4, and IFN-γ, but many more can be added to the list, including proinflammatory cytokines such as TNF-α and IL-1β.

To comprehend the importance of co-stimulatory help, it is important to recall that normal healthy individuals possess T and B cells that are specific and responsive to a variety of autoepitopes.

Conceivably, signal 1 for these pre-existing autoreactive lymphocytes is readily available; once an immune response to a foreign antigen occurs, these autoreactive cells may also become activated through induction of co-stimulatory help that initially is provided to help the immune response to that foreign antigen. As mentioned previously, this process of epitope spreading, in which co-stimulation might be crucial, has been shown to occur in the case of mercury(II) chloride-induced autoimmunity in mice (see section 8.6.1).

The role of co-stimulation has been the focus of many studies in disease and therapy and also investigated in relation to chemical-induced immune effects. Recently, it has been shown that co-stimulatory interactions (CD40-CD154 and the B7 molecules CD80 and CD86) are crucial for sensitization induced by the model autoimmunogenic drugs D-penicillamine and diphenylhydantoin (Nierkens et al., 2002). Also, in the case of contact hypersensitivity responses (Tang et al., 1998; Nuriya et al., 1996) and mercury(II) chloride-induced autoimmune effects in Brown Norway rats (MacPhee et al., 2001), co-stimulation appeared to be decisive for the development of clinical effects.

7.2.5.2 Induction of signal 2

Current knowledge suggests that expression of signal 2-providing receptors and molecules by antigen-presenting dendritic cells is induced by activation of innate danger-recognizing molecules, such as Toll-like receptors (Matzinger, 1994, 2002; McFadden & Basketter, 2000; Seguin & Uetrecht, 2003) or other pattern recognition receptors (Janeway & Medzhitov, 2002; Hoebe et al., 2004). Engagement of pattern recognition receptors (such as Toll-like receptors) will trigger intracellular responses, such as activation of NF-κB, NF-IL-6, or interferon regulatory factor (IRF), which, in turn, stimulates expression of co-stimulatory receptors and proinflammatory cytokines (such as TNF-α) (Sato et al., 2003; Iwasaki & Medzhitov, 2004).

Ligands of the Toll-like receptors described to date include a range of molecules, including lipoproteins (TLR2), double-stranded RNA (polyI:C) (TLR3), lipopolysaccharides (TLR4), heat shock proteins (TLR4), polysaccharides (TLR4), bacterial DNA (CpG stretches, TLR9), and many more structures known to be of microbial origin. Also, a number of synthetic imidazoquinolines are recognized by Toll-like receptors; these include loxoribine, bropirimine, resiquimod (R-848), and imiquimod (approved to treat genital warts) (Sato et al., 2003).

Endogenous molecules have also been shown to induce co-stimulatory activity of dendritic cells. These molecules, such as uric acid (Shi et al., 2003), may, for instance, originate from necrotic cells (Sauter et al., 2000; Shi & Rock, 2002).

With regard to chemical-induced autoimmunity and allergy, induction of co-stimulatory molecules may result from pattern recognition receptor engagement on dendritic cells by components of damaged cells. In this case, the chemical needs to be reactive in a sense that it induces cell death. However, chemicals may also directly bind to pattern recognition receptors, as shown for the imidazoquinolines. This concept is the basis of the danger hypothesis to explain how chemicals may induce co-stimulatory help (Seguin & Uetrecht, 2003).

Limited information exists on the possible role of the danger hypothesis in chemical-induced autoimmune-like derangements. Interestingly, poly I:C has been shown to increase the incidence and severity of D-penicillamine-induced autoimmunity in Brown Norway rats (Sayeh & Uetrecht, 2001).

7.2.6 Immunoregulation

Evidently, being an aggressive defence mechanism and potentially autoreactive, the immune system has to be kept under control so as to tolerate those antigens that pose no threat. In addition, immune responses need to be quantitatively and qualitatively optimal and eventually cease to be operational when the antigen vanishes. A properly balanced immune response is accomplished by a range of regulatory mechanisms, including a variety of regulatory cells (innate as well as adaptive) (Bach, 2003; Morelli & Thomson, 2003; von Herrath & Harrison, 2003; Raulet, 2004; Rutella & Lemoli, 2004), the complement system (Carroll, 2004), activation-induced cell death mechanisms (Green et al., 2003), complement-mediated antibody clearance (Gatenby, 1991), and neuroendocrine–immune interactions (Ligier & Sternberg, 1999).

Mechanisms of Chemical-Associated Autoimmune Responses

Chemically induced autoimmune diseases are often transient, resolve spontaneously, and cannot be induced again in the same animal. For instance, in Brown Norway rats, mercury(II) chloride induces autoimmune phenomena (immune complex glomerulonephritis, phenotypic alterations in immune organs) that peak around day 10 after the last of five subcutaneous injections. Twenty days later, immune alterations are again mostly at control levels, and the effects on the kidney (for instance, proteinuria) are clearly less than on day 10 (Aten et al., 1988). In addition, low-dose pretreatment of Brown Norway rats with mercury(II) chloride prevents the development of adverse immunity. Transience of autoimmune effects as well as low-dose protection may both be due to the development of regulatory immune cells. In the case of mercury(II) chloride, these cells have been identified as either IFN-γ-producing $CD8^+$ regulatory T cells (Pelletier et al., 1987; Szeto et al., 1999) or $RT6.2^+$ T cells (Kosuda et al., 1994). Low-dose pre-exposure to D-penicillamine also induced tolerance in Brown Norway rats (Donker et al., 1984). It appeared in this case that low-dose pretreatment prevented all clinical signs of autoimmunity in 60–80% of rats that were subsequently treated with a high and usually pathogenic dose of D-penicillamine. Recently, this has been shown to be immune mediated and possibly mediated by the regulatory cytokines TGFβ and IL-10, which were found to be produced predominantly by CD4 lymphocytes isolated from spleen (Masson & Uetrecht, 2004). Interestingly, low-dose tolerance to D-penicillamine was prevented by poly I:C or lipopolysaccharide treatment (Masson & Uetrecht, 2004).

The exact phenotype of the regulatory T cells in the case of low-dose D-penicillamine tolerance is not known, and non-lymphoid cells probably play a role as well. In another example of drug-induced autoimmune responses, the phenotype of regulatory T cells was identified as $CD4^+CD25^+$ (Layland et al., 2004). In this study, $CD4^+CD25^+$ cells isolated from mice (A/J strain) exposed to procainamide, mercury(II) chloride, or gold salts were capable of preventing antinuclear antibody formation in similarly treated recipient mice, but also in mice subsequently treated with one of the other two chemicals.

Dose regimen, however, is not the only factor influencing the regulation of autoimmunity. The inherent characteristics of the species or strain are important, not only for disease occurrence, but also for the type of immune effect. This is also apparent from studies on mercury(II) chloride-induced autoimmunity. In contrast to Brown Norway rats, Lewis rats are resistant to mercury(II) chloride-induced autoimmunity, but instead demonstrate an overall state of immunosuppression mediated by $CD8^+$ T cells (Pelletier et al., 1990). This suppression is not antigen-specific, as mercury(II) chloride-treated Lewis rats are also protected against experimental allergic encephalomyelitis (Pelletier et al., 1988). Even when regulatory $CD8^+$ cells (Pelletier et al., 1990) or RT6.2 cells (Kosuda et al., 1994) are eliminated, Lewis rats do not develop autoimmune phenomena, possibly because they lack the susceptible genotype. The relation between genotype and the type of response to mercury(II) chloride has been extensively studied by comparing various inbred and F1 strains (Aten et al., 1991); results show that MHC as well as non-MHC genes are involved in the susceptibility.

7.3 Other mechanisms

Other mechanisms that may contribute to the adverse influence of chemicals on autoimmune processes include the stimulation of MHC class II expression by cells that do not normally express class II molecules, as a consequence of IFN-γ induction.

Most drugs are natively not chemically reactive, which means that they cannot form hapten–carrier complexes with proteins or induce release of sequestered or cryptic epitopes (Uetrecht, 1990). They may also be incapable of causing cell damage and inducing subsequent inflammatory signals to stimulate dendritic cells to raise their co-stimulatory molecules or produce stimulatory cytokines. The present thought is that many drugs that cause sensitization undergo bioactivation by metabolizing enzymes (Uetrecht, 1990; Naisbitt et al., 2001). This can be accomplished by P450 enzymes, but also by oxidative metabolic routes in phagocytic cells of the immune system, such as polymorphonuclear neutrophils. These cells contain myeloperoxidases that have been shown to be able to convert non-haptenizing chemicals into haptenizing derivatives. However, neutrophils are usually not in close proximity to where sensitization may occur.

8. CHEMICAL/PHYSICAL AGENTS AND AUTOIMMUNITY

This chapter provides a number of examples of chemicals and physical agents that have been associated with or are suspected of being associated with autoimmunity. The list of chemicals dealt with is not comprehensive, nor are the individual examples all exhaustively described. The rationale behind selection of the examples is to show the range of agents that are potentially associated with autoimmunity, debates that have been going on for certain agents (e.g. silicone, which eventually was concluded not to have any association with autoimmunity), types of studies that have been done using human and animal models, and mechanisms that may underlie potential autoimmunity. Although the emphasis is on environmental chemicals, some drugs are exemplified to further address and in fact illustrate the potential autoimmune effects of environmental agents.

8.1 Toxic oil syndrome

In 1981–1982, an epidemic spread across Spain, which was eventually labelled the toxic oil syndrome by the World Health Organization (WHO). In less than two years, at least 20 096 people were afflicted by and 356 people died from toxic oil syndrome (Philen et al., 1997; Philen & Dicker, 2000). Women, especially those less than 40 years of age, were affected more severely than men; 61% of the victims and 66% of the deaths were women (Sanchez-Porro Valades et al., 2003). Toxic oil syndrome has striking similarities to autoimmune diseases, particularly scleroderma. In addition, it resembles eosinophilia myalgia syndrome and diffuse fasciitis with eosinophilia. Toxic oil syndrome-associated manifestations evolved from initiating vasculitis to eosinophilia in the acute phase and then sicca syndrome, neuropathy, scleroderma, Raynaud phenomenon, and musculoskeletal inflammation in the chronic phase (Kaufman & Krupp, 1995). More than 70% of toxic oil syndrome patients presented with eosinophilia, regardless of age or sex.

Several potential etiologies were investigated, including infectious agents, pet-borne vectors, contaminated food, organophosphate pesticide exposure, and vinyl chloride contamination from food containers, before a link was made between the new disease and the consumption of adulterated cooking oil. Chemical analysis of the case-associated oil identified brassicasterol, a marker for rapeseed oil, trace amounts of aniline, oleyl anilide, and other fatty acid anilides and contaminants (Aldridge, 1992; Posada de la Paz et al., 1996; Ruiz-Mendez et al., 2001). The toxin or toxins appear to be stable in oil, since consumption of toxic oil one year after the main epidemic led to development of the disease.

8.1.1 Clinical features of toxic oil syndrome

Toxic oil syndrome was a three-phase, multisystem disease with a four- to seven-day interval between ingestion of the adulterated oil and the onset of symptoms. Subjective estimates suggest that the degree of illness varied proportionately with the amount and frequency of intake; however, this has not been validated. The initial event is believed to be a form of vasculitis, a non-necrotizing endothelial damage in vessels of multiple organs. In the acute phase (0–2 months), patients exhibited endothelial lesions (endovasculitis), eosinophilia, pulmonary infiltrates and oedema, pneumopathy, myalgias, fever, rash, and high IgE levels (Hard, 2000; Gelpi et al., 2002; Sanchez-Porro Valades et al., 2003). Aniline was detected in pleural effusion in approximately 50% of the victims (Tabuenca, 1981). Rash was more frequent in children under 15 years of age (21.8% of cases) than in adults (Philen et al., 1997). The primary cause of death for patients in this phase was respiratory failure. Approximately 60% of the patients progressed to the intermediate phase (2–4 months), characterized by myalgias, eosinophilia, cachexia, liver disease, dermal infiltration/oedema, pulmonary hypertension, sicca syndrome, and hypertriglyceridaemia. The primary causes of toxic oil syndrome-related death in this phase were thromboembolism and pulmonary hypertension. Finally, 10–15% of the original toxic oil syndrome cohort have been estimated to progress to the chronic phase (Weatherill et al., 2003). In the early stage of the chronic phase (4 months to 2 years), patients developed sicca syndrome, neuropathy, liver disease, scleroderma, and pulmonary hypertension, and then (>2 years) musculoskeletal pain, lung disease, carpal tunnel syndrome, Raynaud phenomenon, and hyperlipidaemia were common. The primary causes of toxic oil syndrome-related death in the chronic phase were respiratory failure, central nervous system infection, and pulmonary hypertension. While a number of treatments were tested, none successfully controlled the disease, although corticosteroids and diphenylhydantoin did ameliorate some of the symptoms (Gomez de la Camara et al., 1997).

The initial chemical analyses identified oleyl anilide as the primary contaminant and marker for case-associated oils, but the number of anilides and unidentified contaminants suggested that other compounds may also be involved (Posada de la Paz et al., 1989; Aldridge, 1992; Diggle, 2001). No common refinery products, additives, or contaminants were known to induce symptoms and pathological findings consistent with toxic oil syndrome (Hard, 2002). Recently, several anilino-propanediol derivatives that may be associated with the disease, in particular 3-(N-phenylamino)-1,2-propanediol (PAP) and two of its esters, 3-oleyl-ester (MEPAP) and 1,2-di-oleyl ester (DEPAP), were identified by liquid chromatography/mass spectrometry. The oleyl anilide and propanediols were formed by the reaction of aniline with the oleyl side-chain of fatty acids that are abundant in rapeseed oil. Although fatty acid anilides were detected in all tested oil samples, the PAP derivatives were present only in case-associated oil samples. DEPAP was the dominant form and is now considered to be the most likely candidate as the etiological agent (Gelpi et al., 2002).

8.1.2 Immune markers in toxic oil syndrome

Analysis of the sera from 98 toxic oil syndrome patients in the acute phase of the disease showed no differences in IgG, IgM, IgA, specific IgG/IgE antibody, GM-CSF, IL-4, IL-6, or TNF levels, compared with controls. Soluble IL-2 receptor (sIL-2R) and eosinophil granule MBP levels were significantly increased, whereas the 2- to 3-fold increases in IgE and sCD23 levels were not significant (Brostoff et al., 1982; Gallardo et al., 1994; Lahoz et al., 1997; Gelpi et al., 2002). Elevated IgE levels were subsequently confirmed. Positive immunohistochemical examination of skin biopsies from toxic oil syndrome patients were positive for IL-4. B cells and $CD8^+$ T cells were also elevated in toxic oil syndrome patients, but the $CD4^+$ population was not affected (Kammuller et al., 1988; Kaufman & Krupp, 1995). An increase in antiDNA, antilymphocyte, anticollagen, and antimuscle autoantibodies was also observed, but inconsistently. Inconsistencies may reflect differences in the stage of the disease at the time of testing. Post-mortem analysis did not find any difference in IL-1α, GM-CSF, or CD25 gene expression in lung tissue from 26 toxic oil syndrome patients with pulmonary hypertension and oedema compared with controls in either the acute or chronic phase. There was a 2-fold increase in the expression of CD23. Both Th1 (IL-2 and IFN-γ) and Th2 (IL-4 and IL-5) cytokines were upregulated in toxic oil syndrome patients, but there was a predominantly Th2 versus Th1 response.

Cardaba et al. (1999) found no association with the expression of HLA class II genes in 117 survivors of the disease, but 73% of 34 chronic-phase victims in whom toxic oil syndrome was the major cause of death had an increased expression of HLA-DR2 in lung tissue. This is consistent with another study in 29 patients with a history of atypical pneumonia symptoms in the acute phase who had elevated HLA-DR2 in the chronic phase (Arnaiz-Villena et al., 1982). Vicario et al. (1982) reported an increase in HLA-DR3 and HLA-DR4 in female toxic oil syndrome patients, but this study lacked adequate controls. Acetylation via acetylglucosaminyltransferase is linked to chromosome 6, as are the HLA-D antigens. Polymorphism of this enzyme determines whether acetylation proceeds at a fast or slow rate. Toxic oil syndrome was suggested to be lethal in the acute phase via Th1 mechanisms involving slow acetylation; in the chronic phase, Th2 mechanisms associated with fast acetylation led to autoimmune disease (Cardaba et al., 1999). There was an increase in variant alleles of arylamine N-acetyltransferase-2 in 73 toxic oil syndrome patients (Ladona et al., 2001). Different expression of haptoglobin α (Hp) isoforms was observed in toxic oil syndrome patients compared with controls; the most frequent phenotype in controls was Hp2-2, and the most frequent phenotypes in toxic oil syndrome patients were Hp2-1s and Hp1-1s. The haptoglobin protein binds free haemoglobin during hepatic recyling of iron, acts as an antioxidant, has antibacterial activity, and is involved in the acute-phase immune response. The Hp2 allele has been reported to have greater immune reactivity than the Hp1 allele (Quero et al., 2004).

8.1.3 Experimental studies of toxic oil syndrome

A wide variety of species have been treated with both case-associated and reconstituted oils, with only a few reports that some of the classical symptoms have been observed in mice (eosinophilia and elevated IgE) and rats (lung oedema, respiratory difficulties, splenomegaly). Possible explanations for the generally negative results in animal models are that toxic oil syndrome may be a uniquely human disease, animals may have a lower sensitivity to toxic oils, the dose used may not have been adequate, and multiple agents, genetic factors, and biochemical alterations may be involved in disease development.

Since many autoimmune diseases require both genetic susceptibility and an environmental trigger, mice genetically prone to developing autoimmune disease have been employed in toxic oil syndrome research. MRL/lpr (H2s) mice develop idiopathic autoimmune diseases due to a fatal deletion in the Fas gene and are also prone to a high degree of apoptosis (Hard, 2002). The administration of case-associated, reconstituted, and canola oils to MRL/lpr mice by oral gavage suppressed the progression of glomerulonephritis. Serum IgE levels were reduced and serum autoantibodies increased by all three experimental oils compared with levels in naive mice. However, due to many positive responses in mice treated with the canola oil control, this model is generally considered to be unsuitable for the study of toxic oil syndrome (Koller et al., 2001, 2002; Weatherill et al., 2003). A.SW mice, an H2s strain susceptible to autoimmunity but requiring environmental or infectious induction to develop the disease, failed to develop toxic oil syndrome. Body and organ weights, autoantibody titres, and IgG1, IgG2, and IgE serum levels were unaffected by treatment with case-associated and reconstituted oils (Weatherill et al., 2003).

To evaluate the role of specific aniline derivatives in the induction of an autoimmune response, animals were exposed to purified anilides and PAP esters. Oleyl and linoleyl anilides were found to be toxic to the rat lung (Tena, 1982), and anilides induced elevated IgE levels and T cells in mice (Lahoz et al., 1997). Neither PAP nor its monoester induced overt toxicity in Lewis and LAC rats or MF1 mice, but PAP induced mesenteric and pulmonary thromboembolism in rats (Gelpi et al., 2002). Most anilides possess a functional group para to the amino group that has been shown to induce allergy and autoimmunity. The aniline derivatives nitrosobenzene (which does not possess a para substituent), N-hydroxylaniline, linoleic anilide and linolenic anilide, and a mixture of PAP esters all induced a primary T cell-dependent proliferation in the popliteal lymph node cells of Balb/c mice following injection into the footpad. Involvement of B cells was indicated by the increased percentage of B cells in the total cell population. Aniline, nitrobenzene, p-aminophenol, N-acetyl-p-aminophenol, linoleic acid, linolenic acid, and triolein did not induce such a response. Only challenge with nitrosobenzene stimulated a secondary popliteal lymph node response following priming with either nitrosobenzene or linolenic anilide (Wulferink et al., 2001).

Bell and co-workers (Bell, 1996; Bell et al., 1999) developed a toxic oil syndrome model in B10.S, C57BL/6, and A/J mice. Administration of toxic oil syndrome-related test chemicals by intraperitoneal injection resulted in the most severe symptoms and the highest mortality (30–50% for all anilide-treated groups); intraperitoneal delivery by osmotic pump induced disease symptoms, with survival of most of the animals until completion of the study. In both B10.S (H2s, fast acetylator) and A/J (H2a, slow acetylator) mice, oleyl anilide was more toxic than linoleyl anilide and linoleic DEPAP. None of the mice that received linoleyl anilide by osmotic pump developed any symptoms. Linoleic DEPAP induced significant weight loss, lethargy, eosinophilia, and pulmonary congestion in both strains. In addition, B10.S mice exhibited thromboses and haemorrhages in the lungs, while A/J mice developed emphysema. Following osmotic pump injection of oleyl anilide, B10.S mice did not exhibit overt clinical symptoms. However, serum levels of IgE, IgG1, and IgM, mRNA expression of IL-1β and IL-6 in spleen, the number of IgG- and IgM-positive splenocytes, and autoantibodies for denatured DNA, histones, and rheumatoid factor were elevated. In vitro restimulation of splenic lymphocytes by oleyl anilide resulted in elevated secretion of IL-10, but decreased cell proliferation and increased apoptosis (Bell et al., 2002). Similarly, C57BL/6 (H2b, fast acetylator) mice did not exhibit overt symptoms following treatment with oleyl anilide, but serum IgE and IgM levels were elevated. Gene expression analysis showed that TNF-β and IL-1β mRNA expression were suppressed in the spleen compared with control animals, whereas IL-1α, IL-10, TGFβ, TNF-α, IL-4, IL-2, IL-3, IL-5, and IFN-γ gene expression and autoantibody production were unaffected. The only histopathological alteration was splenomegaly (Bell, 1996; Berking et al., 1998). The A/J strain of mice was the most severely affected by oleyl anilide exposure. Fifty to sixty per cent of the mice died within five days of severe cachexia, and another 20% within two weeks of exposure. Only 20% remained asymptomatic. These mice exhibited increased serum IgE, IgG, and IgM and upregulation of IL-10, IL-1α, IL-6, and IFN-γ mRNA in the spleen. There was no effect on IL-1β, TGFβ, TNF-α, TNF-β, or IL-4 expression. In vitro restimulation of splenic lymphocytes by oleyl anilide resulted in elevated secretion of TNF-α, but not of IL-10. Both cell proliferation and apoptosis were increased. T cells isolated from spleens of oleyl anilide-treated mice required the presence of antigen-presenting cells to initiate a proliferative response to oleyl anilide restimulation in vitro (Bell et al., 2002).

The difference in the responses of the various strains of mice tested indicates a genetic component in susceptibility to toxic oil syndrome (Bell, 1996; Weatherill et al., 2003). The early and drastic response to oleyl anilide by A/J mice (haplotype H2a) resembled the toxic oil syndrome acute phase, whereas B10.S mice and, to a lesser extent, C57BL/6 mice (haplotypes H2s and H2b) exhibited symptoms similar to the chronic phase. Consistent with toxic oil syndrome symptoms in affected patients, the serological and gene expression changes in all three strains suggest a Th2-mediated mechanism with possible Th1 involvement in the acute phase and a humoral immune response with polyclonal B cell activation in the chronic phase (Bell, 1996; Berking et al., 1998). It has been proposed that slow acetylator A/J mice process toxins through metabolic pathways that result in the rapid accumulation of reactive immunogenic metabolites (Bell et al., 2002). Some aniline derivatives are similar in structure to diacylglycerol components of cell membranes. If the contaminating anilides, esters, or their metabolites penetrated cell membranes, they could induce membrane destabilization and collapse and an immunological response (Gallardo et al., 1997; Schurz et al., 1997). Fast acetylator mice such as C57BL/6 and B10.S often can eliminate toxins, for example procainamide, by acetylation to stable products that are quickly excreted. The continuing exposure to small amounts of remaining active metabolites can eventually lead to a chronic hyperimmune condition.

DEPAP, but not aniline or other 3-(*N*-phenylamino)-1,2-propanediol derivatives, induced both apoptosis and necrosis in human peripheral blood lymphocytes in vitro in a time- and concentration-dependent fashion. In short-term cell cultures, possibly representative of the toxic oil syndrome acute phase, DNA degradation occurred rapidly. Apoptosis preceded membrane damage. In longer-term cultures, cytotoxicity was characterized by necrosis. As the cells die, abnormal forms of autoantigens are released, activating autoreactive lymphocytes, which could ultimately initiate autoimmune disease (Gallardo et al., 1997; Lahoz et al., 1997).

8.2 TCDD (dioxins)

Dioxins are unintended by-products of natural events and human-made processes such as manufacturing, incineration, paper and pulp bleaching, and exhaust emissions. Immunotoxic effects of dioxins have been studied primarily with respect to 2,3,7,8-tetrachlorodibenzo-*p*-dioxin (TCDD), the most toxic congener of dioxins and an important immunotoxicant (Vos & Moore, 1974).

There are two cross-sectional studies that suggest autoimmune responses in dioxin-exposed persons. In inhabitants in Viet Nam exposed to Agent Orange containing TCDD, the concentration of circulating immune complexes and antinuclear antibodies was elevated, with an increased number of circulating lymphocytes (Kozhevnikova et al., 1991). Their elevation was also detected more frequently in 18 TCDD-exposed workers than in 15 matched controls (Jennings et al., 1988). In a larger controlled study on workers in a German pesticide-producing factory, however, there was no significant correlation between autoantibody levels and polychlorinated dibenzo-*p*-dioxin (PCDD) / polychlorinated dibenzofuran (PCDF) concentrations in blood lipids (Jung et al., 1998). There are recent reports also indicating no induction of antinuclear antibodies in patients intoxicated with PCBs and dioxin contaminants in rice oil (Nagayama et al., 2001) and in Korean veterans exposed to Agent Orange (H.A. Kim et al., 2003).

Prenatal exposure of mice to TCDD modulated fetal antigen expression on thymocytes and inhibited thymocyte maturation (Blaylock et al., 1992). In TCDD-treated mice, moreover, thymic epithelium distribution of MHC class II molecules was found (De Waal et al., 1992), but potent autoreactive V beta 6+ cells were not found (De Heer et al., 1995). TCDD also resulted in the appearance of autoimmune nephritis in young male mice exposed monthly to the chemical and reduced the time to postnatal onset of autoimmune nephritis in male offspring of autoimmune-prone mice receiving a single fetal exposure (Silverstone et al., 1998). Thus, it is proposed that TCDD at prenatal exposure may have the potential to cause defective thymocyte–epithelial cell interactions and antigen presentation on thymocytes, thereby altering normal development of self-tolerance and leading to expression of autoimmunity (Holladay, 1999). The proposal was also supported in autoimmune-prone mice (MRL/lpr mice) exposed prenatally to TCDD, which showed a significant dose-related increase of urinary protein and autoantibodies to single-stranded DNA (ssDNA) (Smith & Germolec, 2000). These findings suggest that developmental exposure to dioxins may accelerate the onset of genetic expression of autoimmune predisposition. Repeated TCDD treatment of mice increased serum IL-6 levels accompanied by higher titres of tissue-specific autoantibodies (H.J. Kim et al., 2003). However, before any firm conclusion on an association of TCDD exposure with autoimmunity or autoimmune disease can be drawn, additional evidence is required.

8.3 Pesticides

8.3.1 General

Pesticides are widely used worldwide in agriculture, public health, and several indoor conditions. Current evidence related to pesticide autoimmunogenic potential is summarized in Table 8. Hexachlorobenzene is the most intensively studied pesticide in the context of autoimmunity, and it will therefore be addressed separately at the end of this section.

There is some evidence, either in animal models or following human exposure, that several pesticides used currently or in the recent past can cause slight changes that could be interpreted as "autoimmune-like effects". However, data supporting this hypothesis are scarce. In some cases, the mere inclusion of observed changes as indicative of autoimmunity is even questionable, whereas in other cases, results of one study have not been confirmed by a subsequent study. Only few compounds that are no longer in use today (i.e. mercury derivatives, hexachlorobenzene) have been shown to induce more marked changes suggesting the potential for causing autoimmune disease.

Table 8. Studies of autoimmunogenic potential of pesticides

Active ingredient	Type of exposure	Observed effects	Reference
Aminocarb	Experimental; animals	Increase of antibody responses to sheep; increased expression of MHC class II antigens	Bernier et al. (1988, 1995)
Carbaryl	Experimental; animals	Increased antibody response to sheep red blood cells	Andre et al. (1983)
Chlordane/ heptachlor	Indoor application (termiticide)	Elevated CD28 cells; antimyelin, anti-smooth muscle, antiparietal cell, antibrush border, and antinuclear antibodies	Broughton et al. (1990); McConnachie & Zahalsky (1992)
Chlordecone	Experimental; animals	Acceleration of lupus-like disease	Sobel et al. (2005)
Chlorpyrifos	Indoor application	Presence of auto-antibodies; lupus-like syndrome	Thrasher et al. (1993)
Hexachloro-benzene	Occupational; accidental poisoning	Increased serum IgM and IgG levels	Queiroz et al. (1998a, 1998b)
Lindane	Experimental; animals	Increase of sheep red blood cells induced antibody response; glomerulonephritis with deposition of immune complexes	Meera et al. (1992); Khurana & Chauhan (2002)
Malathion	Experimental; animals	Antinuclear antibodies production; glomerulo-nephritis in mice; increase of lymphocyte prolifera-tion; increase of antibody responses to sheep erythrocytes; increase of phagocytic capability and production of inflamma-tory mediators; non-specific macrophage activation	Rodgers et al. (1986); Rodgers & Ellefson (1990); Rodgers (1997); Rodgers & Xiong (1997); Cooper et al. (2002)

Table 8 (Contd)

Active ingredient	Type of exposure	Observed effects	Reference
Mancozeb	Occupational exposure	Increase of proliferative response to mitogens	Colosio et al. (1996); Corsini et al. (2005)
Mixture of pesticides	Lifelong exposure	Antinuclear antibody positivity	Rosenberg et al. (1999)
Paraquat	Single case report, occupational	Autoantibodies against basal membrane of the renal glomerulus	Stratta et al. (1988)
Pentachlorophenol	Environmental and indoor	Higher frequency of autoantibodies than expected[a]	McConnachie & Zahalsky (1991)

[a] Finding not confirmed by other studies (Colosio et al., 1993).

The interpretation of human data is difficult, not only because only slight and subclinical effects were observed, but also because human subjects usually are exposed to a mixture of several pesticides, thus making the identification of the role of a single ingredient very difficult. Some studies examined antinuclear or other autoantibodies in subjects exposed to pesticides in occupational settings. It is difficult to interpret studies using these measures if an appropriate comparison group is not included, given the prevalence of autoantibodies that has been reported in studies of healthy, unexposed subjects (Tan et al., 1997). Another major problem in data interpretation is the uncertainty in the extrapolation of animal findings to humans. One such example is the interpretation of enhanced antibody response to sheep red blood cells (Burns et al., 2000).

In conclusion, the body of data available shows an equivocal association between pesticide exposure and autoimmunity. However, since doubt still persists, further investigation in the field is needed.

8.3.2 Hexachlorobenzene

Hexachlorobenzene (C_6Cl_6) is a low molecular weight compound that has been used in the past as a fungicide for seed grains. In the 1970s, such a use was prohibited in most countries, but hexachlorobenzene is still generated as a by-product of several industrial processes. Although emission of hexachlorobenzene has decreased substantially compared with the 1970s, residues can still be found throughout the environment due to its chemical stability, lipophilicity, high persistence, and re-emissions of hexachlorobenzene accumulated in soil and water.

8.3.2.1 Accidental poisoning in Turkey

The toxic effects of hexachlorobenzene on humans were first noted in the eastern part of Turkey between 1950 and 1959. Seed grain treated with hexachlorobenzene was unfortunately used as food, resulting in the poisoning of approximately 3000–5000 people. Victims developed a syndrome that has been called porphyria turcica, characterized by hepatic porphyria (Cam, 1958). Other clinical features were skin lesions in sun-exposed areas, caused by photochemical activation of accumulated porphyrins (Bickers, 1987), painless arthritis, enlarged liver, spleen, lymph nodes, and thyroid, and neurological symptoms (Gocmen et al., 1986; Peters et al., 1987). Histology of skin biopsies showed hyperkeratosis and infiltrations of lymphocytes and macrophages. Other clinical symptoms were fever, diarrhoea, hepatomegaly, and pulmonary infiltrates. Follow-up studies among 204 victims 20–30 years after the poisoning have shown that arthritis, enlarged thyroid, and neurological and dermatological symptoms still persisted (Cripps et al., 1984).

8.3.2.2 Adverse immune effects of hexachlorobenzene

In humans, immunotoxic effects have been clearly seen among the victims of the poisoning in Turkey and also in workers exposed occupationally to hexachlorobenzene in a chemical plant in Brazil. In these workers, impaired functions of neutrophilic granulocytes and increased serum IgM and IgG levels were observed (Queiroz et al., 1998a, 1998b).

Oral exposure of rats to hexachlorobenzene results in a dose-dependent increase in the number of peripheral neutrophilic and basophilic granulocytes and monocytes and of spleen and lymph node weights. Histopathology shows increased marginal zones and follicles and extramedullary haematopoiesis in the spleen and increased numbers of high endothelial venules in mesenteric lymph nodes and popliteal lymph nodes (Vos et al., 1979a, 1979b, 1983; Michielsen et al., 1997). These immune effects were more obvious in Brown Norway rats than in Lewis or Wistar rats (Michielsen et al., 1997), but effects in Brown Norway and Lewis rats were not opposite, as has been seen in studies of mercury(II) chloride. Table 9 summarizes the immunotoxic effects of hexachlorobenzene in the Brown Norway rat.

Table 9. Immunotoxic effects of hexachlorobenzene in the Brown Norway rat[a]

Parameter	Dose[b]	References
Increased spleen weight	150, 450	Michielsen et al. (1997)
Increased popliteal, axillary, and mandibular lymph node weight	450	Michielsen et al. (1997, 2002)
Increased number of high endothelial venules in popliteal lymph nodes	150, 450	Michielsen et al. (1997)
Granuloma formation in the mandibular lymph nodes	450	Michielsen et al. (1997)
Inflammatory skin lesions: hyperplasia epidermis, activated dermal vessels, infiltrates of neutrophils, macrophages, and eosinophils	150, 450	Michielsen et al. (1997, 1999b)
Inflammatory lung lesions: focal accumulations of macrophages, granuloma formation, perivascular eosinophilic infiltrates, high endothelial-like venules	150, 450	Michielsen et al. (1997)
Increased total serum IgM and IgE levels	450	Michielsen et al. (1997)
Increased total serum IgG levels	150, 450	Michielsen et al. (1997)
Increased serum IgM levels against ssDNA	150, 450	Michielsen et al. (1997)
Increased in vitro and in vivo airway hyperresponsiveness	450	Michielsen et al. (2001, 2002)
Decreased IL-2 mRNA expression	150[c]	Vandebriel et al. (2000)
Increased IL-10 mRNA expression	50[c]	Vandebriel et al. (2000)

[a] Brown Norway rats were exposed to hexachlorobenzene via the diet for three or four weeks. The table contains only significant changes.
[b] Dietary hexachlorobenzene concentration in milligrams per kilogram diet.
[c] In this study, rats were exposed to hexachlorobenzene for six weeks.

In a perinatal toxicity study, the primary and secondary IgM and IgG responses to tetanus toxoid and the delayed-type hypersensitivity reactions to ovalbumin were increased at 4 mg of hexachlorobenzene per kilogram diet, the lowest dose tested (Vos et al., 1979a). Schielen et al. (1993) showed that hexachlorobenzene increases the number of ED3+ macrophages in the spleens of Wistar rats. These macrophages are associated with experimentally induced autoimmune diseases such as rheumatoid arthritis (Dijkstra et al., 1987, 1992) and are thought to be capable of activating B-1 cells (Damoiseaux et al., 1991). B-1 cells are known to produce natural antibodies, such as anti-DNA antibodies, and both serum IgM levels against such autoantigens and the number of splenic B-1 cells are increased after hexachlorobenzene exposure (Schielen et al., 1993, 1995). This finding combined with other observations, including histological data, indicated that hexachlorobenzene induced an autoimmune-like pathology.

A number of studies have focused on assessing to what extent hexachlorobenzene has a true autoimmune-based etiology. It was not until recently that it appeared that hexachlorobenzene acts probably as a sort of adjuvant chemical, by directly activating macrophages and other inflammatory cells, and that the compound does not act by creating hexachlorobenzene (or hexachlorobenzene metabolite)-containing neoantigens. For instance, cyclosporin treatment delayed the development of hexachlorobenzene-induced skin lesions and prevented the increase in spleen weight. Furthermore, increases in axillary lymph node weight, lung eosinophilia, and humoral responses were prevented completely in hexachlorobenzene-exposed rats treated with cyclosporin. However, macrophage infiltration was independent of T cells (Ezendam et al., 2004a). Results of studies with hexachlorobenzene in which macrophages were eliminated using clodronate liposomes (Ezendam, 2004) further strengthened the idea that macrophages indeed play a more important role in hexachlorobenzene-induced immune effects than T cells. Remarkably, studies performed to further assess the functional role and specificity of T cells did not provide any evidence for the presence of T cells specific for the hexachlorobenzene metabolite tetrachlorohydroquinone, nor did cytochrome P450 inhibition decrease hexachlorobenzene-induced immune effects (Schielen et al., 1993). Moreover, hexachlorobenzene-induced immune effects could not be adoptively transferred to naive recipients. In addition, a recent study applying gene expression profiling in hexachlorobenzene-exposed rats provided further evidence that hexachlorobenzene induces a systemic inflammatory response, accompanied by oxidative stress and an acute-phase response (Ezendam et al., 2004b).

In conclusion, although hexachlorobenzene induces an autoimmune-like disorder in humans and rats, neoantigen formation and direct elicitation of autoreactive T cells are probably not involved. Rather, hexachlorobenzene, by activation of inflammatory cells such as macrophages, exacerbates autoimmunity above a level at which autoimmune phenomena and systemic inflammatory responses become apparent. This cascade of reactions is depicted in Figure 2 and illustrates the complexity of the etiology of immune derangements induced by hexachlorobenzene.

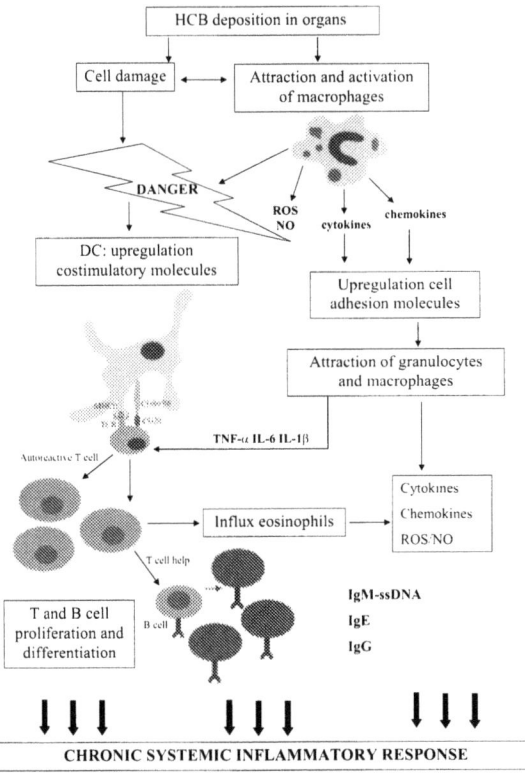

Fig. 2. Proposed mode of action of hexachlorobenzene-induced adverse immune effects (HCB = hexachlorobenzene; ROS = reactive oxygen species; NO = nitric oxide; DC = dendritic cells) (from Ezendam, 2004).

8.4 Ultraviolet radiation

A well known effect of ultraviolet radiation is the exacerbation of lupus erythematosus (Angotti, 2004). Apoptosis in keratinocytes induced by ultraviolet B radiation appears to play a role in exacerbation, probably by inducing release of fragmented autoantigens (Pablos et al., 1999). In fact, occurrence of enhanced skin lesions after skin exposure to ultraviolet radiation is a diagnostic criterion.

A characteristic of some autoimmune disorders is the strong geographical variation. There seems to be a clear latitude gradient in incidence of autoimmune diseases, also indicating the effect of sun exposure. This is well known for multiple sclerosis but has now also been described for diabetes mellitus type 1 and polymyositis. A similar gradient is seen both north and south of the equator (Staples et al., 2003), with the incidence of these diseases rising as one moves away from the equator. In this situation, ultraviolet radiation would be protective against some autoimmune disorders (McMichael & Hall, 1997; Ponsonby et al., 2005).

A prime effect of ultraviolet radiation is on Langerhans cells in the skin, inducing them to leave the skin and affecting their functionality (Schwarz et al., 2000), resulting in dendritic cells that support tolerance rather than activation. Thus, ultraviolet radiation-induced damage in the skin plays a role in the stimulation of the autoimmune disease systemic lupus erythematosus.

Besides exerting local effects in the skin, ultraviolet radiation may, through the production of circulating mediators, also cause systemic immunosuppression. This could be an explanation of the suppression of autoimmune conditions, such as multiple sclerosis and diabetes mellitus type 1, noted to occur less frequently in those countries with abundant sun.

8.5 Silica

8.5.1 Introduction to epidemiological studies of silica exposure

Crystalline silica or silicon dioxide (SiO_2), the most abundant mineral in the earth's crust, is found in rock, sand, and soil. Most studies of silica and autoimmune disease have focused on occupational exposures within the traditional "dusty trades", which include work in mines, quarries, foundries, roadway and other construction sites, masonry, sandblasting, and the production of pottery, glass, and tile. At least three recent studies of silica and autoimmune disease have shown associations with farm work (Parks et al., 2002; Lane et al., 2003; Olsson et al., 2004), including one showing stronger associations with specific dusty tasks and sandy soils (Lane et al., 2003). Iannello et al. (2002) reviewed other types of occupational exposure to silica and reported a case of a dental technician exposed to ceramic silica dust who developed an autoimmune disorder. This technician was diagnosed with a rheumatoid syndrome with lung interstitial disorder and HLA haplotypes associated with autoimmune disease susceptibility. The condition was reversed after six months of protection from exposure to the occupational silica source.

Acute high-level silica exposures may be associated with natural and other disasters, such as earthquakes, volcanic eruptions, and building collapse. High-level exposure to respirable silica dust (particles <5 m) can cause chronic inflammation and fibrosis in the lungs and other organs. Silica exposure in humans has also been associated with increased production of autoantibodies, serum immunoglobulins, and immune complexes.

Studying the association of silica-related autoimmune effects in occupational settings is complicated by the fact that most autoimmune diseases are fairly rare outcomes, particularly in men, who are the dominant workforce in the dusty trades. Similarly, the role of silica in autoimmune diseases is also difficult to assess in a population-based setting, given the female predominance seen in many autoimmune diseases (e.g. 90% of patients with systemic lupus erythematosus are women). Occupational silica exposure may be difficult to assess in case–control studies because of the diversity of sources of exposure encountered in the general population. Studies in women may present an even greater challenge, since exposure assessment techniques for women's occupations are not well developed (Greenberg & Dement, 1994).

The association between occupational exposure to crystalline silica and rheumatoid arthritis, scleroderma, the small-vessel vasculitides (e.g. Wegener granulomatosis), and systemic lupus erythematosus has been examined in recent reviews (Parks et al., 1999;

Mulloy, 2003). The cohort, nested case–control, and registry linkage studies of highly exposed occupational groups (e.g. miners, granite workers) and silicosis patients have generally reported strong associations (i.e. relative risks of 3.0 and higher, with some studies reporting more than a 10-fold increased risk) with these diseases (Sluis-Cremer et al., 1985, 1986; Klockars et al., 1987; Sanchez-Roman et al., 1993; Rosenman & Zhu, 1995; Conrad et al., 1996; Brown et al., 1997; Mehlhorn et al., 1999; Rosenman et al., 1999). Although higher risks are generally seen in silicosis patients, there are now several studies that have reported associations between silica exposure, in the absence of silicosis, and risk of rheumatoid arthritis, scleroderma, and other systemic autoimmune diseases (Klockars et al., 1987; Mehlhorn et al., 1999; Parks et al., 2002).

8.5.2 Occupational silica exposure and systemic autoimmune diseases

The association between occupational exposure to silica dust and rheumatoid arthritis was initially described in the 1950s by Caplan (1953) in a study of rheumatoid features in the lungs. Other cohort studies were conducted in South African gold miners in the 1980s (reviewed in Parks et al., 1999) (Table 10). With the exception of the nested case–control study among pottery workers (Turner & Cherry, 2000), all of the studies of silica exposure and rheumatoid arthritis have reported odds ratios of 2.0 or higher, with some associations in the most highly exposed groups much higher than this. The pottery worker study matched cases and controls by date of birth and date on which employment began, making it difficult to detect differences in cumulative silica exposure.

There have also been several cohort and case–control studies of silica exposure and scleroderma (Table 10) and six case–control studies of silica exposure and various forms of systemic small-vessel or ANCA-associated vasculitis. As with rheumatoid arthritis, almost all of these studies have reported a 2- to 3-fold increased risk of these diseases with silica exposure.

Until recently, the evidence relating silica exposure to lupus was limited to case-reports, mostly of male lupus patients with silicosis and a history of exposure to very high levels of silica. Since 1995, three epidemiological studies in different populations (uranium miners in Germany, silicosis patients in Sweden, and a population-based case–control study in the southeastern United States) have been reported (Table 10). Each of these studies supports the hypothesis that occupational silica dust exposure is associated with risk of this disease.

Table 10. Recent (1985–2005) epidemiological studies of occupational silica exposure and risk of autoimmune diseases

Disease and design	Sex $(n)^a$ / Occupation	Exposure classification and results[b]	References
Rheumatoid arthritis			
Nested case–control	M (157, 157) Gold miners	Silicosis and definite or probable rheumatoid arthritis: OR 2.8 ($P <$ 0.01); higher association seen with definite disease and with rheumatoid factor	Sluis-Cremer et al. (1986)
Cohort–registry linkage	M (35, 1026) Quarry workers	RR 5.1 (3.3, 7.8)	Klockars et al. (1987)
Nested case–control	M + F (58, 8325) Pottery workers	No association with duration, cumulative exposure,[c] or mean silica concentration	Turner & Cherry (2000)
Cohort–registry linkage	M (44, 1130) Silicosis patients	RR 8.1 (5.9, 10.9)	Brown et al. (1997)
Cohort–registry linkage	M (24, 463) Silicosis patients	OR 2.7 (1.7, 4.1)	Rosenman et al. (1999)
Cohort–registry linkage	M (3, 155) Silicosis patients	OR 3.2 (1.1, 9.4)	Rosenman & Zhu (1995)
Case–control	M (176, 630) F (339, 627)	Men: mineral dust – job/exposure history OR 1.8 (0.6, 5.5), $P <$ 0.05 for trend with duration; no association seen in females	Olsson et al. (2004)
Case–control	M (276, 276)	Job/task history (e.g. rock drilling, stone crushing, stone dust) OR 2.2 (1.2, 3.9)	Stolt et al. (2005)

Table 10 (Contd)

Disease and design	Sex (n)[a] / Occupation	Exposure classification and results[b]	References
Systemic sclerosis			
Nested case–control	M (79, 79) Gold miners	Higher cumulative exposure and intensity of exposure in cases	Sluis-Cremer et al. (1985)
Cohort study (incidence rate) and nested case–control	M (10, 486) Gold miners (incident cases)	High incidence (8.2 per 100 000 person years), but no difference in exposure measures between cases and controls	Cowie (1987)
Cohort study (incidence rate)	M (103, 242 900) Uranium miners	High exposure RR 7.8 (6.5, 9.5) Silicosis RR 97 (75, 125) High exposure, no silicosis RR 3.1 (2.2, 4.3)	Mehlhorn et al. (1999)
Cohort–registry linkage	M (5, 1130) Silicosis patients	RR 37.0 (11.9, 86.3)	Brown et al. (1997)
Case–control	M (56, 56)	Possible or probable OR 1.0 (0.13, 7.2)	Silman & Jones (1992)
Case–control	M + F (21, 42)[d]	OR 2.1 (0.34, 13.6)[d]	Bovenzi et al. (1995)
Case–control	M + F (55, 171)[d]	OR 1.7 (0.4, 7.6)[d]	Bovenzi et al. (2004)
Case–control	F (274, 1184)	Silica job OR 1.5 (0.76, 2.9)	Burns et al. (1996)
Case–control	M (160, 83)	Definite or probable OR 3.9 (1.8, 8.5)	Englert et al. (2000)
Case–control	M + F (80, 160)	Ever OR 5.6 (1.7, 18.4); high cumulative exposure score[c] 3.7 (1.1, 13.2)	Diot et al. (2002)
ANCA-related vasculitis			
Case–control	M (16, 32)	Job/task history OR 14.0 (1.7, 114)	Gregorini et al. (1993)
Case–control	M + F (16, 32)	Job/task history OR 5.0 (1.4, 11.6)	Nuyts et al. (1995)
Case–control	M + F (65, 65)	Task history OR 4.4 (1.4, 13.4)	Hogan et al. (2001)

Table 10 (Contd)

Disease and design	Sex (n)[a] / Occupation	Exposure classification and results[b]	References
Case–control	M + F (31, 58)	OR 2.4 ($P = 0.04$)	Stratta et al. (2001)
Case–control	M + F (75, 273)	High – job/task history – ever OR 1.4 (0.7, 2.7)	Lane et al. (2003)
		Year before onset OR 3.0 (1.0, 8.4)	
Case–control	M + F (60, 120)	Job/task history OR 3.4 (1.1, 9.9); dose–response across exposure score[c]	Beaudreuil (2005)
Systemic lupus erythematosus			
Cohort study (prevalence rate)	M (28, 300 000) Uranium miners	Prevalence 10 times expected	Conrad et al. (1996)
Cohort–registry linkage	M (8, 1130) Silicosis patients	RR 23.8 (10.3, 47.0)	Brown et al. (1997)
Case–control	M + F (265, 355)	Job/task history – medium OR 1.7 (1.0–3.2); high OR 3.8 (1.2–11.6); $P < 0.05$ for trend across dose levels	Parks et al. (2002)

[a] For cohort studies, n = number of cases, total cohort size in cohort studies; for case–control studies, n = number of cases, number of controls. M = male, F = female.
[b] Risk ratio (RR) or odds ratio (OR) and 95% confidence interval.
[c] Based on probability, intensity, frequency, and duration measures.
[d] Combining the two studies, the odds ratio was 2.4 for men, 1.5 for women, and 2.4 for the combined sample.

8.5.3 Experimental studies of immune- and autoimmune-related effects of silica

Silica has been shown to have an adjuvant effect in a variety of animal models and disease states. Respirable silica particles are phagocytosed by alveolar macrophages, leading to cellular activation and the release of soluble mediators such as chemokines, proinflammatory cytokines including TNF-α and IL-1, lysosomal enzymes, and reactive oxygen and nitrogen species. These soluble mediators act to recruit and activate additional inflammatory cells that may lead to increased antigen processing and accelerated antibody production. The effect is not limited to the lung. Migration of silica-containing macrophages to the lymph nodes and increased systemic immunoglobulin production have also been shown to occur (Huang et al., 2001; Weissman et al., 2001). In murine models, silica has been shown to increase the levels of antigen-specific antibodies in the lung following intranasal or intratracheal instillation (Granum et al., 2001) and in the blood following intravenous administration (Pernis & Paronetto, 1962). In a genetically susceptible murine model of lupus, silica exposure exacerbated development of autoimmune disease (i.e. increased autoantibody production, immune complexes, proteinuria, and glomerulonephritis) (Brown et al., 2003). Autoantibodies from these mice recognized specific epitopes on apoptotic macrophages (Pfau et al., 2004). In a rat model for multiple sclerosis, administration of silica up to one month prior to or concurrent with spinal cord homogenates increased the incidence and severity and advanced the onset of disease (Levine & Sowinski, 1980).

Increased cytokine production may also play a role in silica-induced autoimmune vascular disease. Adhesion molecule expression is elevated on vascular endothelial cells in response to TNF-α and IL-1. Adhesion molecules such as endothelial leukocyte adhesion molecule-1 (ELAM-1) and intercellular adhesion molecule-1 (ICAM-1) recruit inflammatory cells to specific sites on the vascular endothelium, and it has been hypothesized that vascular pathology following silica exposure may be the result of this interaction (Nowack et al., 1998). IFN-γ is expressed at elevated levels by lymphocytes in silicotic thoracic lymph nodes and may be responsible for the long-lasting inducible nitric oxide synthase (iNOS) expression in these tissues (Friedetzky et al., 2002). The increase in IFN-γ may also cause a shift towards a dominant Th1 response, contributing to the maintenance of a chronic inflammatory state in silica-containing lymph nodes (Garn et al., 2000).

In vitro studies also provide important evidence that silica's properties as an adjuvant may be relevant in silica-induced autoimmunity. Incubation of silica and silicate with isolated human T cells caused polyclonal lymphocyte activation, which in vivo could lead to a breakdown of tolerance via nonspecific stimulation of autoreactive T cell clones (Ueki et al., 1994).

Studies of particulate air pollutants indicate that silica particles stimulate a Th1-type response, with increased production of IFN-γ and increased levels of antigen-specific IgG2a (van Zijverden et al., 2000). Silica also reacts with water to form hydroxyl radicals that further react with cell membranes, resulting in lipid peroxidation and production of additional reactive oxygen species that can activate transcription factors and lead to increased cytokine production (Vallyathan et al., 1988; Ghio et al., 1990). The skewing towards a Th1 response and release of reactive oxygen species promote the continued secretion of proinflammatory cytokines, resulting in chronic macrophage activation. In fact, one hallmark of silica-induced lung injury is its self-perpetuating nature. In alveolar macrophages, the intracellular release of proteolytic enzymes in response to phagocytosis of silica particles leads to cell death. Silica is released from the dying cells and is reingested by other macrophages, creating a cyclical process of inflammation and necrotic cell death. Silica has also been shown to induce apoptosis in human alveolar macrophages and peripheral blood lymphocytes in culture (Iyer et al., 1996; Aikoh et al., 1998). Fas is a well known cell surface molecule that is involved in the apoptosis pathway belonging to the TNF receptor family. Soluble Fas is produced as an alternatively spliced product of the Fas gene and protects cells from apoptosis by blocking the binding the interaction between membranous Fas and Fas ligand. In silicosis patients, soluble Fas message was dominantly expressed compared with membranous Fas expression, although the relative expression levels of the Fas and Fas ligand genes were not significantly altered (Otsuki et al., 1998).

The mechanisms of renal pathology appear to differ among the various autoimmune diseases that may be associated with silica exposure. Silica particles can accumulate in the kidney, leading to localized inflammatory responses and fibrotic lesions similar to those observed in pulmonary silicosis (Slavin et al., 1985). Alternatively, circulating autoantibodies may deposit in the kidney, resulting in immune complex glomerulonephritis. Autoantibodies against the specific antigens proteinase 3 and myeloperoxidase are associated with ANCA-associated glomerulonephritis. The antigens are seldom detected in alveolar macrophages, and Gregorini et al. (1997) hypothesized that following silica inhalation, proteinase 3 and myeloperoxidase are released by activated polymorphonuclear leukocytes, taken up by the alveolar macrophages, and subsequently released into circulation when these cells are destroyed. The circulating antigens then stimulate production of the characteristic antineutrophil cytoplasmic autoantibodies of ANCA-associated glomerulonephritis.

8.5.4 Summary

In conclusion, silica may have immediate and latent effects, suggesting that risk assessment scenarios may need to consider a wide window of silica exposure for autoimmune effects. There is little information on the duration of exposure and dose required for silica-related autoimmune effects, and it is not currently known whether peak or cumulative dose is more predictive of disease development. Silica exposure may often occur in the presence of other exposures that may interact mechanistically to modify the risk of developing autoimmune disease. For example, even trace contamination of quartz dust with iron particles may augment inflammatory effects in the lung (Castranova et al., 1997). Smoking is another common exposure in many silica-exposed workers and has been shown to modify the association of high- and moderate-level silica exposure for risk of systemic lupus erythematosus (Parks et al., 2002). Silica dust exposure may be associated with a wide range of autoimmune diseases and immune abnormalities. Although some studies have explicitly focused on only one disease, several indicate an increased occurrence of several different diseases within the same study population. In addition to exploring the possibility of shared mechanisms, risk analyses should consider the impact of silica dust exposure across multiple diseases. There is also a need to consider the potential for effect modification by genetic or sex differences in disease susceptibility, as well as the modifying effects of other environmental exposures (e.g. metals, smoking). Polymorphisms in tumour necrosis factor and other cytokine genes may be related to severity of silicosis in humans (Corbett et al. 2002; Yucesoy et al., 2002). As allelic variation in these genes has also been linked to other autoimmune diseases, it is plausible that differences in silica-related autoimmunity might be modified by these factors as well. Given that women have higher rates of many autoimmune diseases compared with men, it will be important to learn if they are more or less vulnerable to the effects of silica.

8.6 Heavy metals

It is notable that cadmium as well as mercury and gold can initiate or aggravate autoimmune manifestations in normal or autoimmune-prone animals, respectively. It would seem likely that these heavy metals have the same effects on humans, presumably by a similar mechanism. Autoimmune manifestations induced by heavy metals include lupus-type nephritis, autoimmune haemolytic anaemia, and skin diseases, such as pemphigus and scleroderma-like lesion. Some manifestations of immune-mediated nephritis and elevation of circulating autoantibodies have been noted in case-studies of persons exposed to gold and cadmium as well as mercury (Ohsawa, 1993; Bigazzi, 1994, 1999).

8.6.1 Mercury

The presence of mercury in fish, thermometers, dental amalgams, vaccine preservatives, and the atmosphere has increased public health concerns about adverse health effects in humans exposed to relatively low levels of mercury. The lack of a clear correlation between mechanistic research on mercury toxicity and sublethal non-cytotoxic effects and lack of consideration of mercury-induced immunotoxicity as an important health outcome have limited the application of science-based risk assessment on this issue (Silbergeld & Devine, 2000).

Occupational exposure to mercury, in spite of immunological changes described even in workers with relatively low urinary mercury concentrations (Queiroz et al., 1994; Dantas & Queiroz, 1997; Queiroz & Dantas, 1997), does not usually result in autoimmune response or disease (Bigazzi, 1999). The suggestion that mercury may cause autoimmune response and disease in humans is based mainly on several cases of nephrotic syndrome associated with mercury-containing drugs that were in use until the mid-20th century, in which renal histopathological lesions and the presence of autoantibodies bound to the renal membrane in kidney biopsies were reported.

The use of mercury for the production of dental silver amalgam restorations and the subsequent release of mercury have been a matter of concern over the last 30 years (Clarkson et al., 2003).

Various claims have been made about possible associations with neurological and/or autoimmune diseases. In a recent epidemiological study of 20 000 people (84% males) with detailed exposure data, a consistent level of amalgam treatment across the cohort, and investigation of a wide range of possible health outcomes, an association was evidenced only with multiple sclerosis, and this association was relatively weak (adjusted hazard ratio of 1.24; 95% confidence interval: 0.99–1.53) (Bates et al., 2004). Additional epidemiological studies are needed to fully address the question of autoimmune-related health effects of dental amalgams (Weiner et al., 1990; DHHS, 1993; Cuttres, 1997).

The organic alkylmercury compound thimerosal (sodium ethylmercury thiosalicylate) is another modern facet of mercury. Rare cases of systemic hypersensitivity with skin (Zenarola et al., 1995) and respiratory (Maibach, 1975) manifestations as well as acrodynia (Matheson et al., 1980) have been reported. Thimerosal in vaccines is discussed more in chapter 9.

Mercury has two types of immunotoxic effects, both of which have been described in humans, primates, and rodents. First, in rodents, subtoxic doses of mercury may induce a characteristic systemic autoimmune syndrome associated with three major pathological sequelae: lymphoproliferation, hypergammaglobulinaemia, and the development of autoimmunity. Autoimmunity is manifested as the formation of antinuclear antibodies and highly specific antinucleolar autoantibodies, which are deposited within the kidney and eventually disrupt renal function, causing clinical disease (Bagenstose et al., 1999a, 1999b; Bigazzi, 1999; Pollard et al., 1999; Silbergeld & Devine, 2000). The mechanism for mercury-induced autoimmunity probably involves the modification of the autoantigen fibrillarin by mercury followed by a T cell-dependent immune response driven by the modified fibrillarin (Arnett et al., 2000; Nielsen & Hultman, 2002). Antinucleolar antibodies present a virtually identical specificity of response to that of autoantibodies found with high titres in sera of patients with systemic scleroderma, the human autoimmune disease most often associated with exposure to environmental agents (Takeuchi et al., 1995; Arnett et al., 1996; Yang et al., 2003). The second type of mercury immunotoxic effects is immunosuppression, which occurs at relatively low doses of mercury and methylmercury that directly impair Th1 responses and augment Th2 responses (Lawrence & McCabe, 1995; Silbergeld &

Devine, 2000; Bagenstose et al., 2001). Apoptosis has been suggested as a possible mechanism for immunosuppression (Shenker et al., 1998; Whitekus et al., 1999). Mercury-induced immunotoxic alterations are observed not only after parenteral application of mercury(II) chloride, but also after oral or epicutaneous exposure to mercury salts, implantation of dental amalgam, and exposure to mercury vapour (Eneström & Hultman, 1995; Schuppe et al., 1998).

Rodent susceptibility to the systemic autoimmunity induced by mercury(II) chloride is genetically controlled (see chapter 7). Both MHC class II genes and non-MHC genes determine responsiveness (Hultman et al., 1996; Hanley et al., 1998; Schuppe et al., 1998; Abedi-Valugerdi & Möller, 2000; Hultman & Nielsen, 2001). The induction and development of autoimmune responses in susceptible strains vary across species. Rats become resistant to mercury-induced autoimmunity after a subsequent challenge, whereas mice do not show resistance to subsequent mercury exposures (see also chapter 10).

The preferential activation of Th2 cells in several rat and mouse strains susceptible to mercury-induced systemic autoimmune disease compared with a Th1 response after mercury treatment in resistant strains led to the assumption that Th2 cells mediate induction of the syndrome and that Th1 cells or $CD8^+$ T cells (see chapter 7) are responsible for the resolution of the disease (reviewed in Bagenstose et al., 1999b). However, recent examination of the role of these cytokines has demonstrated that IL-4 production is not required for mercury-induced disease. The question remains whether Th1 cells participate in both the induction and the regulation of the disease (Bagenstose et al., 1998a). Treatment with IL-12, a Th1-promoting cytokine, does not fully prevent mercury-induced autoimmunity (Bagenstose et al., 1998b; Gorrie et al., 2000). Moreover, some studies have suggested that IFN-γ and therefore Th1 cells are required for the development of mercury-induced disease (Dubey et al., 1993; Kono et al., 2000). Recent studies on the contribution of co-stimulatory signals (see chapter 7) for the activation and expansion of autoreactive T cells demonstrated that complete blockade of the immune response inhibitory pathway CD28/CTLA-4:B7-1/B7-2 prevented mercury-induced disease in susceptible mice. These findings point to the presence of independent mechanisms in the regulation of the various manifestations of the mercury-induced syndrome. The requirements for co-stimulatory molecules, adherent cells, and mature T cells argue that mercury(II) chloride-induced T cell proliferation possesses the property of an antigen-induced response (Pollard & Landberg, 2001; Bagenstose et al., 2002).

Recent studies have raised the possibility that both genetic and environmental factors act synergically at several stages of autoimmunity pathogenesis. These studies predict that individuals susceptible to spontaneous autoimmunity should be more susceptible following xenobiotic exposure by virtue of the presence of predisposing background genes (Cooper et al., 1999; Pollard et al., 1999). In this regard, recent discussions regarding the autoimmune effect of mercury are not only, or even mainly, concerned with the risk of inducing de novo autoimmune conditions, but further the possibility that mercury might accelerate or aggravate spontaneously occurring systemic autoimmune conditions (Havarinasab et al., 2004).

Rowley & Monestier (2005) reviewed mechanisms of the induction of autoimmunity by the heavy metal mercury in the rat and mouse. In contrast to the rat autoimmune model, in the mouse model for autoimmunity induced by mercury, the autoantibody response is specifically targeted towards nucleolar antigens and is associated with induction of antifibrillarin autoantibodies. Second, exposure to low doses of mercury can dramatically worsen the development of autoimmune responses in lupus mouse models. A third difference is the nature of the interaction of heavy metals such as mercury with thiol groups and the role of this affinity in the availability of certain thiol-containing molecules for immature cells.

Fournie et al. (2001) addressed the immunological disorders induced by mercury. They examined data available that suggest that mercury can behave as an adjuvant and trigger autoimmunity responses. This supports the notion that mercury acts by promoting differentiation of autoreactive T cells towards pathological pathways through a "bystander effect". The importance of genetic factors in the triggering and development of this Th1- and/or Th2-mediated effect and related immune responses (e.g. T cell cytokine expression, IL-4 response) is demonstrated by differences in susceptibility to development of immunotoxicity following mercury exposure in different rat strains (e.g. Brown Norway versus Lewis rats). The role and expression of certain chromosome loci are hypothesized as possible explanations or contributors to this genetic difference in susceptibility to development of immunological disorders.

8.6.2 Gold

Gold medication (i.e. organic gold therapy of rheumatoid arthritis) is well known to often induce autoimmune glomerulonephropathy (refer to section 8.11.6). Despite the adverse effects of gold therapy, it is not known whether environmental or occupational exposure to gold causes renal pathology in humans. However, progressive interstitial lung fibrosis was found in goldsmiths (Kirchner et al., 1997), as well as in patients on gold therapy (Smith & Ball, 1980).

Proteinuria and associated glomerular lesions were observed in rabbits fed with a gold oxide-containing diet (Nagi & Khan, 1984). Fournie et al. (2001) proposed that gold, like mercury, can act as an adjuvant, resulting in autoimmunity due to a bystander effect. Genetic susceptibility in the induction of autoimmune reactions and immunological disorders is suggested from the differing outcomes seen with exposure to gold in different rat strains. These genetic-based responses are associated with certain chromosome loci that are implicated in control of T cell polarization to either Th1- or Th2-type immune responses.

8.6.3 Cadmium

Occupational and environmental exposure to cadmium causes renal damage indicated by increased levels of protein in the urine. The renal dysfunction in workers and the general population exposed to high levels of cadmium is characterized as the tubular-type nephritis. Chronic exposure of humans to cadmium has, however, frequently resulted in the tubular and glomerular mixed-type nephritis associated with the development of glomerular damage (Bernard et al., 1976; Lauwerys et al., 1984; Mueller et al., 1992). Circulating antilaminin antibodies (Bernard et al., 1987) were also found in workers exposed to cadmium, but there is no definitive evidence that cadmium-induced glomerular nephritis in human subjects is caused by autoimmune mechanisms.

The accumulated evidence indicates clear renal toxicity in animals exposed to cadmium as well as in humans and also a variety of immunotoxic effects, including suppression or potentiation of antibody production and cellular immune responses. Chronic injections of cadmium chloride were earlier found to cause glomerular amyloidosis in rabbits (Castano, 1971). Early studies in Sprague-Dawley rats showed that chronic oral exposure to cadmium via the drinking-water (100 or 200 mg/l) caused immune complex nephritis (Joshi et al., 1981). Similarly, the chronic exposure of Sprague-Dawley rats, but not Brown Norway rats, to cadmium (20 or 100 mg/l in drinking-water) induced production of autoantibodies against two components of glomerular basement membrane — i.e. laminin and type IV procollagen (Bernard et al., 1984). A significant induction of antinuclear antibodies was seen in ICR mice exposed to cadmium at 30 mg/l in the drinking-water for 10 weeks (Ohsawa et al., 1988), but Balb/c mice were less susceptible. In vitro cadmium can enhance the proliferative responses of lymphocytes and antibody production without antigen priming. Thus, autoantibodies could be induced by polyclonal activation of B cells due to cadmium. Although these autoantibodies may be involved in autoimmune renal pathogenesis, no direct evidence is available. Exposure to cadmium also accelerated the age-dependent production of anti-DNA antibodies in male MRL-lpr/lpr mice (Ohsawa et al., 1990). In NZB/NZW mice, exposure to cadmium at 10 mg/l in the drinking-water exacerbated immune complex deposition in the kidney and proteinuria after four weeks of exposure (Leffel et al., 2003). Moreover, interstitial nephritis with mononuclear cell infiltration was produced in SJL/J mice given daily cadmium injections of 1.25 mg/kg for 13 weeks (Weiss et al., 1994). In this latter case, T cells isolated from nephritic kidneys of mice given cadmium were reactive to the heat shock protein HSP-70.

8.6.4 Other heavy metals

A variety of immune alterations have been reported in humans and laboratory animals exposed to other heavy metals, depending on the dose, duration, and route of exposure and genetic susceptibility (Koller, 1980; Ohsawa, 1993; IPCS, 1996). In many studies of subchronic or chronic exposure, non-essential heavy metals such as cadmium, lead, and mercury were immunosuppressive in animals and consequently decreased host resistance to infectious agents and tumours. Immunostimulation has also been shown to occur at levels of exposure lower than those associated with immunosuppression, presumably linking to allergic or autoimmune responses.

Some other heavy metals may cause autoimmune responses in humans and animals. Pemphigus was found in a worker exposed to chromium (Tsankov et al., 1990), but no firm conclusions can be drawn. Multiple sclerosis was suggested to be associated with occupational exposure to zinc (Stein et al., 1987). Various autoantibodies were also found in human subjects exposed to heavy metals. Antioxidized DNA base autoantibodies were detected with a significant increased titre in nickel–cadmium battery workers heavily exposed to these metals and with an increasing trend in workers exposed to welding fumes containing manganese, nickel, and chromium (Frenkel et al., 1994). Female SJL/N mice implanted in the peritoneal cavity with silver alloy not containing mercury for 10 weeks or 6 months developed autoantibodies to nucleoprotein fibrillarin and systemic immune complex deposition in a time- and dose-dependent manner (Hultman et al., 1994). It is noteworthy that induction of autoantibodies to neural proteins can be caused by heavy metal exposure. For example, antibodies to nervous system structural proteins were induced in workers in a nickel–cadmium battery factory (Evans et al., 1994); antibodies to lead-altered neuroproteins were observed in mice immunized with the proteins (Waterman et al., 1994); and antibodies to glutamate receptors were found in rats with cobalt-induced epilepsy (Dambinova et al., 1998). It is also reported that autoantibodies against nucleoplasmic proteins can be induced in mice treated with hexachloroplatinate (Chen et al., 2002). Although contribution of these autoantibodies to autoimmune pathogenesis is proposed, direct relevance of these autoantibodies to autoimmunity induced by individual heavy metals has not been established.

Similar to mercury and cadmium, lead has the potential to accelerate expression of autoimmune predisposition: lead accelerated the death of male, but not female, NZB/NZW mice due to spontaneously developing autoantibodies and glomerulonephritis (Lawrence et al., 1987) and exacerbated the susceptibility of NZ mixed strains to develop lupus-type nephritis (Hudson et al., 2003). This potential contribution of lead to autoimmune disease remains a valid concern.

8.7 Solvents

Beginning in the early 1960s, a number of case-reports established a linkage between occupational exposure to vinyl chloride and the development of a scleroderma-like disease characterized by skin thickening, Raynaud phenomenon, acroosteolysis (shortening of the terminal digital phalanges due to bone resorption), and a number of other clinical features, such as hepatomegaly, hypothyroid, and pulmonary involvement (Suciu et al., 1963; Wilson et al., 1967; Dodson et al., 1971; Czernielewski et al., 1979). It has been suggested that susceptibility to disease is increased in individuals expressing HLA-DR5 and that HLA-DR3 antigens favour progression of the disease, similar to that observed in classical scleroderma (Black et al., 1983, 1986).

Vinyl chloride has also been shown to produce highly reactive metabolites, chloroethylene oxide and chloroacetaldehyde, that have a high affinity for sulfhydryl groups on proteins (Chiang et al., 1997) and may result in the covalent modification of these proteins, leading to self-recognition. It has also been suggested that oxidation of intracellular thiols, via binding to sulfhydryl groups, may lead to preferential inactivation of cytotoxic T lymphocytes (Yoshida & Gershwin, 1993). The loss of suppressor cell activity as a result of this inactivation could lead to a breakdown in self-tolerance and be a contributing factor in the autoimmune response (Powell et al., 1999). Administration of vinyl chloride increased the number of circulating microchimeric white blood cells and the collagen content in the skin of retired breeder Balb/cJ mice (Christner et al., 2000). Dermal inflammation and fibrosis similar to that observed in skin from patients with systemic sclerosis or graft versus host disease were observed in vinyl chloride-treated retired breeders, but not in vinyl chloride-treated virgin females or untreated retired breeders. Fetal DNA and microchimeric cells have also been identified in the skin lesions of female patients with systemic sclerosis (Artlett et al., 1998).

The association between systemic sclerosis (scleroderma) and solvent exposure (primarily in occupational settings) has been investigated in more than a dozen studies to date (Table 11). These studies have fairly consistently reported a 2- to 3-fold increased risk of disease with various forms of solvent exposure. However, a clear consensus has not developed on specific exposures or classes of chemicals or on the extent to which similar findings are seen in other autoimmune diseases. Some studies on rheumatoid arthritis, systemic small-vessel vasculitis, and multiple sclerosis also demonstrate associations with occupational exposure to solvents, but no association was seen in a large population-based case–control study of systemic lupus erythematosus (Table 11).

Table 11. Epidemiological studies of solvent exposure[a] and risk of autoimmune disease

Disease and design	Sex (n)[b]	Results[c]	Reference
Systemic sclerosis			
Meta analysis of eight studies (1989–1998)	M + F (722 total cases)	Any: OR 2.9 (1.6, 5.3)	Aryal et al. (2001)
Case–control	M + F (178, 200)	Any solvent-oriented hobbies: no association	Nietert et al. (1999)
		High cumulative exposure: OR 2.5 (1.1, 5.9)	
Case–control	M + F (80, 160)	Any: OR 2.7 (1.4, 5.2); similar results for specific solvent and groups and for high cumulative exposures	Diot et al. (2002)
Case–control	F (63, 95)	Any: OR 2.6 ($P <$ 0.05)	Czirjak & Kumánovics (2002)
Case–control	F (660, 2227)	Any: OR 2.0 (1.5, 2.5); similar results seen with paint thinners and trichloroethylene	Garabrant et al. (2003)
Case–control	M + F (93, 206)	Any: OR 3.2 (1.6, 6.6)	Maitre et al. (2004)
Case–control	M + F (55, 171)	Any (organic): OR 2.3 (1.0, 5.4)	Bovenzi et al. (2004)
Case–control	M + F (21, 42)	Any (organic): OR 9.3 (1.1, 244)	Bovenzi et al. (1995)

Table 11 (Contd)

Disease and design	Sex (n)[b]	Results[c]	Reference
Undifferentiated connective tissue disease			
Case–control	F (205, 2095)	Paint thinners OR 2.7 (1.8, 4.2), mineral spirits OR 1.8 (1.1, 3.0), associations with solvent-related jobs also seen	Lacey et al. (1999)
Rheumatoid arthritis			
Record linkage	M + F (total 1525 cases)	Spray painters, lacquer workers OR 2.4 (1.1, 5.4) (men)	Lundberg et al. (1994)
Case–control Incident cases Plus prevalent cases (pooled analysis)	M + F (235, 752) (515, 1257)	Men: OR 1.5–3.0 for various solvent-related occupations Women: OR > 3.0 for printmakers and engravers	Olsson et al. (2004)
Systemic lupus erythematosus			
Case–control	M + F (265, 355)	High: OR 1.0 (0.57, 1.9) Moderate: OR 1.0 (0.60, 1.6)	Cooper et al. (2004)
Primary systemic vasculitis			
Case–control	M + F (75, 220)	Any: ORs > 2.5	Lane et al. (2003)
Multiple sclerosis			
Meta-analysis of nine studies	M + F (27 total cases)	OR 2.6 (CI 1.2, 3.3)	Landtblom et al. (1996)
Registry linkage	M (3241 total cases)	Solvent-related jobs OR 0.9 (0.7, 1.1)	Mortensen et al. (1998)
Cohort	11 542 painters (9 cases)	OR 2.0 (0.9, 4.5)	Riise et al. (2002)

[a] Occupational exposures, except as noted in the study by Nietert et al. (1999).
[b] M = male, F = female; n cases, n controls.
[c] Risk ratio (RR) or odds ratio (OR) and 95% confidence interval.

Studies in laboratory animals have helped elucidate the mechanisms through which exposure to particular solvents may influence the development or progression of autoimmune disease. Antibodies to malondialdehyde, a product of the oxidative degradation of polyunsaturated fatty acids, have been demonstrated in patients with systemic lupus erythematosus and scleroderma (Vaarala et al., 1993) and in MRL +/+ and MRL lpr mice following trichloroethylene exposure (Khan et al., 2001). In addition to increased levels of autoantibodies, these lupus-prone mice show elevated levels of Th1 cytokines and activated $CD4^+$ T cells (Khan et al., 1995; Griffin et al., 2000a). T cell activation and secretion of IL-4 can be blocked with inhibitors of CYP2E1, suggesting that metabolic activation of trichloroethylene may be important in the disease process (Griffin et al., 2000b). Biotransformation of trichloroethylene results in the generation of metabolites such as highly reactive aldehydes and oxides. These reactive intermediates can be strong acylating agents, binding to hydroxyl groups and inducing lipid peroxidation. Trichloroacetaldehyde, a primary metabolite of trichloroethylene, has been shown to serve as a costimulatory factor for T cell proliferation in vitro, upregulating CD28 and activating components of the AP-1 signal transduction cascade (Gilbert et al., 2004). Other metabolites of trichloroethylene have been shown to directly activate T cell responses following in vivo exposures and alter susceptibility to activation-induced cell death (Blossom et al., 2004). It has been postulated that solvent-induced lipid peroxidation leads to the formation of reactive intermediates, which can covalently bind to endogenous proteins, resulting in the generation of neoantigens and stimulating an autoimmune response (Chiang et al., 1997; Khan et al., 2001). Alternatively, reactive aldehydes may activate T cells through Schiff base formation, a transient interaction between the carbonyl and amine groups in physiological systems (Rhodes et al., 1995; Gilbert et al., 2004). Schiff base-forming compounds have been shown to induce cell activation independent of TCR signalling (Guo & Rhodes, 1990).

8.8 Tobacco smoke

Tobacco smoke has been demonstrated to have multiple effects on the immune system. Some effects are seen in the lung, such as an increased number, but decreased functional ability (e.g. antibacterial phagocytosis), of alveolar macrophages. Other effects include impaired secretion of proinflammatory cytokines and decreased activity of NK cells. These and other mechanisms contribute to an immunosuppressive effect of smoking and an increased susceptibility to infections (Sopori, 2002).

Considerable research has focused on tobacco use in relation to autoimmune diseases, including inflammatory bowel diseases, thyroid diseases, multiple sclerosis, rheumatoid arthritis, and systemic lupus erythematosus. The association between tobacco use and the risk of inflammatory bowel disease is quite interesting, in part because of the differences seen with respect to ulcerative colitis and Crohn disease (Table 12). An inverse association has been observed between smoking and the risk of ulcerative colitis (i.e. a reduced risk is seen among current smokers compared with never smokers), with a summary odds ratio of 0.42. Among former smokers, however, disease risk is higher than among never smokers (odds ratio 1.6). There is some evidence of a dose–response with the amount smoked (cigarettes per day) for both the inverse association among current smokers and the positive association among former smokers (Calkins, 1989). Smokers also showed reduced severity of ulcerative colitis, as assessed by self-reported symptoms, hospitalizations, or medication use (Loftus, 2004). In Crohn disease, however, most epidemiological studies have shown an increased risk among current and former smokers.

Vestergaard (2002) reported results from a meta-analysis of 25 studies pertaining to smoking history and Graves disease (hyperthyroidism), Graves disease with ophthalmopathy, and various forms of hypothyroidism. Current smoking was strongly associated with risk of developing Graves disease (odds ratio 3.3), but the association in former smokers was much weaker (Table 12). One study showed an increasing risk with increasing number of cigarettes per day in current smokers. Some studies were limited to women; in other studies, the number of men was relatively small (20% of the total sample). Nevertheless, there was some indication in the two studies that allowed sex-specific analyses that the association was stronger in women than in men. Stronger associations for never smokers and current smokers were seen with Graves disease with ophthalmopathy (for never smokers, the odds ratio was 4.4), particularly in patients with the more advanced form of this disease. The only study that presented sex-specific analyses reported a stronger effect in women than in men. Fewer studies are available regarding smoking and hypothyroidism (defined as Hashimoto thyroiditis, clinical hypothyroidism, subclinical hypothyroidism, or autoimmune thyroiditis), and the overall association with hypothyroidism was weaker (odds ratio around 1.5) than with Graves disease.

Table 12. Epidemiological studies of smoking and risk for specific autoimmune diseases

Disease and design	Associations with smoking[a]	References
Ulcerative colitis		
Meta-analysis and review	Current OR 0.41 (0.34, 0.48)	Calkins (1989); Loftus (2004)
	Former OR 1.64 (1.36, 1.98)	
Crohn disease		
Meta-analysis and review	Current OR 2.00 (1.65, 2.47)	Calkins (1989); Loftus (2004)
	Former OR 1.80 (1.33, 2.51)	
Graves disease (hyperthyroidism)		
Meta-analysis	Ever: OR 1.90 (1.42, 2.55)	Vestergaard (2002)
	Current: OR 3.30 (2.09, 5.22)	
	Former: OR 1.41 (0.77, 2.58)	
Graves disease with ophthalmopathy		
Meta-analysis	Ever: OR 4.40 (2.88, 6.73)	Vestergaard (2002)
Hypothyroidism		
Meta-analysis	Ever: OR 1.56 (1.07, 2.28)	Vestergaard (2002)
Multiple sclerosis		
Cohort study	Ever: RR 1.6 (1.1, 2.9)	Riise et al. (2003)
Cohort study	Former RR 1.5 (0.6, 3.3)	Villard-Mackintosh & Vessey (1993)
	Current RR 1.6 (0.8, 3.1)	
	Current RR 1.8 (0.8, 3.6)	
Cohort study	Current RR 1.6 (1.2, 2.1)	Hernán et al. (2001)
	Former RR 1.2 (0.9, 1.6)	
Rheumatoid arthritis		
Review	ORs 1.1–4.4 reported, generally higher in rheumatoid factor-positive cases and in men	Albano et al. (2001); Stolt et al. (2003)
Systemic lupus erythematosus		
Meta-analysis	Current: OR 1.5 (1.1, 2.1)	Costenbader et al. (2004)
	Former: OR 0.98 (0.75, 1.3)	

[a] OR = odds ratio or RR = risk ratio and 95% confidence interval.

Several prospective studies provided data regarding the risk of developing multiple sclerosis in relation to smoking history in women (Table 12). The largest study is based on the Nurses Health

Study cohorts in the United States, which reported an increased risk among current smokers (relative risk 1.6), with some evidence of a dose–response with pack-years (Hernán et al., 2001). Villard-Mackintosh & Vessey (1993) also found an association with smoking history and multiple sclerosis in the Oxford Family Planning Association cohort. In a small study using self-reported multiple sclerosis in a population-based study in Norway, the overall association with ever smokers (risk ratio 1.8) was higher in men (2.8) than in women (1.6) (Riise et al., 2003).

Two recent reviews have summarized studies of smoking history in relation to risk of developing rheumatoid arthritis (Albano et al., 2001; Stolt et al., 2003), although neither calculated combined measures of association across studies. Approximately half of the studies included men. The association with smoking history appears to be stronger in patients positive for rheumatoid factor than in patients negative for rheumatoid factor and stronger in men than in women. Smoking has also been associated with the production of rheumatoid factor in the general (non-diseased) population, and an interaction between the HLA-DRB1 genotype and current smoking was seen among rheumatoid factor-positive rheumatoid arthritis cases in Sweden (odds ratio 7.5, 95% confidence interval 4.2–13.1 for this combination of genes and exposure, compared with an odds ratio of 2.4 for smoking in the absence of the genes) (Padyukov et al., 2004). There is also some evidence of associations with pack-years or smoking duration, but more variable effects have been seen with the amount smoked per day (Albano et al., 2001; Stolt et al., 2003). The severity of rheumatoid arthritis may be increased in smokers, as evidenced by increased disability and risk of extra-articular manifestations, including vasculitis and interstitial lung disease, but not of joint swelling (Albano et al., 2001; Harrison, 2002).

A recent meta-analysis examined the association between smoking and the risk of systemic lupus erythematosus in seven case–control and two cohort studies (Costenbader et al., 2004) (Table 12). The combined estimate showed a weak association with current smoking (OR = 1.5), but no association with past smoking (OR = 0.98).

Larger studies specifically designed to assess sex differences are needed to understand the effect of smoking across the spectrum of autoimmune diseases. Because smoking habits differ between men and women (e.g. age at smoking initiation, amount smoked), detailed information pertaining to duration and intensity of smoking needs to be collected to separate biological from non-biological explanations for the observed associations.

8.9 Ethanol

There is increasing evidence that many patients with alcoholic liver disease have unique antigen-driven immune responses that target self-proteins.

Autoantibodies directed towards alcohol dehydrogenase, HSP-65, hepatocyte plasma membranes, and hydroxyethyl free radicals that cross-react with CYP2E1 and CYP3A4 have been reported in patients with alcoholic liver disease (Paronetto, 1993; Lytton et al., 1999; Viitala et al., 2000; Albano, 2002; Vidali et al., 2003). Although a positive correlation between alcohol intake and the degree of liver injury has been reported, there is a high degree of variability in the development and severity of disease between individuals with similar levels of abusive ethanol consumption, and only a small percentage of alcoholic patients develop cirrhosis or hepatitis. Heavy drinkers without significant liver disease had significantly lower titres of IgA antibodies against acetaldehyde-modified erythrocyte protein and IgG antibodies against oxidized- or malondialdehyde-modified low-density lipoproteins, compared with patients with alcoholic liver disease (Viitala et al., 2000). These studies suggest that multiple mechanisms or genetic factors may be involved in the disease process. In support of this, two studies using the National Academy of Sciences – National Research Council twin registry in the United States concluded that there was genetic predisposition to organ-specific complications of alcoholism based on the significant concordance rates in monozygotic twins (Hrubec & Omenn, 1981; Reed et al., 1996). Gene polymorphisms encoding for the enzymes responsible for ethanol metabolism, oxidative stress, and proinflammatory/immune responses have been investigated (Bataller et al., 2003).

The primary enzymes that metabolize alcohol in the human liver are alcohol dehydrogenase and CYP2E1. Acetaldehyde, a primary metabolite of ethanol, may have direct fibrogenic activity, and genetic polymorphisms in the ADH2, ADH3, ALDH2, or CYP2E1 genes, which affect the rate of acetaldehyde production, have been suggested as a mechanism to explain some of the differences in disease rate and severity (Friedman, 1999; Bataller et al., 2003). A genetic analysis of individuals participating in a study evaluating liver disease in northern Italy suggested that heavy drinkers with cirrhosis or alcoholic liver disease had a higher frequency (0.33 and 0.19, respectively) of the C2 allele in the promoter region of CYP2E1 than did healthy heavy drinkers (0.06; Monzoni et al., 2001). A study in alcoholic patients in Japan reported an increase in the frequency of individuals homozygous for the C1 allele in men with alcoholic cirrhosis (Yamauchi et al., 1995). Grove and colleagues (1998) demonstrated that in Caucasian men, possession of the mutant C2 allele of CYP2E1 increases the risk of alcoholic liver disease at a given level of cumulative alcohol consumption. This risk appears to be particularly strong in individuals carrying the ADH3*2 allele. In contrast, there was no difference in either C1 or C2 allelic distribution in an earlier study conducted in Caucasian men (Carr et al., 1995). Associations between liver disease and ADH genes were also documented in both the Italian and Japanese study populations, although in Japanese men, the ADH2*2/ADH2*2 genotype was more prevalent in patients with cirrhosis, while the ADH3*2/ADH3*2 genotype was associated with alcoholic liver disease in heavy drinkers from specific geographic areas (Yamauchi et al., 1995; Monzoni et al., 2001).

Cytokine gene polymorphisms have also been suggested to play a role in the pathogenesis of alcoholic liver disease. Among heavy drinkers, possession of the C→A allelic polymorphism at position 167 within the IL-10 promoter is associated with an increased risk of advanced liver disease (Grove et al., 2000). Individuals with the A allele are believed to secrete lower levels of IL-10, a cytokine that has both antifibrotic and anti-inflammatory properties. The same laboratory found a significant excess of the rare allele TNFA-A (G (−238) → A), which results in increased production of tumour necrosis factor, in patients with biopsy-proven alcoholic liver disease (Grove et al., 1997). Polymorphisms in the IL-1β gene have been associated with a number of autoimmune diseases. Takamatsu et al. (2000) investigated two polymorphisms in the IL-1β gene. The IL-1β −511 allele 2/+3953 allele 1 haplotype was significantly associated with the development of alcoholic cirrhosis. The −511 allele 2 was found at a higher frequency in patients with cirrhosis than in heavy drinkers without liver disease. A C→T (−159) CD14 gene polymorphism has also been investigated. Jarvelainen and colleagues (2001) demonstrated that in Finnish males, expression of one T allele was associated with both alcoholic hepatitis and cirrhosis. The CD14 cell surface receptor, which binds bacterial endotoxin, is overexpressed in individuals who possess copies of the T allele. The overall age-adjusted risk for cirrhosis in individuals with the homozygous TT genotype was 4.17. In several European studies, patients with alcoholic liver disease expressed the mutant CTLA-4 G allele at a higher frequency than did controls (Vidali et al., 2003; Valenti et al., 2004). This specific mutation has been shown to increase the risk of developing autoantibodies towards CYP2E1 (Clot et al., 1996; Vidali et al., 2003). There is conflicting evidence as to whether variations in the genes encoding for manganese superoxide dismutase represent a risk factor for alcoholic liver disease (Degoul et al., 2001; Stewart et al., 2002).

The data on cytokine and metabolic enzyme gene polymorphisms in the human population as well as experimental studies with ethanol-fed rodents are indicative of the importance of inflammation, oxidative stress, and endotoxin in the pathogenesis of alcohol-induced liver damage. In rodents, ethanol-induced liver injury is mediated, at least in part, by increased secretion of TNF-α by Kupffer cells (Yin et al., 1999). Altering TNF-α secretion via inactivation of Kupffer cells, antibody binding, or gene/receptor knockouts ameliorates alcohol-induced liver injury (Adachi et al., 1994; Yin et al., 1999). Chronic ethanol exposure has been associated with the formation of alcohol-modified proteins, leading to autoantibody formation and immune-mediated damage to the liver. In patients with alcoholic liver disease and ethanol-fed rats, titres of anti-CYP2E1 antibodies correlated with the severity of alcohol-induced liver damage (Lytton et al., 1999; Vidali et al., 2003). Circulating antibodies recognizing acetaldehyde–malondialdehyde adducts have been found in Wistar rats fed an ethanol-containing liquid diet (Xu et al., 1998). Immunization with acetaldehyde adducts in conjunction with ethanol feeding stimulated ex vivo lymphocyte proliferation in B6 mice, but not in several other strains (Shimada et al., 2002), and malondialdehyde–acetaldehyde haptenated proteins have been shown to induce high-titre antibody responses in Balb/c mice and enhance T cell proliferative responses in vivo and in vitro (Willis et al., 2002, 2003; Thiele et al., 2003). The antibodies generated by these alcohol-modified proteins may also respond to unmodified self-proteins, leading to a breaking of tolerance and autoimmune pathology.

8.10 Iodine

Three animal models have been used to demonstrate the effect of iodine in promoting thyroiditis. Obese strain chickens spontaneously develop a disease very similar to Hashimoto thyroiditis. They were the first model that showed that exposure to iodine affects the course of disease. Depletion of iodine after hatching, achieved by injections of potassium chlorite, reduced thyroid infiltration. In contrast, the onset of spontaneous thyroiditis was hastened by adding sodium iodide to the diet. This effect, however, was reduced by administration of antioxidants, suggesting that reactive oxygen intermediates are one mechanism by which iodine contributes to cell injury.

The Biobreeding/Worcester rat has been widely used as a model for studying spontaneous diabetes mellitus, but it also develops autoimmune thyroiditis. Administration of excess iodine accelerates the appearance of the lymphocytic infiltration of the thyroid and the production of thyroid-specific autoantibodies.

The NOD.H2^{h4} mouse model of autoimmune thyroiditis was selected by cross-breeding the classical NOD strain (which spontaneously develops diabetes) with the B10.A (4R) mouse, a good responder to thyroglobulin. The incidence of diabetes is very low, but many of the animals develop autoimmune thyroiditis. The prevalence and severity of the disease rise if dietary iodine is increased. Iodinated thyroglobulin is more antigenic than the same molecule lacking iodine, suggesting another mechanism by which iodine enhances thyroiditis.

Several studies have evaluated the effects of excessive iodine intake in humans, and antithyroid antibodies and iodine-induced hypo- and hyperthyroidism have been reported following long-term iodine treatment for endemic goitre (Boyages et al., 1989; Kahaly et al., 1997, 1998).

8.11 Therapeutic agents

Therapeutic agents are a frequent and underestimated cause of adverse immune-mediated reactions (Bachot & Roujeau, 2001; Demoly & Bousquet, 2001). Although a few epidemiological analyses have been published, they are often confounded by the absence of a clear-cut diagnosis. Clinical outcomes can be the result of immunoallergic, pseudoallergic, or autoimmune-like mechanisms.

8.11.1 General

Therapeutic agents are one of the main causes of chemically induced autoimmunity (Olsen, 2004). However, a comprehensive review of adverse autoimmune responses and autoimmune diseases associated with therapeutic agents is beyond the scope of this monograph, and only a few examples will be discussed below. Table 13 provides an abbreviated list of therapeutic drugs that have reportedly been associated with autoimmune reactions.

When considering drug-induced autoimmunity, it is important to differentiate two situations. On the one hand, treatments with potent immunostimulatory agents, such as rIL-2 and IFN-α, can be more often associated with a wide variety of autoimmune diseases closely similar to spontaneous diseases (Vial et al., 2002). On the other hand, one given agent is associated with only one given type of autoimmune disease. In the latter case, the disease can be organ-specific and then closely mimic the spontaneous disease, except that cessation of the offending agent leads to the progressive recovery of clinical and then biological manifestations of the disease. The disease can also be systemic and consists of clinical manifestations and biological/immunological changes markedly different from those of spontaneous diseases.

Interestingly, drug-induced systemic autoimmune-like reactions often resemble systemic hypersensitivity reactions, and this further illustrates overlapping mechanisms between immunoallergic and autoimmune-like reactions. One example is the so-called drug hypersensitivity syndrome or DRESS (for drug rash with eosinophilia and systemic symptoms) (Bocquet et al., 1996). Many early clinical case-reports described lupus syndromes associated with anticonvulsant drugs, such as diphenylhydantoin and carbamazepine, but it is now well established that an appropriate diagnosis is anticonvulsant hypersensitivity syndrome, or DRESS (Knowles et al., 1999). It is worth emphasizing that most therapeutic agents found positive in the popliteal lymph node assay (see chapter 9) have been reported to induce DRESS in human patients.

Table 13. Examples of therapeutic agents associated with autoimmune disease

Therapeutic agent	Autoimmune disease(s)/reaction(s)
Acebutolol	Lupus syndrome
Alpha-methyl-dopa	Autoimmune haemolytic anaemia
Captopril	Pemphigus
Carbimazole	ANCA-associated vasculitis
Chlorpromazine	Lupus syndrome
Dihydralazine	Autoimmune hepatitis
Fludarabine	Autoimmune haemolytic anaemia
Hydralazine	Lupus syndrome, ANCA-associated vasculitis
Infliximab	Lupus syndrome
Interferons-alpha	Wide range of autoimmune diseases
Iproniazid	Autoimmune hepatitis
Isoniazid	Lupus syndrome
Nomifensine	Autoimmune haemolytic anaemia
Penicillamine	Myasthenia, dermatomyositis
D-Penicillamine	Anti-GBM (Goodpasture) disease
Practolol	Oculocutaneomucous syndrome
Procainamide	Lupus syndrome
Propylthiouracil	ANCA-associated vasculitis
rIL-2	Autoimmune thyroiditis
Simvastatin	Lupus syndrome
Tienilic acid	Autoimmune hepatitis
Tryptophan contaminants	Eosinophilia myalgia syndrome (see section 9.3.5)
Zimeldine	Guillain-Barré syndrome

8.11.2 *Hydralazine*

Hydralazine is an antihypertensive agent that can cause a lupus-like syndrome characterized by serosal inflammation, arthralgias, and rash (Hari et al., 1998). Hydralazine inhibits the covalent binding reaction of the complement protein C4, and susceptibility to hydralazine-induced lupus, as in idiopathic systemic lupus erythematosus, may depend partly upon genetically determined C4 levels (Sim & Law, 1985; Speirs et al., 1989). Hydralazine inhibits T cell DNA methylation, increases lymphocyte function-associated antigen-1 (LFA-1) (CD11a/CD18) expression, and induces autoreactivity in T cell lines. Adoptive transfer of T cells made autoreactive by treatment with either hydralazine or procainamide causes a lupus-like disease (Yung et al., 1997). In contrast to procainamide, hydralazine has no direct effect on DNA methyltransferase (DNMT) activity. Instead, hydralazine inhibited extracellular signal-regulated kinase (ERK) pathway signalling, thereby decreasing DNMT1 and DNMT3 mRNA expression and DNMT enzyme activity similar to mitogen-activated protein kinase inhibitors (Deng et al., 2003). T cells from patients with active lupus have impaired ERK pathway signalling, decreased DNMT mRNA and enzyme activity, hypomethylated DNA, and overexpression of LFA-1 on an autoreactive T cell subset (Richardson et al., 1990, 1992; Deng et al., 2003). It has been suggested that hydralazine inhibition of T cell ERK pathway signalling could contribute to the pathogenesis of drug-induced lupus through effects on DNA methylation by a mechanism resembling that in idiopathic human lupus (Deng et al., 2003).

8.11.3 *Procainamide*

Procainamide, widely used in the treatment of ventricular and supraventricular arrhythmias in the past, recently had its use restricted to short-term treatments due to the induction of autoimmunity and the development of drug-induced lupus (Ayer et al., 1993; Kretz-Rommel & Rubin, 1999). It has been suggested that procainamide-induced autoimmunity is characterized predominantly by an antihistone and anti-denatured DNA immune response (Rubin et al., 1986; Rubin, 1992; Mongey & Hess, 2001). Mechanistic studies have revealed that procainamide is a competitive DNMT inhibitor of some, but not all, nuclear methyltransferase activity (Scheinbart et al., 1991; Richardson, 2003).

The possibility of a lupus-inducing effect of the drug on T cell development in the thymus has been suggested (Quddus et al., 1993; Yung et al., 1996, 1997; Kretz-Rommel et al., 1997; Kretz-Rommel & Rubin, 2000, 2001; Rubin et al., 2001). Interference of procainamide-hydroxylamine, a reactive metabolite of procainamide, with self-tolerance mechanisms following T cell maturation in the thymus resulted in the emergence of chromatin-reactive T cells followed by humoral autoimmunity (Kretz-Rommel et al., 1997). Studies of the specificities of B cells that respond to chromatin-reactive T cells at the initiation of this autoimmune process demonstrated a rapid and robust expansion of anti-chromatin-secreting B cells, thus indicating the presence of a normal immune repertoire that includes non-tolerant autoreactive B cells that respond to strong T cell drive and are readily manifested if Fas-mediated activation-induced cell death is inhibited (Ayer et al., 1993).

8.11.4 D-Penicillamine

D-Penicillamine, which is structurally related to the amino acids valine and cysteine, is used as an anti-inflammatory drug in the treatment of rheumatoid arthritis, cystinuria, and Wilson disease. Because of a high incidence of adverse events and the strong association with several autoimmune-like phenomena, including myasthenia, pemphigus, and Goodpasture disease, the clinical use is limited. Patients with HLA-DR3 haplotype as well as those with inherited impaired sulfoxidation status are at increased risk (Emery & Panayi, 1989).

The adverse effects of D-penicillamine in animals are similar to those observed in humans. A study on the effects of D-penicillamine in various strains of mice indicated that D-penicillamine facilitates the induction of autoantibodies in animals with an inherent susceptibility to autoimmunity (Brik et al., 1995). Studies using the popliteal lymph node assay demonstrated that D-penicillamine is capable of inducing an antigen (i.e. compound)-specific T cell response controlled by non-MHC as well as MHC-linked genetic loci (Hurtenbach et al., 1987).

In rats, particularly Brown Norway rats, D-penicillamine induces a disease characterized by dermatitis, vasculitis, production of antinuclear antibodies, formation of circulating immune complexes, and IgG deposits along the glomerular basement membrane (Donker et al., 1984; Tournade et al., 1990). In D-penicillamine-treated Brown Norway rats, a preferential increase in IgE mediated by IL-4 was observed as well, and this suggested that D-penicillamine preferentially stimulates Th2 cells. Interestingly, low-dose pretreatment of D-penicillamine-treated Brown Norway rats was found to induce complete tolerance to a subsequent pathogenic dose of the drug (Donker et al., 1984). This tolerance could be transferred by T cells and accompanied by increased expression of TGFβ and IL-10, which is indicative of the presence of regulatory T cells (Masson & Uetrecht, 2004).

8.11.5 Zimeldine

Zimeldine is an antidepressant drug withdrawn from the market shortly after its introduction in the early 1980s because some patients developed Guillain-Barré syndrome (Dexter, 1984; Fagius et al., 1985). The syndrome was preceded by influenza-like symptoms, such as fever, headache, muscle and joint pains, and myalgia, which generally started within 6–17 days after starting zimeldine treatment. The British Department of Health and Social Security reported that 400 out of 100 000 patients displayed similar adverse responses to zimeldine. Four of these patients died, but no causal link was established.

A number of experiments performed thereafter were supportive for the immune-based etiology of zimeldine-induced adverse effects (Kristofferson & Nilsson, 1989). Three individuals occupationally exposed to zimeldine developed allergy to the compound and showed positive patch and skin prick tests and positive response to zimeldine in the lymphocyte transformation test. Patients with a history of zimeldine-induced disease showed marked lymphocyte transformation test responses to zimeldine as well as two metabolites (norzimeldine and CPP200). These findings indicate that zimeldine may be immunogenic; indeed, zimeldine has been shown to be positive in the popliteal lymph node assay, based on cell numbers and including germinal centre formation and production of IgM and IgG antibodies (Thomas et al., 1989).

8.11.6 Gold drugs

Gold drugs, such as aurothioglucose, gold sodium thiomalate, and auranofin, have long been used in the treatment of rheumatoid arthritis. The most common adverse effects associated with gold therapy appeared in skin and mucous membranes (about 15% of all patients) and kidneys (about 5–10%), mostly as proteinuria.

Gold drugs induce membranous glomerulonephropathy (Tonroth & Skrifvars, 1974). Gold-induced autoimmune manifestations involve MHC in humans. Gold-treated rheumatoid arthritis patients with HLA-DR3 are more susceptible to developing autoimmune renal manifestations (Wooley et al., 1980; Bardin et al., 1982; Gran et al., 1983; Berger et al., 1984). Other autoimmune manifestations in gold-treated rheumatoid arthritis patients also seem to be associated with certain HLA-DR haplotypes (Rodriguez-Perez et al., 1994; Evron et al., 1995). It is suggestive, moreover, that progressive interstitial lung fibrosis was found in gold therapy (Smith & Ball, 1980), possibly with an autoimmune pathogenesis. Gold therapy occasionally causes autoimmune haemolytic anaemia (Hunziker, 1978), autoimmune thrombocytopenia (Kotsy et al., 1989), and pemphigus (Bagheri et al., 2002).

Early studies showed that injections of gold thiomalate caused renal lesions, immune complex nephropathy, and proteinuria in Wistar rats (Nagi et al., 1971), rabbits (Nagi & Khan, 1984), and guinea-pigs (Ueda et al., 1986). The histology of these lesions can be characterized as either interstitial nephritis or glomerulonephritis, with specific diagnosis dependent on the presence of specific autoantibodies. Recent works using inbred animals have provided additional information on the pathogenesis of gold-induced renal autoimmunity. Inbred A.SW mice (H2s haplotype) treated with gold thiomalate produced autoantibodies to nucleolar antigens (Goter-Robinson et al., 1986; Schuhmann et al., 1990), with elevation of serum levels of IgE, IgG, and IgM (Pietsch et al., 1989). Autoimmunity induced by gold as well as mercury in mice appears dependent on MHC class II (Stiller-Winkler et al., 1988). As autoantibody production was induced in response to Au^{III} but not to Au^{I} after chronic treatment of mice with Au^{I}, the oxidation state of gold seems to contribute to induction of autoimmune responses (Schuhmann et al., 1990). Brown Norway rats treated with gold compounds developed autoimmune membranous glomerulopathy and developed autoantibodies against glomerular basement membrane, laminin 1 (an extracellular matrix component), and other components, including nuclear antigens, double-stranded DNA, thyroglobulin, actin, myosin, and tubulin (Tournade et al., 1991). These findings indicate that gold compounds appear to cause polyclonal B cell activation to induce a variety of autoantibodies, but detailed mechanisms have not been established.

8.11.7 Biopharmaceuticals

Biopharmaceuticals or biologicals are pharmaceutical products consisting of (glyco)proteins and/or nucleic acids that have evolved into a new and important category of therapeutic agents, in particular since the development of recombinant DNA technology.

Biopharmaceuticals include recombinant cytokines (interferons, IL-2, GM-CSF), blocking antibodies (such as the anti-TNF-α drug infliximab), and vaccines, as well as products not directly related to the immune system, such as blood clotting factors and hormones (Factor VIII, erythropoietin, heparin), enzymes, and hormones (Crommelin et al., 2003).

The main difference between classical low molecular weight pharmaceuticals and biopharmaceuticals is that biopharmaceuticals are large molecules that can be recognized directly by the immune system, without the need of metabolism or haptenation. Indeed, it has become clear that nearly all biopharmaceuticals induce antibodies, although many are of human origin and thus immunologically tolerated (Schellekens, 2003). The formed antibodies may have no effect at all or are neutralizing, but occasionally adverse reactions may occur. For instance, erythropoietin has been shown to induce autoimmune anaemia in macaques (Chenuaud et al., 2004), and a number of patients developed antibody-mediated pure red cell aplasia during treatment with recombinant human erythropoietin (Swanson et al., 2004).

Additionally, a number of biopharmaceuticals, or immunotherapeutics, such as the interferons-alpha or anti-TNF-α drugs, are intended to modulate the immune system or components thereof.

Treatments with recombinant therapeutic cytokines occasionally induce autoimmune phenomena. In particular, IFN-α may cause or exacerbate autoimmune effects, in particular thyroiditis, but also autoimmune thrombocytopenia or autoimmune hepatitis, and systemic lupus erythematosus has been reported. Relationships between IFN-α treatment and dermatomyositis (Dietrich et al., 2000) and diabetes mellitus (Fabris et al., 2003) have been observed. In addition, increased levels of various autoantibodies have been found in patients receiving IFN-α (Vial et al., 2002). Monzani et al.

(2004), Prummel & Laurberg (2003), and Ward & Bing-You (2001) examined the development of thyroid abnormalities during IFN-α therapy. Identified risk factors included the female sex, presence of pre-existing autoimmune thyroiditis, the treated disease (e.g. hepatitis B or C, multiple sclerosis, malignancies), along with genetic and environmental factors. The mechanism of the adverse thyroid effects induced by IFN-α has not yet been elucidated, but it appears to involve immune enhancement or dysregulation.

Anti-TNF-α drugs have recently been approved for the treatment of a number of autoimmune diseases, including rheumatoid arthritis and Crohn disease. A number of adverse consequences, including the development of antinuclear antibodies and anti-dsDNA antibodies and the autoimmune diseases leukocytoclastic vasculitis and systemic lupus erythematosus, have been reported following treatment with anti-TNF-α drugs (Hyrich et al., 2004).

8.11.8 Diethylstilbestrol

8.11.8.1 Diethylstilbestrol-induced immune alterations

Modifying influences on immune responses have been reported for the sex steroids 17β-estradiol and testosterone. 17β-Estradiol and synthetic non-steroidal estrogenic compounds such as diethylstilbestrol are potent modulators of immunity. The effects observed in rodents include thymic atrophy, suppression of thymus-dependent cellular immune responses, acceleration of autoimmune diseases, suppression of NK cell activity, myelotoxicity, and stimulation of the mononuclear phagocyte system (see Luster et al., 1984; Holladay, 1999). However, the immune effects described for diethylstilbestrol depend largely on the age of the animals at treatment, exposure to diethylstilbestrol, and sex.

Short-term exposure of mice to diethylstilbestrol has been described as inducing differential immunological effects, depending upon the dose of hormone and sex (Calemine et al., 2002). Aged mice appear especially sensitive to diethylstilbestrol treatment, as highly significant alterations were seen in the thymus and bone marrow of aged 21-month-old mice exposed subacutely to diethylstilbestrol. Severe thymic hypocellularity develops in treated mice following five consecutive days of intraperitoneal injection with diethylstilbestrol.

Upon neonatal treatment of mice with diethylstilbestrol, the delayed-type hypersensitivity response to oxazolone was similar in controls and diethylstilbestrol-treated animals at eight weeks, increased in treated females and males at six months, but reduced in treated females at one year (Forsberg, 2000). In the same study, the levels of serum IgG and IgM antibodies to cardiolipin showed age-dependent fluctuations but were similar in controls and diethylstilbestrol-treated females; however, the IgG antibodies in diethylstilbestrol-treated females were qualitatively different from those in controls with respect to sensitivity to bovine serum (a source of β_2-glycoprotein I), although these antibodies are not associated with autoimmune disease. In contrast to the situation with females, diethylstilbestrol-treated males had higher levels of these antibodies than controls (Forsberg, 2000).

A potential role of diethylstilbestrol in autoimmunity is also demonstrated by enhanced autoantibody production both in vitro and in vivo. BWF1 mice, a murine model for systemic lupus erythematosus, implanted with diethylstilbestrol after orchidectomy developed murine lupus, characterized by IgG anti-DNA antibody production and IgG deposition in the glomeruli in the kidney. Plaque-forming cells producing autoantibodies specific for bromelain-treated red blood cells were significantly increased in mice implanted with diethylstilbestrol. IgM antibody production by B1 cells in vitro was also enhanced by diethylstilbestrol treatment. Estrogen receptor expression was upregulated in B1 cells in aged BWF1 mice that developed lupus nephritis. The authors suggested that diethylstilbestrol modulates autoantibody production by B1 cells and may be an etiologic factor in the development of autoimmune diseases (Yurino et al., 2004). A number of studies have also demonstrated that perinatal exposure to diethylstilbestrol in mice produces profound thymus atrophy; although a direct cause–effect relationship has not been established, this has the potential to influence negative selection processes and subsequently influence autoimmune diseases.

8.11.8.2 Immune effects of diethylstilbestrol in humans

Although a substantial number of animal data demonstrate numerous immune alterations following in utero exposure to diethylstilbestrol, including abnormal B cell and T cell responses and diminished NK cell activity, limited data are available on long-term immune effects in humans following in utero diethylstilbestrol exposure. Evidence for immunostimulation was reported from increased lymphoproliferative responses to the mitogens PHA (phytohaemagglutinin) and PWM (pokeweed mitogen) in eight women with reproductive tract abnormalities and evidence of cervical and/or vaginal adenosis (Ways et al., 1987). Another small study of daughters with reproductive tract changes consistent with in utero diethylstilbestrol exposure suggested possible altered function of NK cells (Ford et al., 1983). In a follow-up study, using two different groups of diethylstilbestrol-exposed women and an appropriate control group for each, no differences in the prevalence or serum titre of antibodies to five common viral diseases and six less common ones were observed. However, an increased prevalence was found in diethylstilbestrol-exposed women of a relatively rare immunological hyperreactivity, rheumatic fever, subsequent to microbial infection (strep throat) (Blair et al., 1992). In a further study (Blair, 1992), sera of diethylstilbestrol-exposed and non-exposed women were examined for the presence of factors associated with autoimmune diseases. In addition, immunoglobulin levels were determined. The study demonstrated that the incidence of high antibody titres to red blood cell antigen was higher in the diethylstilbestrol-exposed females than in the controls. Also, serum IgA values were significantly increased. Blair (1992) concluded that, in general, humans exposed prenatally to diethylstilbestrol do not exhibit severe defects in basic immune function, but their propensity to develop autoimmune disease and other diseases associated with defects in immune regulation is increased.

There are relatively few data pertaining to risk of specific autoimmune diseases in relation to in utero diethylstilbestrol exposure, although some studies suggest an increased rate of respiratory tract infections, other infectious diseases, or allergies (Noller et al., 1988; Wingard & Turiel, 1988; Vingerhoets et al., 1998). However, in a follow-up study of the children born as part of a randomized clinical trial that had been conducted in the 1950s, there was little difference in the rates of reported symptoms or specific diagnoses of infectious, allergic, or autoimmune conditions in diethylstilbestrol-exposed individuals (253 sons and 296 daughters) compared with the controls (241 sons, 246 daughters) (Baird et al., 1996). Even with this sample size, however, the statistical power to assess the risk of specific autoimmune diseases was very limited.

8.11.8.3 Conclusion

Studies performed in laboratory animals demonstrate numerous immune alterations following exposure to diethylstilbestrol, notably thymus toxicity and alterations in thymus-dependent immunity, that appear mediated by estrogen receptor-induced alteration of thymic hormones in thymic epithelial cells. However, the immune effects of diethylstilbestrol depend largely on the age of the animals at treatment, dose of diethylstilbestrol, and sex. Immune effects following in utero exposure can persist for the lifetime of the animal. Aged animals appear especially sensitive. Recent studies also indicate a potential role of diethylstilbestrol in autoimmunity, as demonstrated in mice, including a study in a murine model for systemic lupus erythematosus. Also, studies in humans indicate that individuals exposed prenatally to diethylstilbestrol do not exhibit severe defects in basic immune function, but their tendency to develop autoimmune disease and other diseases associated with defects in immune regulation is increased. This warrants continuing surveillance of humans exposed in utero to diethylstilbestrol for diseases related to immune dysregulation.

8.12 Silicones

8.12.1 Introduction

In the early 1990s, serious concern was raised about health risks associated with silicone breast implants, both in the scientific literature and in the lay press. The concern was especially focused on systemic adverse effects resulting from the potential immune stimulation and interaction with silicones, resulting in some form of autoresponse eventually leading to the fulmination of autoimmune connective tissue diseases. For silicone-related complaints, several terms were used, including, among others, "undifferentiated connective tissue disease", "human adjuvant disease", "silicone poisoning", "siliconosis", and "(silicone) associated connective tissue disease". Evidence for an association between silicone breast implants and such a syndrome is lacking, however (Noone, 1997; Todhunter & Farrow, 1998).

The right use of the terminology for silicones is important in order to avoid misunderstanding with regard to the chemical characteristics of silicones. Silicon, silicones, and silica sound very similar, but are different entities (Williams, 1996). Silicon is the tetravalent element that has strong affinity to oxygen. The basis for naturally occurring and synthetic silicon-based product is the silicon–oxygen bond, which is referred to as siloxane. Polymers with repeating siloxane units, the silicon–oxygen couplet, are called polysiloxane or silicone. Addition of organic groups gives polydimethylsiloxane, which is a liquid when it forms linear chains (silicone fluids or silicone oils). Cross-linking results in the formation of so-called silicone gels (low level of cross-linking) or silicone elastomers (high level of cross-linking). Silica is the silicon dioxide, which can exist in crystalline (quartz) or amorphous form.

Silicone breast implants consist of an elastomeric outer shell blended with amorphous silica for reinforcement and silicone gel as filler. Also, for saline implants or hydrogel implants, the outer shell is a silicone elastomer. Thus, even when an implant has a non-silicone filling, there is exposure to the silicone elastomeric shell. Silicone is considered to be a biologically inert material. However, residues and contaminants may be present in the silicone gel that can migrate from the implant. Such low molecular mass species and small cross-linked molecules as intermediates of the production process can easily migrate through the elastomeric silicone shell, as there is a high similarity in chemical composition between the residues and the silicone shell. This phenomenon of gel bleeding is not uncommon for silicone breast implants and cannot be completely avoided, as these low molecular weight residues are extremely difficult to remove (Williams, 1996). In addition, residues of catalysts, such as platinum, may leak from the implants (Lykissa et al., 1997; Flassbeck et al., 2003; Maharaj, 2004). Also, local adverse effects and trauma resulting in implant rupture leading to massive exposure to the content of the implant (silicone gel) will remain a potential hazard for breast implant recipients.

8.12.2 Silicone breast implants and systemic disease

There have been case-reports of a confirmed diagnosis of systemic sclerosis, rheumatoid arthritis, or systemic lupus erythematosus in patients with silicone breast implants (Silverstein et al., 1992; Sanchez-Guerrero et al., 1994; Cuellar et al., 1995; Field & Bridges, 1996). However, no association between silicone breast implants and connective tissue disease has been seen in more than

10 large epidemiological studies (Gabriel et al., 1994; Sanchez-Guerrero et al., 1995; Hennekens et al., 1996; Hochberg et al., 1996; Silverman et al., 1996; Friis et al., 1997; Edworthy et al., 1998; Miller et al., 1998; Nyren et al., 1998; Brown et al., 2001; Fryzek et al., 2001; Kjoller et al., 2001; Gaubitz et al., 2002) conducted in the past 10 years. For women with extracapsular silicone from ruptured silicone breast implants, an association was observed for fibromyalgia in one study (Brown et al., 2001), but this was not observed in a subsequent study (Holmich et al., 2003). Systematic reviews of the scientific literature (Perkins et al., 1995; Hochberg & Perlmutter, 1996; Noone, 1997; Gerszten, 1999; Janowsky et al., 2000; Brown, 2002) and a court-appointed national science panel (Tugwell et al., 2001) conclude that there is ample evidence for the *lack* of a relation between the presence of a silicone breast implant and systemic disease.

Besides antisilicone antibodies, the presence of antipolymer antibodies has also been claimed in silicone breast implant recipients (Tenenbaum et al., 1997a) and fibromyalgia patients (Wilson et al., 1999b). There has been criticism of the methodology employed by Tenenbaum et al. (1997a) (Angell, 1997; Edlavitch, 1997; Everson & Blackburn, 1997; Korn, 1997). The chemical structure of the polymerized polyacrylamide used as antigen in the antipolymer antibodies assay is unrelated to that of silicone. No evidence has been put forward for the antigen-specific nature of the immunoglobulin binding, and a possible cross-reactivity between silicones and acrylamide was explained by structural similarity for the low molecular weight fractions (Tenenbaum et al., 1997b). So, the antigen specificity of the immunoglobulin binding in the antipolymer antibodies assay in terms of "antipolymer antibody" remains a question. The prevalence of the antipolymer antibodies was reported to be highest in silicone breast implant recipients and fibromyalgia patients with severe symptoms (Tenenbaum et al., 1997b; Wilson et al., 1999b). Although a diagnosis cannot be made on the basis of the presence of these antipolymer antibodies alone, the value of such an assay would be the objectivity of a laboratory test. However, in two independent studies, the results of Tenenbaum et al. (1997a) could not be confirmed (De Jong et al., 2002, 2004). In another study, a weak positive association was observed for antipolymer antibodies and fibromyalgia (Jensen et al., 2004). In view of the rather long exposure time to silicone breast implants in this particular study (more than 15 years), it was concluded that long-term exposure to silicones did not result in antipolymer antibody formation. Recently, autoantibodies were described against proteins attached to a silicone ventricular-peritoneal shunt (VandeVord et al., 2004). A high proportion of these patients were also positive in the antipolymer antibodies assay, with highest antibody levels in patients with infection-associated malfunction. The antibody binding to the antipolymer antibodies test polymer was found to be specific for partially polymerized polyacrylamide (VandeVord et al., 2004). For both the autoantibody responses to the silicone-adherent proteins and the antipolymer antibodies responses, the clinical significance is unknown and remains to be determined.

Antinuclear antibodies were demonstrated in women with silicone breast implants, although no association with disease status was noted (Constant et al., 2000; De Jong et al., 2002; Gaubitz et al., 2002). In women both with and without complaints, antinuclear antibodies were described, with women with silicone breast implants showing a higher proportion of positives compared with normal non-silicone breast implant controls. In another study, antinuclear antibodies in women with silicone breast implants were comparable to those in healthy control women (Karlson et al., 1999). Fibromyalgia patients without silicone breast implants showed positivity similar to that of the silicone breast implant recipients (Bridges et al., 1996). In symptomatic women with silicone breast implants, an increase in various types of autoantibodies was observed (Zandman-Goddard et al., 1999). In general, no clear association of the presence of various antibodies with either the presence of a silicone breast implant or disease could be established.

8.12.3 Conclusion

In conclusion, although silicones may be chemically inert, as for all implants, there is a host response against silicone implants. Silicone itself does not induce autoimmune disease in the animal models investigated, although in one animal model it enhanced the induction of disease by the eliciting antigen/adjuvant combination. Large-scale epidemiological studies did not reveal a role for silicone in autoimmune diseases or autoimmune-like syndromes in women with (a history of) silicone breast implants.

9. NON-CHEMICAL FACTORS IN AUTOIMMUNITY

In this chapter are described factors that could induce or influence autoimmune outcomes, as well as factors that have been suspected of being associated with autoimmune phenomena.

9.1 Infections: cause of autoimmunity, and immune programming

Almost all autoimmune disorders have had an infectious agent raised as a possible etiological agent. The topic is extensively reviewed in Shoenfeld & Rose (2004). Animal models suggest that both genetic and environmental factors such as infections are important in co-morbidity; of particular interest is the way in which environmental factors can modify genetic susceptibility. NOD mice develop thyroiditis and sialoadenitis in addition to autoimmune diabetes (Skarstein et al., 1995). This expression of autoimmune disorders is modified by the degree of microbial contamination of the environment (Rossini et al., 1995) and by early life exposure to filarial worms (Imai et al., 2001). In both cases, early immune stimulation leads to lower incidence of diabetes, showing how genetic susceptibility to multiple autoimmune disorders may be disguised by environmental factors. Infections are also important as a secondary feature of autoimmune diseases themselves; thus, diabetes mellitus type 1 leads to markedly increased susceptibility to infection.

There are autoimmune diseases in which infection clearly plays the key role and others where the evidence is less certain. Examples are given below, and Table 14 illustrates the range of autoimmune diseases with a putative infectious etiology.

Table 14. Infections associated with autoimmune diseases

Autoimmune disease	Associated infections
Antiphospholipid syndrome	Pneumonia, urinary tract infection, hepatitis C virus, human immunodeficiency virus, cytomegalovirus
Bechcet syndrome	Herpes simplex virus, streptococci
Chagas disease	*Trypanosoma cruzi*

Table 14 (Contd)

Autoimmune disease	Associated infections
Diabetes mellitus type 1	Coxsackie virus, enteroviruses, cytomegalovirus
Gastric autoimmunity	Helicobacter pylori
Guillain-Barré syndrome	Campylobacter jejuni, Haemophilus influenzae, cytomegalovirus
Idiopathic thrombocytopenic purpura	Herpes simplex virus, hepatitis C virus, varicella zoster virus, Epstein-Barr virus, cytomegalovirus, Helicobacter pylori
Inflammatory bowel disease	Clostridium difficile, Mycobacterium paratuberculosis, measles virus
Liver disease (primary biliary cirrhosis, autoimmune hepatitis, primary sclerosing cholangitis)	Hepatitis C virus, hepatitis D virus, herpes simplex virus, enteric bacteria
Myocarditis	Coxsackie virus
Multiple sclerosis	Herpes virus type 6, measles, rubella, paramyxovirus, coronavirus, varicella zoster virus, mumps, retrovirus
Paediatric autoimmune neuropsychiatric disorders	Streptococcus
Pemphigus	Herpes simplex virus, human herpes virus-8, Epstein-Barr virus, human immunodeficiency virus, cytomegalovirus
Polymyositis/ dermatomyositis	Coxsackie virus, parvovirus, enterovirus, human T-lymphotropic virus, human immunodeficiency virus, Toxoplasma, Borrelia
Reiter syndrome	Shigella, Chlamydia
Rheumatic fever	Streptococcus
Systemic lupus erythematosus	Epstein-Barr virus
Systemic sclerosis	Parvovirus B19, cytomegalovirus, Epstein-Barr virus, endogenous retrovirus, Helicobacter pylori
Thyroid disease	Yersinia enterocolitica, enteroviruses, retroviruses
Vasculitis	Hepatitis B virus, hepatitis C virus, Staphyloccocus aureus, parvovirus B19

9.1.1 Streptococcus and rheumatic fever

Rheumatic fever classically follows pharyngeal infection with a few specific M serotypes of group A streptococcus. While the diagnosis of rheumatic fever may be problematic, since there is no single pathognomic feature, the use of standardized criteria such as the Jones criteria has permitted extensive epidemiological description. The disease has been in decline for over 100 years, with an accelerated decline seen since the availability of antibiotics. However, it continues to be a feature of communities that suffer from poverty, and specifically some of Polynesian ancestry. The disease is clearly associated temporally with pharyngeal infection, and epidemics are seen from time to time. Yet the organism has rarely been isolated from the affected tissues. A number of strands of evidence suggest that the mechanism is in fact autoimmune:

1. Patients with rheumatic fever have heart-reactive antibodies in their sera. In addition, these antibodies are at higher titre than in people with streptococcal infection and no rheumatic fever. In addition, they persist for up to three years following an acute attack — the period of time at which patients are at risk of recurrence. A rise in antibodies is seen at the time of second attacks when these are associated with endocarditis.

2. Patients also have antibodies to myosin, which cross-react with the M protein of the streptococcus.

3. In those patients who develop chorea, the typical neurological complication of rheumatic fever, antibodies against the caudate nucleus of the central nervous system are present. These antibodies correlate with clinical disease activity.

In addition to these antibody patterns, both lymphocytes and macrophages aggregate at the site of tissue damage in the heart.

The weight of this evidence strongly suggests that rheumatic fever, and subsequent rheumatic heart disease, is an autoimmune disorder triggered by cross-reactive proteins in particular strains of group A streptococci.

9.1.2 Hepatitis C virus

The hepatitis C virus, which is predominantly transmitted by contaminated needles and blood products, leads to persistent infection in >80% of those infected. Those persistently infected have been found to have a high prevalence of autoantibodies, antinuclear antibody and rheumatoid factor being those most commonly detected. The exact prevalence of these varies from series to series — for example, the prevalence of antinuclear antibodies has been reported to be in the range of 4–41% of patients with hepatitis C. This variation is most probably dependent on the variability in methods used for their detection. Nevertheless, it is well above the range seen in healthy individuals (2–3%). One intriguing aspect of this association is that it appears to vary geographically; a recent study found a gradient of prevalence in antinuclear antibodies among patients infected with hepatitis C virus, with a higher prevalence in southern Europe than in northern Europe (Yee et al., 2004).

Autoimmune disease may be associated with these antibodies. Vasculitis is a well recognized complication of persistent hepatitis C infection and is associated with cryoglobulinaemia. The presence of anticardiolipin antibodies in association with clinical thrombosis has been reported in these patients. The true incidence of these events has not been determined. Glomerulonephritis has a well described association with hepatitis C virus. These patients frequently have hypocomplementaemia and circulating cryoglobulins. More controversial is a putative association with Sjögren syndrome, with some authors claiming that 10–20% of patients may be affected and others refuting this. Anti-Ro and anti-La antibodies do not appear to be markedly increased in subjects infected with hepatitis C virus, but there is a suggestion that sialoadenitis, occasionally with sicca symptoms, does occur at increased frequency. Similarly, there are discrepant reports concerning the association between infection with hepatitis C virus and the occurrence of thyroid disease, although it is clear that autoimmune thyroid disease is associated with the IFN-α therapy that many of these patients receive.

In summary, autoantibodies are clearly increased in subjects with persistent hepatitis C virus infection. The true incidence of autoimmune diseases in comparison with an appropriate control group is yet to be determined, although there is good evidence to suggest that some associations do exist.

9.1.3 Epstein-Barr virus

There has been considerable interest in the role of Epstein-Barr virus in the etiology of several autoimmune diseases, particularly systemic lupus erythematosus and multiple sclerosis. Epstein-Barr virus is a common infection. Most people (90% or more) are infected, without symptoms or with only mild, nonspecific symptoms, during childhood. When people are exposed as teenagers or as adults, however, infection may result in mononucleosis. Of importance with respect to autoimmune diseases, Epstein-Barr virus infects B cells and results in a latent infection. A close similarity between a peptide sequence in the Epstein-Barr nuclear antigen-1 and a sequence in the Sm autoantigen, one of the autoantibodies seen in systemic lupus erythematosus, has been reported (Sabbatini et al., 1993). In addition, several epidemiological studies have demonstrated strong associations between exposure to Epstein-Barr virus, as demonstrated by virus-specific IgG or IgA antibodies, and risk of systemic lupus erythematosus in children (James et al., 1997) and adults (James et al., 2001; Parks et al., 2005).

With respect to multiple sclerosis, Martyn et al. (1993) showed that there was a markedly elevated risk of multiple sclerosis among patients who both were positive for Epstein-Barr infection and reported acute glandular fever in adolescence. A strong association between Epstein-Barr exposure, as determined serologically, and risk of multiple sclerosis was reported in a review of eight case–control studies (Ascherio & Munch, 2000), with a summary odds ratio of 13.5 (95% confidence interval: 6.3–31.4). This association has also been examined in prospective studies in the Nurses Health Study cohort (Ascherio et al., 2001) and in using the sera repository of the United States armed services, with an increasing risk seen with increasing antibody titres (Levin et al., 2005).

9.1.4 Other infections

Most hypotheses relating infection to autoimmunity have assumed that infection has a direct causal role. However, an alternative is that infection prepares the ground for the seed that is the actual cause of disease. Infections are known to be critical to current immune responsiveness. Human immunodeficiency virus (HIV) is an obvious example, but measles virus, Epstein-Barr virus, and many others are known to modify the immune response both in the short term and over longer periods. Infections also appear to influence the immune system qualitatively; the strong epidemiological evidence for a shift in Th1/Th2 balance related to early life infection is now receiving direct biological support from the measurement of cytokines (von Hertzen, 2000), although the exact mechanisms and influences that programme the immune system need to be clarified (Hall et al., 2002), as do relationships between programming and cumulative risks. One method for examining the role of early life programming in autoimmunity is co-morbidity studies. Here there is controversy; some authors (Tremlett et al., 2002) claim an inverse relationship between allergic and autoimmune disorders at the individual level, whereas others find no relationship (Sheikh et al., 2003).

Multiple sclerosis is perhaps the autoimmune disorder par excellence that has been purported to result from an infection. It has a striking age incidence curve, beginning in the late teens, rising to a peak in the early 30s, and then falling to virtually zero by middle age. It has been proposed that this represents a shift of the age incidence curve of childhood infections into adult life — i.e. that the disease is a result of a common childhood infection in a susceptible individual with long latency. The list of agents that have been proposed at one time or another is long, including human herpes virus type 6, measles virus, rabies virus, paramyxovirus, coronavirus, varicella zoster virus, rubella virus, mumps virus, and retroviruses (Murray, 2002). Even bacteria have been proposed, including *Chlamydia pneumoniae* and *Borrelia burgdorferi*.

9.1.5 Absence of infections: the hygiene hypothesis

Concomitant with the increasing incidence of immune disorders over the past 50 years has been a decrease in the incidence of infectious diseases and a shift to a later age of acquisition (Bach, 2002). In 1989, the "hygiene hypothesis" was proposed (Strachan, 1989). It asserted that a downshift in early life infection may contribute to the increase in hayfever over time. The initial interpretation of the hygiene hypothesis was a lack of shift from a perinatal Th2 immune profile to a Th1 immune profile, due to inadequate exposure to antigenic stimulation in a hygienic environment (missing immune deviation) (Romagnani, 2004).

However, the increasing incidence over time of Th1-related disorders (diabetes mellitus type 1, Crohn disease, multiple sclerosis) has also been suggested to be more likely to be due to an alternative possible mechanism — reduced immune suppression and effect on regulatory T cells (Tedeschi & Airaghi, 2001).

If the protective effect of infection depended on the type of exposure and this varied across populations, a differing role for infection could explain the differential validity of the hygiene hypothesis across diseases and countries (Bach, 2005).

In summary, it is highly likely that infection plays a role in many autoimmune disorders, although the agent and mechanism may differ from one to another. Chemical agents may play an important role in interacting with infections — an area that has hardly been studied. Whether or not this is so, infection must be controlled in any epidemiological study, since it is a potential confounding factor in any association between chemical agents and autoimmune diseases.

9.2 Vaccine-related factors

9.2.1 Vaccines themselves

While there is considerable theoretical basis for vaccination triggering autoimmune phenomena — in many of the same ways as natural infection — the main interest in this area has arisen from public concern (Offit & Hackett, 2003). There is a general concern regarding the relationship between autoimmune diseases and vaccination, but large-scale studies have been performed on only two diseases — multiple sclerosis and diabetes mellitus type 1.

The concern with multiple sclerosis arose with hepatitis B vaccination in France. The original concern came from a case-series in a specialist neurological centre. Subsequently, case–control studies and cohort studies, particularly utilizing computerized prescription databases, failed to demonstrate any association. The evidence was reviewed at a meeting at WHO, and the conclusion reached was that there was no association (Hall et al., 1999).

The association between vaccination and diabetes mellitus type 1 arose from the observation that diabetes mellitus type 1 is rising, and this is associated with increasing use of vaccination in the general population. Some small studies suggested a link. However, a recent major Danish record linkage study conclusively showed no relationship between the two (Hviid et al., 2004).

Arthritis has been described following administration of hepatitis B, rubella, mumps and measles, influenza, diphtheria–pertussis–tetanus, and typhoid vaccine. These are rare occurrences, and causality is difficult to establish. However, it does appear that rubella vaccination may, in genetically susceptible individuals, lead rarely to an arthropathy.

Guillain-Barré syndrome was particularly associated with "swine flu" vaccine in 1976. It has rarely been associated with other vaccines — tetanus toxoid, BCG, rabies, smallpox, mumps, rubella, hepatitis B, diphtheria, and polio (Wraith et al., 2003).

9.2.2 Vaccine additives

Mercury is clearly immunomodulatory in sufficient doses. Since it is a constituent part of thimerosal, which is used as a preservative in killed vaccines, concern has been raised with regard to its role in immune-mediated diseases and autism (Clarkson, 2002). Thimerosal is primarily present in the tissues as ethylmercury. This compound has caused illness and several deaths due to erroneous handling when used as a disinfectant or as a preservative in medical preparations. Madsen et al. (2003) found no correlation between thimerosal-containing vaccines and autism in a study with 956 Danish children. The authors also reported that the discontinuation of thimerosal-containing vaccines in Denmark in 1992 was followed by an increase in the incidence of autism. In contrast, epidemiological evidence, based upon tens of millions of doses of vaccine administered in the United States, that associates increasing thimerosal from vaccines with neurodevelopmental disorders was reported by Geier & Geier (2003). An analysis of the Vaccine Adverse Events Reporting System database showed statistical increases in the incidence rate of autism, mental retardation, and speech disorders with the use of thimerosal-containing diphtheria, tetanus, and acellular pertussis vaccines in comparison with thimerosal-free vaccines.

The ongoing debate on thimerosal in vaccines has revealed a lack of information on the toxicology of this compound, and conclusions were to a large extent arrived at by making an analogy with the toxicology of methylmercury (Stratton et al., 2001).

Alum is used as an adjuvant in several vaccines. It is a poor inducer of cell-mediated immunity, and there is no epidemiological evidence of it leading to autoimmunity. Recently, some concern has been raised in France in patients where aluminium hydroxide-induced persistent macrophagic myofasciitis is present. It has been hypothesized that the persistence of this lesion may be associated with a higher incidence of a syndrome with arthralgias, myalgias, and chronic fatigue (Gherardi et al., 2001; Gherardi & Authier, 2003). However, these observations are still controversial (Rivas et al., 2005).

Kuroda et al. (2004) reported autoimmunity induced by adjuvant hydrocarbon oil components of some human and veterinary vaccines. This study showed that an injection of certain adjuvant hydrocarbon oils (pristane, incomplete Freund's adjuvant, or squalene) induced lupus-related autoantibodies to nuclear ribonucleoproteins (nRNP)/Sm and Su in non-immune Balb/c mice.

9.3 Dietary factors

There is considerable interest in research on the influence of dietary factors on autoimmune diseases. This is a broad area that includes caloric intake, specific nutrients and foods, and dietary supplements. Coeliac disease is an example of an autoimmune disease with a clear dietary link — the immunological response to specific proteins in wheat, barley, and rye producing autoantibodies directed against tissue transglutaminase and mucosal damage in the small intestine. The role of iodine in autoimmune thyroid diseases is discussed in chapter 8 (section 8.10). The following summary of dietary factors focuses on experimental studies using animal models and human studies of the etiology and progression of multiple sclerosis, diabetes mellitus type 1, inflammatory bowel diseases, rheumatoid arthritis, and lupus. The basis for much of this research is the general immunomodulating effect of dietary components, particularly with respect to cytokine production and inflammation. Other effects are more relevant to specific diseases (e.g.

demyelination, platelet aggregation). In general, data from studies in humans are more limited and less consistent than the data from animal studies.

9.3.1 Caloric restriction and leptin

The hormone leptin is produced by adipocytes and is involved in the regulation of food intake and obesity. Periods of caloric restriction inhibit production of leptin. Fasting can improve symptoms in some patients with rheumatoid arthritis (possibly through an anti-inflammatory effect of fasting mediated through leptin), but the effects are not sustained when the fasting period is over (Muller et al., 2001). In mouse models of multiple sclerosis (experimental autoimmune encephalomyelitis) and diabetes mellitus type 1, leptin secretion was closely linked to disease onset (Matarese et al., 2002; Sanna et al., 2003). Recent studies report an effect of leptin on T cell stimulation and production of proinflammatory cytokines (Sanchez-Margalet et al., 2003). Caloric restriction in lupus mouse models inhibits the disease process and prolongs survival (Leiba et al., 2001).

9.3.2 Dietary fat and fatty acid content

The type and amount of fat in foods are important aspects of nutrition, with implications for atherosclerosis, cardiovascular disease, and obesity, as well as for immune-mediated diseases. The fatty acid composition of foods is determined by the length of the carbon chain and the number and location of double bonds. The "n-3" or "omega-3" fatty acids are those with one or more double bonds, the first of which is located at the third carbon from the omega end of the carbon chain. The essential fatty acids are those that cannot be synthesized and so are available only from foods or supplements. Animal fats are a source of arachidonic acid (an omega-6 fatty acid), and fish is a source of the omega-3 fatty acids ecoisapentaenoic acid (EPA) and docosahexaenoic acid (DHA). EPA can also be converted from α-linoleic acid, found in green leafy vegetables, flaxseed, and canola oils. Arachidonic acid and EPA are the specific fatty acid precursors for the synthesis of specific prostaglandins (PGE) and leukotrienes (LTE), respectively. The relative balance of different prostaglandins and leukotrienes affects the inflammatory response. Arachidonic acid is converted to PGE_2 and LTE_4, which are proinflammatory, stimulating NK cell activity and proinflammatory cytokines (e.g. IL-1 and TNF-α). EPA is converted to the more anti-inflammatory compounds PGE_2 and LTE_5 (Calder, 1997; Simopoulos, 2002).

Because of the potential effects on inflammation and immune-mediated function, there has been considerable interest in the potential therapeutic role of omega-3 fatty acids in autoimmune disease. Most studies in humans have been on patients with rheumatoid arthritis. The randomized clinical trials tend to be relatively small, but there is some evidence of improvement in terms of reduced joint count and morning stiffness in trials of fish oil supplementation (Fortin et al., 1995). There have also been some small trials ($n < 30$) of omega-3 supplementation in patients with systemic lupus erythematosus, but these studies were conducted before the adoption of standardized measures of disease activity and damage. In general, some improvements in lipid profiles and inflammatory measures have been seen, but there are mixed results with respect to improvements in clinical status (Leiba et al., 2001). In a large observational (non-randomized) study in Japan, there was no association between intake of total fat, type of fat, or omega-3 fatty acids and subsequent disease activity among 216 lupus patients (Minami et al., 2003). In ulcerative colitis and Crohn disease, trials of omega-3 (fish oil) supplements have reported improvements in terms of decreased steroid dosage, decreased disease activity, prolonged periods of remission, and increased weight gain, but there are inconsistencies between observed effects among studies, and long-term benefits have been difficult to demonstrate (Belluzzi, 2002).

Relatively few studies have been conducted examining fats and fatty acid intake in relation to risk of developing specific autoimmune diseases. In a recent analysis of risk of multiple sclerosis in two large cohorts of women, no association was seen with total fat, monounsaturated fat, or total n-6 or total n-3 polyunsaturated fats (Zhang et al., 2000). There is some suggestion from case–control studies of a protective effect of fish or omega-3 fatty acids on risk of developing rheumatoid arthritis (Pattison et al., 2004), but there are currently no prospective studies analysing dietary intake of fats in relation to the risk of developing rheumatoid arthritis, systemic lupus erythematosus, or inflammatory bowel diseases.

9.3.3 Antioxidants

The influence of antioxidants (e.g. vitamin E or α-tocopherol, vitamin C or ascorbic acid, and carotenoids, including β-carotene and lycopene) on autoimmune diseases has not been extensively studied. There is some evidence that damage induced by reactive oxygen species contributes to the destruction of pancreatic beta cells, brain tissue, and joints seen in diabetes mellitus type 1, multiple sclerosis, and rheumatoid arthritis, respectively. However, there are few prospective studies of antioxidant intake and risk of autoimmune diseases. Although there is some evidence of a reduced risk of rheumatoid arthritis and lupus with higher intake or serum levels of antioxidants, there are inconsistent findings with respect to which antioxidants or foods are involved (Comstock et al., 1997; Knekt et al., 2000; Cerhan et al., 2003). Only one prospective study of antioxidants and risk of multiple sclerosis is available, and that study reported no association with intakes of vitamin C, vitamin E, or carotenoids (Zhang et al., 2001).

9.3.4 Vitamin D

Vitamin D can be obtained from some foods, but its major source is through the action of ultraviolet radiation, which converts 7-dehydrocholesterol to cholecalciferol in the skin. Hydroxylation of this compound in the liver produces 25-hydroxycholecalciferol, which is then converted in the kidney to 1,25-hydroxycholecalciferol, the active form of vitamin D. Vitamin D plays a major role in promoting absorption of calcium and maintaining bone mineralization. Recently, research has focused on immunosuppressive effects of vitamin D. The vitamin D receptor has been detected in lymphocytes and the thymus, and vitamin D plays a role in T cell-mediated immune response (Deluca & Cantorna, 2001).

Most of the human studies of vitamin D and autoimmune diseases have focused on diabetes mellitus type 1 and multiple sclerosis. Higher risks of these diseases are generally seen at higher latitudes (e.g. farther north in the northern hemisphere and farther south in the southern hemisphere), which would be areas of relatively low exposure to ultraviolet radiation (Ponsonby et al., 2002). Case–control and prospective studies of maternal and child vitamin D intake have provided some evidence of a protective effect of vitamin D on risk of developing diabetes mellitus type 1

(Hypponen et al., 2001; Fronczak et al., 2003; Zella & DeLuca, 2003). Prospective studies have also reported a reduced risk of multiple sclerosis (Munger et al., 2004) and rheumatoid arthritis (Merlino et al., 2004) in women with higher intakes of vitamin D. The relative contribution of foods and supplements to the protective effects seen in these studies is not clear.

In murine models of experimental autoimmune encephalomyelitis (multiple sclerosis), diabetes mellitus type 1, and inflammatory bowel disease, treatment with 1,25-hydroxycholecalciferol (in conjunction with adequate calcium intake) has been shown to inhibit the development of disease (Froicu et al., 2003; Hypponen, 2004; Van Amerongen et al., 2004). In lupus mouse strains, however, a more complex situation is seen, with some evidence of worsening of disease (particularly with respect to measures of renal damage) with 1,25-hydroxycholecalciferol treatment (Vaisberg et al., 2000).

9.3.5 L-Tryptophan and eosinophilia myalgia syndrome

Eosinophilia myalgia syndrome is a multisystemic, autoimmune disease that was first diagnosed in 1989 and was associated with the use of contaminated L-tryptophan (Hertzman et al., 1990). An essential amino acid and serotonin precursor, L-tryptophan is used to treat depression, premenstrual syndrome, and insomnia. In nine months, 1658 people were diagnosed with the disease in the United States, Germany, and Belgium (Swygert et al., 1990; Andre et al., 1991; Carr et al., 1994). A product recall dramatically reduced the number of new cases reported, although approximately 3% of patients with eosinophilia myalgia syndrome did not use L-tryptophan (Swygert et al., 1990). Rare non-L-tryptophan-associated cases continue to be reported (Margolin, 2003). Although eosinophilia myalgia syndrome was most frequently reported in women (84%), non-Hispanic whites (97%), and residents of western states in the United States (Swygert et al., 1990), statistical analysis showed no correlation with duration of L-tryptophan intake, concurrent medications (Kamb et al., 1992; Carr et al., 1994; Kaufman & Krupp, 1995), sex, or race, since the majority of people using these products are female (60%) and white (80%). There have been associations with dose, age of the patient (average 48 years), and a single supplier that had made changes in the manufacturing process preceding the epidemic (Swygert et al., 1990; Kamb et al.,

1992; Das et al., 2004). The hallmark manifestations of eosinophilia myalgia syndrome are profound eosinophilia (>1000 cells/mm^3) and debilitating myalgia (Swygert et al., 1990); other symptoms include serum antinuclear antibodies targeting lamin C and three unique disease-specific proteins (Kaufman et al., 1991, 1995; Varga et al., 1992), fasciitis, arthralgia, peripheral neuropathy, paresthesias, oedema, scleroderma, pruritic rash, dyspnoea, myopathy, fatigue, muscle cramps, cognitive impairment, increased aldolase levels, and increased liver enzyme levels (Swygert et al., 1990; Hertzman et al., 1995; Kaufman & Krupp, 1995).

Gene expression and protein synthesis of TGFβ1, fibronectin, type IV collagen (Peltonen et al., 1991), and fibroblast type I collagen (Varga et al., 1993; Hitraya et al., 1997) were increased in human tissues and cells affected by eosinophilia myalgia syndrome, compared with controls. These reports suggest that the cytokine TGFβ1, upregulation of collagen genes, and subsequent accumulation of collagen may play a role in the development of connective tissue alterations, especially diffuse fasciitis and cutaneous fibrosis (Peltonen et al., 1991; Varga et al., 1993). Muscle and fascia from patients with eosinophilia myalgia syndrome revealed an inflammatory exudate composed primarily of activated T cells and macrophages at perimysial, endomysial, perivascular, and fascial sites. CD8$^+$ cells were the dominant T cell subpopulation, and MHC class I antigen complex expression was increased on inflammatory and endothelial cells and muscle fibres, indicating a cell-mediated immune response targeting connective tissue. Emslie-Smith et al. (1991) proposed that a contaminant of L-tryptophan haptenates a connective tissue component, forming a stable, immunogenic complex and initiating an autoimmune response that is augmented by the local release of inflammatory cytokines from activated cells; however, the specific cellular target is not yet known.

A higher frequency of the rare variant allele of the CYP2D6 gene, resulting in the poor metabolizer genotype, and the absence of activity in the corresponding enzyme among cases of eosinophilia myalgia syndrome ($n = 27$) indicate that altered xenobiotic metabolism may play a role in the pathogenesis of eosinophilia myalgia syndrome (Flockhart et al., 1994). Animal models also suggest a genetic component to eosinophilia myalgia syndrome susceptibility; autoimmune-prone NZBWF1 mice and Lewis rats have a lower hepatic nuclei binding affinity for case-associated L-tryptophan compared with Swiss mice and Sprague-Dawley rats, respectively (Sidransky & Verney, 1994, 1997).

Two contaminants identified in the tryptophan preparations associated with eosinophilia myalgia syndrome, 1,1'-ethylidene-bis[L-tryptophan] (EBT) and 3-(phenylamino)-L-alanine (PAA), have been the focus of further investigation into the etiologic agent (Mayeno et al., 1992; Hill et al., 1993; Simat et al., 1999; Barth et al., 2001). EBT stimulated gene expression and synthesis of type I collagen in cultured human fibroblasts in a dose-dependent manner, suggesting that EBT may be involved in the fibrosis of eosinophilia myalgia syndrome (Takagi et al., 1995; Zangrilli et al., 1995). In C57BL/6 mice, EBT induced inflammation, fibrosis, increased mast cell proliferation, and degranulation; enhanced gene expression for types I, III, and IV collagen and TGFβ1; and altered metabolism of L-tryptophan by the kynurenine pathway in dermal and subcutaneous tissue (Silver et al., 1994; Suzuki et al., 1996). PAA is chemically similar to PAP, one of the candidate etiologic agents for toxic oil syndrome. In vitro conversion of PAA to PAP and of PAP to PAA has been demonstrated (Mayeno et al., 1995; Schurz et al., 1997), suggesting a possible mechanistic connection between toxic oil syndrome and eosinophilia myalgia syndrome. The true etiologic agent of eosinophilia myalgia syndrome and the mechanism of action remain elusive; however, the prevailing theories support a combination of genetic susceptibility, haptenation of self-proteins by L-tryptophan contaminants and subsequent activation of autoreactive T cells, and a cell-mediated immune response targeting connective tissue.

10. ANIMAL MODELS TO ASSESS CHEMICAL-INDUCED AUTOIMMUNITY

10.1 Introduction

The number of animal models of autoimmunity is extensive. These models represent a variety of systemic and organ-specific diseases and are mostly used to explore etiology and therapeutic possibilities for certain autoimmune diseases. It is important to point out that the nutritional and microbial status of the animals can influence the outcome of the autoimmune diseases (see also chapter 9). Etiology in the various models can be based either on spontaneous, genetically predisposed development or on induction with specific antigens (mostly in combination with an adjuvant), infectious agents, or chemicals (Chernajovsky et al., 2000; Sakaguchi, 2000). Irrespectively of how the disease is induced, most models rely on inbred animals, indicating the importance of genetic background and in accordance with the idiosyncratic nature of many autoimmune diseases.

In the case of spontaneous autoimmune diseases, mice are most frequently used; with the advent of genetically modified mice, the number of genetically predisposed autoimmune models has increased enormously. For systemic lupus erythematosus, about 30 genetically modified mouse models have been described (Chan et al., 1999). New models have been designed using transgenics or gene invalidation techniques for type 1 (insulin-dependent) diabetes, multiple sclerosis, and arthritis (Goverman, 1999; Holmdahl et al., 1999; Wong et al., 1999; Chernajovsky et al., 2000). Modifications of the MHC class II genome are being used to design models of autoimmunity in mice (Taneja & David, 1999; Das et al., 2000; Boyton & Altmann, 2002) and in the rat (Taurog et al., 1999). These new models are primarily used to further study the pathogenesis of disease.

In contrast, chemical-induced autoimmune models are actually uncommon (Table 15). Based on the multifactorial and idiosyncratic nature of autoimmune diseases, it is not surprising that relatively few compounds have been shown to induce clinically apparent autoimmune or autoimmune-like allergic phenomena in animals. The route of exposure may be of significance in relation to interpretation and extrapolation of data from animal models to the development and status of human autoimmune diseases. However, it is important to note that routes of exposure used in many animal models (e.g. intraperitoneal, intramuscular, subcutaneous) may not be relevant or are artificial routes with respect to typical human exposure (primarily oral, but possibly dermal or inhalation, particularly in occupational settings — except for injected vaccines).

Table 15. Examples of chemicals shown to induce autoimmune phenomena in animals

Animal model	Chemical	Autoimmune outcome or marker of autoimmunity
Rat		
Brown Norway	Mercury(II) chloride	Immune complex glomerulonephritis
	Gold salts	Skin pathology; dermatitis
	D-Penicillamine	Polyclonal IgE
	Nevirapine	Autoantibodies (type IV collagen, antinuclear antibodies antiacetylcholine, antithyroglobulin antibodies)
	Hexachlorobenzene	Systemic inflammatory response with autoimmune symptoms
Lewis	Cyclosporin	Alopecia
		Graft versus host disease
Mouse		
Various strains with differences in sensitivity (see text)	Procainamide	Antinuclear antibodies
	D-Penicillamine	Antinucleolar antibodies
	Mercury(II) chloride	Splenomegaly
	Gold salts	Antifibrillarin antibody
	Hydralazine	Anti-insulin antibody
C57BL/Ks	Streptozotocin	Diabetes mellitus type 1
DBA/1 susceptible DBA/2 resistant	Pristane	Pristane-induced arthritis
Neonatal mouse	Cyclosporin	Multiorgan-type inflammation

Table 15 (Contd)

Animal model	Chemical	Autoimmune outcome or marker of autoimmunity
Dog		
Beagle	Procainamide	Antinuclear antibodies
Doberman	Sulfonamides	Multiple symptoms, including skin eruptions (urticaria) and blood dyscrasias
	Radiocontrast media	
	Etoposide	
Cat	6-Propylthiouracil	Systemic lupus erythematosus: antinuclear antibodies, Sm antigen lymphadenopathy, haemolytic anaemia
Chickens		
Obese strain	Iodine	Autoimmune thyroiditis
Monkey	L-Canavanine (alfalfa seeds)	Systemic lupus erythematosus
		Antinuclear antibodies

10.2 Rat models

10.2.1 The Brown Norway rat model

The Brown Norway rat has long been considered to be a valuable model (Donker et al., 1984; Balazs, 1987), as a number of chemicals have been shown to induce clinically manifested autoimmune-like disease in this particular strain of rats. This model has been used extensively in studies of mercury(II) chloride. D-Penicillamine (Tournade et al., 1990), gold salts (Tournade et al., 1991; Qasim et al., 1997), and hexachlorobenzene (Vos et al., 1979a; Michielsen et al., 1999a, 1999b; Ezendam et al., 2004a, 2004b) have been shown to induce clinical effects in the Brown Norway rat model. Captopril (Donker et al., 1984) and also felbamate (Popovic et al., 2004) were tested in Brown Norway rats as well, but effects were not seen with these exposures.

The autoimmune-related effects that have been observed in the Brown Norway rat model are only partly compound specific and include both local (glomerulonephritis, splenomegaly, skin rashes, inflammatory responses in lungs) and systemic effects (hyperimmunoglobulinaemia, in particular IgE, and increased levels of autoantibodies). Derangements in Brown Norway rats are accompanied by polyclonal lymphoproliferation (both T and B cells)

(Hirsch et al., 1982, 1986). However, it is not yet known if these effects are autoimmune mediated. Brown Norway rats are known as so-called Th2-prone animals (e.g. they are activated to produce high levels of IgE and to display many characteristics of type 2 immune response). This property and/or the underlying genetic trait may be responsible for the high susceptibility of this strain to chemical-induced autoimmune effects. This point is often discussed as a limitation of using this strain. However, as for disease-prone mouse strains, it can also be argued that the inherent susceptibility of this rat strain resembles the inherent susceptibility in human cases of chemical-induced autoimmune disorders.

10.2.1.1 Metals

Autoimmune-like phenomena in Brown Norway rats induced by mercury(II) chloride peak around day 10 after the last of five subcutaneous injections. After 20 days, immune alterations are mostly at control level, and the kidney effects (e.g. proteinuria) are clearly less than on day 10 (Aten et al., 1988). In addition, low-dose pretreatment of Brown Norway rats with mercury(II) chloride prevents development of adverse immunity (Szeto et al., 1999), and neonatal injection of mercury(II) chloride in Brown Norway rats renders them tolerant to mercury-induced (but not gold-induced) autoimmune phenomena (Field et al., 2000). These phenomena, transience of autoimmune effects as well as low-dose protection, are shown to be due at least in part to the development of regulatory immune cells. In the case of mercury(II) chloride, these cells have been identified as either IFN-γ-producing $CD8^+CD45RC$ high regulatory T cells (Pelletier et al., 1990; Mathieson et al., 1991; Szeto et al., 1999; Field et al., 2003) or $RT6.2^+$ T cells (Kosuda et al., 1994). In view of this, it is relevant to note that Lewis rats that produce predominantly $CD8^+$ regulatory T cells ("suppressor" T cells) in response to mercury(II) chloride are resistant to mercury-induced autoimmunity and instead display a polyclonal immunosuppressive response (Pelletier et al., 1987). Based on these differences in strain sensitivity, it is clear that susceptibility to mercury-induced autoimmune effects is dependent on MHC class II haplotype (Aten et al., 1991).

Gold salts also induce an autoimmune syndrome in the Brown Norway rat similar to that observed with mercury(II) chloride (and

D-penicillamine), with increased IgE levels and vasculitis (observed in the gut) (Balazs, 1987; Qasim et al., 1997).

10.2.1.2 D-Penicillamine

The Brown Norway rat has also been used to study the adverse immune response to D-penicillamine, with effects similar to those seen in some patients (Tournade et al., 1990). Recently, a series of studies have further explored D-penicillamine-induced autoimmunity in the Brown Norway rat, in particular with respect to immunoregulation (Masson & Uetrecht, 2004). Interestingly, only 60–80% of all treated Brown Norway rats develop the autoimmune disease; in addition, low-dose pretreatment with D-penicillamine has been shown to tolerize the animals to subsequent normally autoimmunogenic doses (Donker et al., 1984; Masson & Uetrecht, 2004). It appeared that the observed tolerance is mediated by immune cells, including T and non-T cells. This again illustrates that idiosyncracy also occurs in animals and moreover that these diseases are subject to regulatory mechanisms.

10.2.1.3 Hexachlorobenzene

The environmental pollutant hexachlorobenzene has also been studied in Brown Norway rats, as well as in Lewis, Wistar, and Sprague-Dawley rats (see section 8.3.2 on hexachlorobenzene). All of these rat strains displayed hexachlorobenzene-induced symptoms reminiscent of an autoimmune-like disease (splenomegaly, increased serum levels of autoantibodies, inflammatory responses in lungs and skin), with the Brown Norway rat the most sensitive (Michielsen et al., 1997). This strain independence indicates that hexachlorobenzene-induced pathology is probably less or not at all idiosyncratic. In addition, a clear role of T cells has not been found, although interference with T cell activation by cyclosporin prevented or delayed a number of T cell-dependent responses, such as levels of IgE and eosinophilia in the lung, and skin lesions (Ezendam et al., 2004a). Further analyses (e.g. adoptive transfer studies) did not reveal an initiating role of T cells. It is currently thought that hexachlorobenzene is probably a general inflammatory rather than an autoimmunogenic chemical (Ezendam et al., 2004b), predominantly activating macrophages and, only secondary to this, by some kind of adjuvant signal, also activating T cells.

10.2.2 Other rat models

Cyclosporin A is able to induce an autoimmune syndrome in Lewis rats, but only when these rats are subjected to lethal (8.5 Gy) X-irradiation and reconstituted with syngeneic or autologous bone marrow (Damoiseaux, 2002). About two weeks after cessation of cyclosporin treatment, which starts on the day of the bone marrow transplantation, the rats start to develop autoimmune disease. Acute symptoms of cyclosporin-induced autoimmunity are similar to those of graft versus host disease, with erythroderma, dermatitis, and alopecia. The chronic phase is characterized by progressive alopecia combined with scleroderma-like skin pathology. Cyclosporin-induced autoimmunity is clearly immune dependent and involves autoreactive T cells (specific for an MHC class II peptide named CLIP) and requires both an intact thymus and absence of regulatory T cells ($CD45RClowCD4^+$ phenotype) (Barendrecht et al., 2002). The effect of cyclosporin on the thymus has been the subject of many studies. Cyclosporin inhibits differentiation of $CD4^+CD8^+$ thymocytes, possibly by interference with activation-induced cell death (Shi et al., 1989). This probably is the cause of the increased release of autoreactive T cells (Kosugi et al., 1989). In line with this and with the protocol required to induce cyclosporin-induced autoimmunity in rat, neonatal administration of cyclosporin in mice also induces a multiorgan-type autoimmune disease (Sakaguchi & Sakaguchi, 1989).

10.3 Mouse models

A number of studies have been performed to induce systemic immunosensitization and autoimmunity (i.e. autoantibody formation or autoreactive T cells) in mice, and, again, occurrence of disease appears to be strain dependent. Robinson et al. (1986) compared in one study a large number of MHC-defined mouse strains with respect to induction of antinuclear autoantibodies by mercury(II) chloride (subcutaneously, detected after 0.5–2 months), gold salts (intramuscularly, detected after 1–5 months), and D-penicillamine (orally, detected after 4.5–5 months) and reported that A.SW mice were high responders to all three chemicals.

10.3.1 Metals

Subcutaneous administration of mercury(II) chloride (Mirtcheva et al., 1989; Kubicka-Muranyi et al., 1995, 1996) or intramuscular treatment with gold salts (Schuhmann et al., 1990) has been shown to induce antinuclear and antinucleolar autoantibodies from around four weeks of exposure, in particular in high-responding A.SW mice (MHC-H2s haplotype). Other H2s mice, such as B10s mice, are also susceptible, but congenic H2d mice (e.g. B10D2) or H2k mice (B10.BR) are resistant to mercury-induced autoimmune effects, indicating the importance of MHC haplotype (Mirtcheva et al., 1989). The response to mercury(II) chloride in A.SW mice is Th2 mediated, involving IL-4 production and increases in IgE and IgG1 levels (Ochel et al., 1991). Interestingly, both H2s and H2d mice responded to mercury(II) chloride exposure with an increase in the number of activated $CD4^+CD45R$ low-effector T cells (van Vliet et al., 1993), implying that the difference between these strains also involves immunoregulatory processes. Mercury(II) chloride given orally via the drinking-water also induced antinucleolar antibodies (IgG-class) in SJL/N (H2s) mice after 10 weeks (Hultman & Enestrom, 1992). Rowley & Monestier (2005) show autoimmune manifestations by mercury exposure in lupus-prone mice (NZB×NZW/F1).

10.3.2 Drugs

The potential to induce autoimmune phenomena in mice has been successfully identified for only a few drugs. D-Penicillamine has been shown to induce anti-ssDNA and anti-insulin antibodies in C57BL/Ks (H2d) and C3H/He (H2k) mice but not in Balb/c or C57BL/6 mice after subcutaneous exposure for four weeks (Brik et al., 1995). Also after oral treatment (for 7–8 months, in the drinking-water), D-penicillamine (and in the same study, also quinidine) induced an increase in autoantibodies in A.SW/Sn (H2s) mice (Monestier et al., 1994).

The antineoplastic drug streptozotocin is capable of inducing type 1 (insulin-dependent) diabetes when administered (intraperitoneally) at low doses on six consecutive days. Important to note is that a strong dependency on strain and/or sex has been observed, with male C57BL/Ks (H2d) mice most sensitive (Leiter, 1982; Herold et al., 1996). Streptozotocin appeared to elicit a typical Th1-

dependent type 1 response, including a strong activation of macrophages, IFN-γ-producing $CD4^+$ and $CD8^+$ T cells, and IgG2a antibodies (Albers et al., 1998; Nierkens et al., 2002).

Procainamide has been found to induce an increase in antinuclear antibodies in A/J mice after eight months of exposure via the drinking-water (Layland et al., 2004). This increase appeared mediated by $CD4^+CD25^-$ T cells and regulated by $CD4^+CD25^+$ regulatory T cells.

Diphenylhydantoin (via drinking-water for six months) was tested in genetically predisposed mice (C57BL/6-lpr/lpr strain) and found to depress levels of autoantibodies (Bloksma et al., 1994). In another study (Okada et al., 2001), a slight shift towards a Th2 response was demonstrated by showing an increase in the keyhole limpet haemocyanin (KLH)-induced production of IL-4 and IgE as measured by direct enzyme-linked immunosorbent assay (ELISA) in a four-week exposure study.

10.3.3 Pristane

Pristane (2,6,10,14-tetramethylpentadecane) is a mineral oil known to induce arthritis, also called pristane-induced arthritis, in an experimental disease model (Wooley & Whalen, 1991). Pristane-induced arthritis is MHC-haplotype dependent. DBA/1 mice, but not DBA/2 mice, are susceptible. The disease is accompanied by a broad spectrum of autoantibodies (rheumatoid factor, anticollagen, antibodies to heat shock protein). Pristane-induced arthritis is clearly immune dependent, since it is not observed in nu/nu mice and irradiated mice (Wooley & Whalen, 1991). $CD4^+$ T cells and polyclonal T cell activation are involved in the disease process (Wooley et al., 1998), and disease can be prevented by $CD4^+$ Th2 cells specific for 65-kilodalton heat shock protein (Beech et al., 1997).

Pristane-induced arthritis is also inducible in rat, with DA rats being susceptible and E3 rats being resistant (Wester et al., 2003). It is controlled by multiple genes, identified as pristane-induced arthritis (pia) loci (Olofsson et al., 2003).

10.4 Genetically predisposed animal models

Chemicals may exacerbate autoimmunity in genetically predisposed animals or in induced animal models (Kammuller et al., 1989a). The rationale behind using autoimmune-prone animal strains for the purpose of studying and predicting the autoimmunogenic potential of chemicals is that, apart from being probably very sensitive for adverse immune effects, exacerbation of disease is considered one of the possibilities by which chemicals may elicit autoimmune phenomena (Pollard et al., 1999). As mentioned also, the Brown Norway rat is a sensitive rat strain for Th2-dependent phenomena, as is the Lewis rat for cyclosporin-induced autoimmunity.

Examples of spontaneous models of autoimmune disease are the BB rat (Mordes et al., 1987; Prins et al., 1991) and the NOD mouse (McDevitt et al., 1996), which develop autoimmune pancreatitis and subsequently diabetes, or the NZB×NZW/F1 or MRL/lpr mouse (Pollard et al., 1999; Shaheen et al., 1999), which spontaneously develop systemic lupus erythematosus-like disease.

In induced models, a susceptible animal strain is immunized with a mixture of an adjuvant and an autoantigen isolated from the target organ. Examples are adjuvant arthritis in the Lewis strain rat (Pearson, 1956) and experimental allergic encephalomyelitis, a model of multiple sclerosis (Ben-Nun & Cohen, 1982). Induced models are often used to study the pathogenesis of and therapeutic venues for relevant autoimmune diseases. These models have been proposed as means to evaluate the immunomodulatory effects of chemicals on ongoing autoimmune diseases in a second tier of immunotoxicity testing.

10.4.1 Systemic lupus erythematosus-prone strains of mice

Several medications are linked to lupus-like symptoms (e.g. drug-related lupus). Although drug-induced lupus differs from systemic lupus erythematosus in certain aspects (Pollard et al., 1999; Shaheen et al., 1999), it has been proposed to use systemic lupus erythematosus-prone strains of mice as model animals to test for the exacerbating and even initiating potential of drugs. Among the mice strains proposed for this purpose are the spontaneous systemic lupus erythematosus models (BWF1, NZB×SWR/F1, MRL/lpr/lpr/Mp,

BXSB/Mp, NZB×NZW/F1, NZM, AKR). Experience with any of these strains is scarce and is restricted mainly to salts of heavy metals such as mercury. Mercury has been clearly shown to have immunostimulatory effects in NZB×NZW/F1 mice (Pollard et al., 1999). In a study examining the immunotoxic effects of diphenylhydantoin (Bloksma et al., 1994), MRL mice were exposed to the drug in the drinking-water for a period of six months; in this case, however, no indications of adverse immune reactions were found. Future studies should include more autoimmunogenic pharmaceuticals and negative controls in order to determine the extent to which systemic lupus erythematosus-prone models are useful to study or predict chemical-induced autoimmunity.

10.5 Other species

Dogs are a species frequently used in toxicity studies. However, there are only few reports in the open literature on dog studies with respect to chemical- or drug-induced hypersensitivity reactions or autoimmune effects, and studies are also often contradictory. For instance, procainamide has been shown to induce mainly an increase in antinuclear antibodies in one study (Balazs & Robinson, 1983), but not in another study with younger dogs (Dubois & Strain, 1972). Similar discrepancies were observed for hydralazine-induced effects in mice (Kammuller et al., 1989a).

More recent reports show clear sulfonamide-induced idiosyncratic responses in dog. The syndrome induced by sulfonamides in dogs (mostly Dobermans) encompasses fever, arthropathy blood dyscrasias (neutropenia, thrombocytopenia, or haemolytic anaemia), hepatopathy, skin eruptions, uveitis, and keratoconjunctivitis sicca (Trepanier, 2004). These symptoms start to occur on average as soon as 12 days after start of exposure. The incidence in dogs (and cats) is as expected from idiosyncrasy, estimated to be around 0.25% (Noli et al., 1995).

Experiments with cats showed that propylthiouracil induces systemic lupus erythematosus-like phenomena (autoantibodies against nuclear antigen, Smith [Sm] antigen, red blood cells, and cytoplasmic components, lymphoadenopathy, weight loss) (Aucoin, 1989). However, important propylthiouracil-induced symptoms, such as agranulocytosis and liver toxicity, observed in humans are not observed in cats (Shenton et al., 2004). The model could also not be reproduced in more recent years for yet unknown reasons, shedding doubt on the usefulness of the propylthiouracil-induced cat model at this moment (Shenton et al., 2004).

Chemical-induced (including diet-mediated) autoimmune effects in other species have also been documented; in most, if not all, cases, however, they are limited to isolated cases (for review, see Kosuda & Bigazzi, 1996). For instance, monkeys fed alfalfa seeds developed antibody-induced anaemia, chickens (Cornell C strain) receiving excess of iodine developed antibodies against thyroid hormones and lymphocytic thyroiditis, halothane-treated rabbits displayed antibodies against a set of five endogenous antigens, and drug-specific antibodies to a number of drugs (including isoniazid and procainamide) were detected in guinea-pigs (upon injection of drug in combination with complete Freund's adjuvant) (Katsutani & Shionoya, 1992; Aida et al., 1998).

10.6 Local and popliteal lymph node assays

10.6.1 Introduction

The local lymph node assay and the popliteal lymph node assay are straightforward animal test models that are used to link direct lymph node reactions to local application (epidermal in the local assay, subcutaneously in the popliteal assay) of potentially immunoactive chemicals. The local lymph node assay is widely used in regulatory toxicology in the testing of contact sensitizing properties of chemicals. The popliteal lymph node assay could also be used to identify sensitizing properties of chemicals involved in either systemic allergy or autoimmunity. In particular, the popliteal lymph node assay has been extensively used to evaluate the potential of certain drugs to stimulate the immune system, and, when proper immunologically relevant parameters are assessed, the popliteal lymph node assay may also identify immunosensitizing potential (Pieters & Albers, 1999).

10.6.2 Primary, secondary, and adoptive popliteal lymph node assays and the lymph node proliferation assay

The primary popliteal lymph node assay, in which lymph node weight, cell number, or proliferation of lymph node cells is used as a measure of immunostimulation, is a straightforward animal model that allows screening of immunostimulatory or sensitizing potential of an array of structurally or functionally related compounds. The popliteal lymph node assay is mostly performed in mice (Gleichmann, 1981; Bloksma et al., 1995; Goebel et al., 1996), but rats (Verdier et al., 1990; Descotes, 1992) have also been used basically to determine changes in the paw-draining lymph node upon subcutaneous injection of a suspected chemical into the footpad. The response, which can be assessed by detecting lymphocyte proliferation or changes in the distribution of leukocyte subsets, cytokine production, or immunohistology, is determined 6–8 days after injection (Ravel & Descotes, 2005).

In the secondary popliteal lymph node assay, pretreated animals are re-exposed to the same chemical or to a metabolite in a dose that itself is incapable of stimulating naive T cells. A measured response to this low dose strongly indicates, but does not formally prove, that memory T cells are present. Proof for the formation of memory T cells can be obtained with the adoptive transfer popliteal lymph node assay in which purified T cells obtained from systemically treated mice are transferred to naive recipients that subsequently receive an injection into the paw of a non-sensitizing dose of the same chemical or a relevant metabolite.

Recently, an inventory study was carried out to evaluate the predictive value of local lymph node approaches for the immunosensitizing potential of drugs (Weaver et al., 2005). Since the footpad injection raises ethical concerns, in some instances, head injection and ear injection with the auricular lymph node as read-out organ were used instead. The head injection protocol, designated the lymph node proliferation assay, showed that 6 out of 10 drugs tested were adequately identified as positive and that negative compounds were supposed to be so, known to require metabolic activation, or too toxic to use in sufficiently high doses.

10.6.3 Reporter antigen popliteal lymph node assay

Recent modifications include the use of reporter antigens in the popliteal lymph node assay (Albers et al., 1997; Gutting et al., 2002a). Reporter antigens can be regarded as bystander antigens, and the response to reporter antigens can be determined fairly easily by the enzyme-linked immunosorbent spot (ELISPOT) assay. Depending on the antigen used, the reporter antigen response can provide information about the way the drug stimulates the immune system. For instance, when a compound is co-injected with TNP-Ficoll, a T cell-independent antigen susceptible to neoantigen-specific T cell help, and an increase of trinitrophenol (TNP)-specific antibody-forming cells of the IgG isotype is detected, it can be concluded that the compound induces T cell sensitization. When using a regular T cell-dependent antigen such as TNP-OVA, a chemical-induced increase in the number of TNP-specific IgG-forming cells merely indicates that the chemical has adjuvant activity (providing the response with TNP-Ficoll is negative). Thus, the use of immunology-based read-out parameters improves the predictability of the popliteal lymph node assay; in addition, such parameters allow the further study of fundamental aspects of chemical-induced sensitization (Albers et al., 1997; Goebel et al., 1999; Wulferink et al., 2001; Gutting et al., 2002a; Nierkens et al., 2002). In a recent study using the reporter antigen protocol with TNP-Ficoll as reporter antigen, ear injection and subsequent detection of specific antibody formation with a range of pharmaceuticals showed comparable results obtained in a reporter antigen–popliteal lymph node assay using footpad injection (Nierkens et al., 2004).

Interestingly, the popliteal lymph node assay technique can be used in combination with relevant route of exposure models. Basically, T cell activation in the popliteal lymph node in response to a subcutaneous injection of a non-immunogenic dose of an appropriate chemical (hapten, relevant metabolite, native autoantigen, or reporter antigen) may allow the assessment of systemic T cell memory and hence systemic immunosensitization in animals that have been exposed to the chemical for a certain period. For example, by combining oral exposure to diclofenac with the reporter antigen–popliteal lymph node assay using TNP-Ficoll, it has been reported that a single oral dose of diclofenac (Gutting et al., 2002b) or D-penicillamine (Nierkens et al., 2005) resulted in an increased IgG1 response to TNP-Ficoll in the lymph node upon co-injection with a non-sensitizing dose of the respective drug in the paw. In addition, it appeared that oral exposure to D-penicillamine, diclofenac, or nevirapine for variable periods of time stimulated the delayed-type hypersensitivity response and/or the antibody responses to the reporter antigen TNP-OVA after 3–4 weeks.

Together, these findings indicate that oral exposure to the drugs may induce T cell responses to bystander antigens, such as reporter antigens or maybe autoantigens. The latter needs to be proven in future experiments.

10.6.4 Popliteal lymph node assay as predictive assay

Approximately 140 compounds have been tested to date in one or more of the types of the popliteal lymph node assay. Those chemicals with known immunostimulating activity in humans were predicted correctly (Kammuller et al., 1989b; Albers et al., 1997; Gutting et al., 1999, 2002a; Pieters & Albers, 1999; Shinkai et al., 1999). This number includes a substantial number of structural homologues of diphenylhydantoin (Kammuller & Seinen, 1988) and zimeldine (Thomas et al., 1989, 1990), and, importantly, compounds that require metabolic conversion turned out to be false negative unless metabolic systems (myeloperoxidase-positive phagocytes, S9 mix) were added as well. However, only about 20 compounds have been tested using the reporter antigen–popliteal lymph node assay (Albers et al., 1997; Gutting et al., 1999; Nierkens et al., 2004). As indicated already, a recent inventory study using a different subcutaneous route of exposure (the lymph node proliferation assay) showed that 6 out of 10 compounds were identified correctly as positive, whereas compounds that were not identified correctly either required metabolic activation or were too toxic (Weaver et al., 2005).

10.7 Testing strategy

Autoimmunogenic (as well as systemic allergenic) effects of compounds are usually missed in regulatory 28-day toxicity studies, in part because animals that are used are outbred, but also because relevant parameters are not evaluated or detected. In addition, outliers are usually discarded from the experiment, whereas it is these outliers that may give an indication of unexpected and idiosyncratic immune effects. Recently, it has been suggested that including histopathology and particular immune parameters (such as detection of immune complex formation, anti-DNA and antihistone antibodies) may substantially improve the predictive value of 28-day studies for detecting the autoimmune potential of a compound.

Together, although a number of models displaying chemical-induced autoimmunity exist, a general model or strategy to assess the autoimmunogenic potential of a wide range of chemicals is lacking.

Because of the multifactorial nature of many of the chemical-induced autoimmune diseases, achieving one standard model for the prediction of these side-effects may be a difficult task. Rather, one might try to design a toolbox approach with a number of models that fit to a two- or multiple-tiered approach. Based on the knowledge that the process leading to hyperreactivity responses or autoimmune diseases may start in many cases with an initial phase of sensitization, the first tier may include one of the local lymph node approaches, such as the popliteal lymph node assay (possibly in combination with a metabolizing system, but preferably with an immunological read-out parameter such as the reporter antigen approach). This first tier would then allow screening for a chemical's potential to stimulate the immune system. It is important to note that the popliteal lymph node assay in any of its forms is a hazard identification test and belongs to the qualitative stage of the risk assessment paradigm. So, at best, although the popliteal lymph node assay (in any of its forms) could be predictive of a sensitizing potential, it is not indicative of the autoimmunogenic potential of a compound as such.

The next tier of testing could include animal models (e.g. either normal or autoimmune-prone animals) using systemic exposure routes (relevant to the drug to be tested) and immunological and preferentially clinical outcomes. The recent studies using the reporter antigen approach in combination with oral exposures (in particular with penicillamine) might serve as an example of combining straightforward local lymph node approaches and oral route of exposure (see above).

In summary, high priority has to be given to the validation of the popliteal lymph node assay (or other local lymph node approaches) and to the further development of predictive animal assays using routes of exposure that are more directly relevant to the human experience. These advancements would significantly enhance the usefulness of animal models and testing strategies for autoimmunity and autoimmune diseases.

11. HUMAN TESTING FOR AUTOIMMUNE DISEASE

11.1 Introduction

Autoimmune diseases are relatively uncommon diseases. In order to make a diagnosis of a particular autoimmune disease, characteristic clinical features of the disease must be present. Early clinical manifestations in some diseases, however, are nonspecific, and in such patients the presence of autoantibodies may be used as a diagnostic marker. In the majority of patients, the diagnosis, however, is reasonably clear after a thorough clinical assessment, and in such patients antibody testing is used to confirm the diagnosis or to make an alternative diagnosis. In many autoimmune diseases, signs of tissue inflammation are present, reflected by elevated levels of c-reactive protein. Furthermore, autoantibodies can be measured. Positive predictive values of these antibodies for certain autoimmune diseases, when tested in a general population, are low, since the diseases are uncommon. In the context of characteristic clinical features, however, the positive predictive value may be sufficiently high. Despite low positive predictive values for diagnosis in an individual patient, autoantibody testing in a population that is exposed to a certain environmental factor may be useful to provide preliminary information for detailed studies of the factor.

Many hundreds of different autoantibodies have been described to date (Peter & Shoenfeld, 1996). These autoantibodies are most often detected in body fluids that are easily obtained (e.g. in serum or plasma). Therefore, autoantibody assays are primarily standardized for measuring autoantibodies in the circulation. The mere demonstration of autoantibodies is not equivalent to diagnosis of an autoimmune disease. For instance, autoantibodies are relatively common in healthy humans, especially in the elderly. Furthermore, there exist so-called natural autoantibodies, being primarily low-affinity IgM antibodies, which may represent a physiological phenomenon and may even have a protective function. Testing for autoantibodies is most often based on the usage of solid-phase autoantigens (Rose et al., 2002). After binding of autoantibodies, visualization is obtained by subsequent binding of labelled anti-human immunoglobulin reagents. Alternatively, precipitation of antigen–antibody complexes, often facilitated by addition of anti-human immunoglobulin reagents, enables the detection of specific autoantibodies.

This chapter primarily discusses the different methods of human autoantibody detection, as well as the implication of the choice of autoantigen preparation and anti-human immunoglobulin reagents for the interpretation of the results obtained. In the context of this document, it should be stressed that these tests are designed as diagnostic tests and not for identifying chemical–disease associations per se. The measurement of immunoglobulin isotypes and subclasses is discussed next, since several autoimmune diseases are characterized by polyclonal B cell activation, resulting in hypergammaglobulinaemia. Quantification of subclasses may be especially important, because environmental chemicals may result in skewing of the immune response, in particular towards a type-2 cytokine response, causing elevated levels of the IgG4 subclass and IgE isotype. Finally, experimental methods that are being explored for antigen-specific immune responses that are elicited upon chemical exposure are alluded to. These tests are mentioned only briefly, as they are poorly validated compared with the diagnostic tests that are in use for human autoimmune diseases.

With respect to autoantibody testing, several health organizations have proposed a testing scheme for preliminary evaluation of individuals exposed to chemicals. The WHO suggests testing for antinuclear antibodies, anti-dsDNA antibodies, antimitochondrial antibodies, and rheumatoid factor (IPCS, 1996). The screening panel recommended by the United States Centers for Disease Control and Prevention and Agency for Toxic Substances and Disease Registry includes antinuclear antibodies, rheumatoid factor, and antithyroglobulin antibodies, whereas the United States National Academy of Sciences recommended, besides the tests suggested by the WHO, also antibodies to red blood cells. However, no advice with regard to the method of detecting these autoantibodies and relevant cut-off values is given, and, as stated in this chapter, this may influence the conclusions drawn from the results obtained.

11.2 Methods of human autoantibody detection

11.2.1 Indirect immunofluorescence technique

The indirect immunofluorescence (IIF) technique is based on the specific binding of circulating autoantibodies to an antigen substrate consisting of tissue sections or cell suspensions. These substrates are attached on a glass slide and are either air dried or incubated with a fixative to facilitate autoantibody binding. Next, the nonspecific antibodies are washed away, and incubation with an anti-human antibody reagent conjugated to fluorescein isothiocyanate enables the visualization of autoantibody binding with the aid of a fluorescence microscope. Knowledge about the tissue distribution or cellular localization of the autoantigen of interest is essential for the proper interpretation, and this requires an experienced microscopist. A distinctive reaction pattern will be obtained by the presence of different types of autoantibodies, but the read-out may be hampered by the presence of multiple autoantibodies reacting with different autoantigens in the same tissue. Although computer-assisted classification of immunofluorescent patterns in autoimmune diagnostics is a promising development, further improvement is required for the usage of such a system in routine diagnostics. IIF on tissue sections and cell suspensions (typically Hep-2 cells or neutrophilic granulocytes) is widely used as a screening assay for the presence of autoantibodies in the case of organ-specific and systemic autoimmune diseases, respectively. The obtained results may require confirmation in antigen-specific assays (see below). Quantification of autoantibodies by IIF is at best semiquantitative. This is most often performed by testing serial, two-step dilutions or, alternatively, by quantitative image analysis of a single dilution of the serum sample. In the latter case, the fluorescence intensity obtained with a patient sample is compared with the intensity of standardized calibrators. The fluorescence intensity is directly converted into an antibody titre.

11.2.2 Counter-immunoelectrophoresis

The method of counter-immunoelectrophoresis (CIE) depends on the formation of immune complexes in an agarose matrix. Insoluble immune complexes are typically formed at the site where an antibody encounters its antigen in an optimal concentration. Both excessive antigen concentration as well as excessive antibody concentration will prevent immune complex formation. Where autoantibodies are present in the serum sample, a precipitation line will form at the point of equilibrium. In the case of CIE, the migration of antibody and antigen towards each other is facilitated by addition of an electrolyte to the agarose matrix and application of an electronic current across the gel. Alternatively, antibody and antigen can migrate only because of diffusion; this assay is referred to as the Ouchterlony assay. For diagnostic purposes, CIE is primarily used for the detection of autoantibodies to extractable nuclear antigens. These antigens are negatively charged in the electrolyte-containing matrix, whereas the autoantibodies are positively charged. Therefore, the former migrate to the anode and the latter reversely towards the cathode. Since thymic extracts of rabbit or bovine origin, which contain multiple antigens, are used, several different precipitation lines may be obtained in a screening assay in the case where distinct antibodies are present in the test serum. Positive samples have to be reanalysed next to antibody preparations of well defined monospecificity in alternating wells. In the case of identity in the precipitating antigen–antibody combination, the immunoprecipitation lines of two neighbouring wells will fuse, whereas non-identical combinations will result in crossing immunoprecipitation lines. It is clear that CIE is only a qualitative screening assay.

11.2.3 *Haemagglutination*

Aggregation of red blood cells can be triggered upon cross-linking surface antigens with a specific antibody. This haemagglutination technology not only is fundamental and widely used in blood group serology, but also can be adopted for autoantibody detection to a whole array of antigens. The so-called Coombs test either detects in vivo autoantibodies (and/or complement) bound to the surface of the red blood cells (direct Coombs test) or detects and/or types circulating autoantibodies directed to erythrocytes (indirect Coombs test). In the case of the direct Coombs test, addition of anti-human globulin reagent will directly agglutinate the erythrocytes if autoantibodies (and/or complement) have bound to their surface. The indirect Coombs test is started with incubation of test red blood cells with patient serum prior to incubation with anti-human globulin reagent. To increase the sensitivity of the indirect Coombs test and to detect IgG antibodies, pretreatment of the red blood cells by addition of colloid, proteolytic enzymes, or low ionic strength saline is required. As already mentioned, the antibody detection system is also widely used to determine the presence of other, red blood cell-unrelated (auto)antibodies. In these assays, the respective autoantigens are bound to the surface of chemically modified erythrocytes. Modification may occur by pretreatment of the erythrocytes with either tannic acid or chromic chloride. Several of these autoantigen-precoated erythrocytes are commercially available. A difference with the Coombs test is the origin of the red blood cells. To prevent false-positive reactions to blood group antigens, xenogeneic, for instance chicken or turkey, red blood cells are used instead of human red blood cells in the Coombs test. If autoantibodies are present, the antigen-coated red blood cells will agglutinate upon incubation of patient serum. This assay can be performed in serial dilutions in microtitre plates to obtain semi-quantitative results when a reference reagent is included. Actually, any type of antigen-coated microspheres that precipitate upon cross-linking can be applied for this type of assay.

11.2.4 *Enzyme-linked immunosorbent assay/fluorescent enzyme immunoassay*

In the ELISA, an enzyme is employed that is conjugated either to anti-immunoglobulin reagents or to antigen-specific antibodies. This immunoassay may detect the presence of antibody or antigen. Furthermore, there exist a multitude of different ELISA systems: direct versus capture ELISAs and competitive versus non-competitive ELISAs. In general, competitive ELISAs are applied for antigen quantification, whereas direct, non-competitive ELISAs are the primary method of choice for autoantibody detection. In this latter assay, microtitre plates are first coated with the antigen, and free binding places are blocked to prevent nonspecific binding of antibodies. Next, antigen-specific autoantibodies are enabled to interact with the antigen. After removal of nonspecific antibodies in a wash step, the microwells are incubated with enzyme (horseradish peroxidase or alkaline phosphatase)-conjugated anti-human immunoglobulin. In the presence of autoantibodies, this will result in the formation of an enzyme-labelled complex of antigen, autoantibody, and anti-human immunoglobulin that converts the finally added substrate to form a coloured end-product. The extent of colour formation is positively correlated with the autoantibody concentration in the test medium. With properly determined cut-off values, the ELISA may be applied as a qualitative assay, revealing only positive or negative results. The ELISA may even give quantitative results in international units if well defined reference standards are available, or in arbitrary units when other standards are used.

Fluorescent enzyme immunoassays (FEIA) are basically similar to the direct, non-competitive ELISAs. The main difference is that a fluorochrome instead of an enzyme is conjugated to the anti-human immunoglobulin. A prerequisite of direct ELISAs or FEIAs is that the autoantigen can be obtained in great purity, since other autoantibodies may react with the contaminants and cause a similar reaction as the autoantibodies to be tested for. Therefore, if autoantigen purification is hampered in any way, a capture ELISA may be more appropriate. In the capture ELISA, an antigen-specific monoclonal antibody is bound to the microwells. Next, the autoantigen will be more or less purified by the capturing antibody, and all other contaminants are removed by washing the microplates. All further steps are essentially the same as in the direct ELISA. Selection of reagents, however, is more delicate, because the anti-human immunoglobulin should not react directly with the capturing monoclonal antibody. Since the autoantigen is presented in a native orientation, the capture ELISA is more sensitive than the direct ELISA. On the other hand, the epitope recognized by the capturing monoclonal antibody is blocked. This seems to be only a minor disadvantage of the capture ELISA, since autoantibody responses are polyclonal and in general directed to multiple epitopes.

11.2.5 Radioimmunoassay

The radioimmunoassay (RIA) is a liquid-phase assay in which a radiolabelled antigen is precipitated by the combination of specific autoantibodies and anti-human immunoglobulin. If the antigen is a receptor (e.g. the acetylcholine receptor), a ligand (e.g. the snake venom α-bungarotoxin) may be radiolabelled instead of the antigen. The extent of radioactivity in the precipitated immune complexes is directly related to the autoantibody concentration in the test sample. Like in ELISA/FEIA, the use of well defined international standards enables the generation of quantitative results. This assay specifically detects high-affinity antibodies, which are considered to be clinically most relevant. This is particularly true in the case of detection of anti-dsDNA antibodies by the so-called Farr assay, which is a somewhat modified RIA. The RIA is hampered by the requirement of pure antigen preparations as well as special facilities for working with radioactive material.

11.2.6 Immunoblotting

The immunoblotting procedure is essentially the same as that for IIF and ELISA. Proteins are bound to membrane carriers by direct application in dots (dot-blot) or lines (line-blot) or transferred from an electrophoresis gel (Western blot). In case of the dot-blot and line-blot, pure antigen preparations are required. Western blotting may apply crude antigen preparations, because the antigens are separated by electrophoresis, and simultaneous blotting of a molecular weight marker enables the identification of the autoantigen by molecular weight characteristics. Alternatively, a well defined mixture of purified or recombinant antigens may be applied. The latter are often commercially available as prepared membranes. After application of the antigen(s) to the membrane, free binding sites are blocked with an irrelevant antigen to prevent binding of nonspecific antibodies. After incubation with the test sample and subsequent removal of nonspecific antibodies by a wash procedure, the blot is incubated with anti-human immunoglobulin conjugated to an enzyme. Incubation with an appropriate substrate will result in an insoluble, detectable reaction product at the site where autoantibodies have bound to their respective antigens. Alternatively, fluorochrome or radioactive labels can be applied. Obviously, blotting procedures will give only qualitative results, as in CIE. Additionally, however, Western blotting enables determination of the molecular weight of the recognized antigen and as such gives an extra indication as to the antigen specificity. A disadvantage of the Western blotting approach is that the proteins are separated by gel electrophoresis in the presence of sodium dodecyl sulfate, resulting in partial denaturation of the proteins and subsequent loss of antigenic epitopes.

11.2.7 Multiplex analysis

Whereas in immunoblotting and, to a lesser extent, also in IIF, several autoantibodies can be detected in qualitative terms in one single test, there is progression towards quantitative detection of multiple autoantibodies in a single fluorescence-based assay. This so-called multiplex immunoassay is based on a mixture of bead subsets that are each labelled with a unique combination of internal fluorescent signal and antigen. In essence, each bead subset represents a separate immunoassay; owing to the distinct internal fluorescent signals, however, many combinations of these assays can be analysed in the same tube. Incubation with the serum sample enables binding of autoantibodies to the beads labelled with the respective antigens. As in other assays, the nonspecific antibodies are washed away. After incubation with fluorescent anti-human immunoglobulins, the presence of autoantibodies can be detected by flow cytometry. Autoantibodies can be quantified from standard curves obtained by measuring the signal intensity of beads coated with well defined amounts of antigens. One disadvantage of this assay is that, depending on the complexity, it may generate positive results that have not been asked for by the clinician. The laboratory should determine in advance how to cope with this type of result.

11.3 Selection of detection method

Since the different methods for autoantibody detection as described above differ in terms of laboratory requirements, the local situation influences the choice of method. For instance, RIA and multiplex analysis require investments in special facilities and equipment. Indirect immunofluorescence tests and, to a lesser extent, immunoblotting require less investment, but demand the availability of properly trained technicians. Also, the results obtained are different in terms of qualitative versus quantitative data and in terms of the immunoglobulin isotype that is recognized by the anti-human immunoglobulin reagent. This type of difference will have an impact on the clinical applicability. Finally, the selection of methods is restricted by the availability of highly purified or recombinant antigens, since several assays (haemagglutination, direct ELISA, FEIA, RIA, and multiplex analysis) cannot be employed with crude antigen extracts.

11.3.1 Autoantigens

The autoantigen used in a test can be of different quality: purified or present in a whole mixture of antigens, native or recombinant, and of human or animal origin. Antibodies tend to recognize conformational epitopes, and therefore the three-dimensional structure of the autoantigen, and in some instances the non-covalent interaction with associated molecules, should be maintained. Obviously, post-translational modifications will be detrimental to the structural organization of the protein. Therefore, the choice of autoantigen will directly influence basic characteristics, such as sensitivity and specificity (see below), of the test system. In particular, IIF, when applied on human cells or tissues, has an optimal source of autoantigen, being species specific, native in origin, and unmodified by isolation procedures. However, in many instances, the structure of the autoantigen is affected by fixation of the tissue/cells. Furthermore, due to many legal regulations and risks of infection, it becomes more and more difficult to obtain human tissue for IIF. Therefore, primate tissues, with almost similar restrictions as human tissues, or even rodent tissues are widely used. It may be clear that this will reduce the sensitivity of the assay. Mixtures of autoantigens, present in crude extracts, are also used in the CIE and Western blotting. In these cases, the three-dimensional structure of the autoantigen may be affected during electrophoresis by the electrolytes and the denaturing conditions, respectively. All other assays utilize purified or recombinant autoantigens. Impurity of the autoantigen preparation is a critical caveat in most assays, but not in the capture ELISA and the Western blot. In the first assay, further purification is achieved during the capturing step with the antigen-specific monoclonal antibody; in the latter assay, the molecular weight of the recognized antigen will enable distinction between autoantigen and contamination, unless of (nearly) similar molecular weight. Recombinant protein technology has provided an alternative to circumvent problems with purification (Schmitt & Papisch, 2002). Recombinant proteins can be species specific and obtained in large and pure preparations. Although purification from the expression system (e.g. *Escherichia coli*, yeast, or baculovirus in insect cells) is still required, the purification can be facilitated by cloning a special tag at the end of the recombinant protein. Nevertheless, depending on the applied expression system, the use of recombinant autoantigens is hampered by differences in post-translational modifications and therefore may result in reduced sensitivity. In the future, this problem may be overcome by co-expression of the relevant processing factors in the expression system.

11.3.2 Anti-immunoglobulin reagents

Anti-human immunoglobulin reagents are required in most, but not all (CIE, haemagglutination), immunoassays for the detection of autoantibodies. There exists a wide array of anti-human immunoglobulin reagents and conjugated reporter molecules. The proper choice is relevant in terms of clinical interpretation of the obtained results. Anti-immunoglobulin reagents may react with all immunoglobulins, with specific isotypes, or even with subclasses. For many autoimmune diseases, the detection of distinct immunoglobulin isotypes is not of equal importance. Overall, autoantibodies of the IgM isotype are diagnostically less specific for autoimmune diseases, since these IgM autoantibodies are typically of low affinity and represent the so-called natural autoantibodies. Some exceptions to this rule include IgM rheumatoid factor and high-titre IgM anticardiolipin antibodies. The first of these two, the IgM rheumatoid factor, may even cause false-positive results for other IgM autoantibodies, since these antibodies may interact with the Fc-chain of an IgG autoantibody and thereby mimic an IgM response. Isotype switching from IgM to IgG or IgA indicates the involvement of T cells, which is considered a hallmark of autoimmune disease. IgA autoantibodies are particularly relevant for autoimmune diseases that affect mucosal tissues; in most other instances, autoantibodies of the IgG isotype are most specific. The quality of the isotype-specific anti-human immunoglobulins is quite diverse. While domestic animals are immunized with purified immunoglobulin isotypes, the obtained anti-human immunoglobulin reagents are not isotype specific. Owing to the presence of light chains common to all immunoglobulin isotypes, antibodies to these light chains will cross-react with all immunoglobulin isotypes. Therefore, further processing of the obtained antisera is required, and this includes depletion of the anti-immunoglobulin antibodies that react with the light chains. Besides the generation of anti-human immunoglobulin reagents in other species, there also exist naturally occurring molecules with the intrinsic capacity to specifically interact with human IgG — for instance, the *Staphylococcus aureus* cell wall protein A or the group G *Streptococcus* cell wall constituent protein G. Both reagents differ in terms of human IgG subclass detection: whereas protein G recognizes all four IgG subclasses, protein A does not recognize the IgG3 subclass. The issues discussed above mainly affect the specificity and clinical relevance of the results obtained. Another part of the anti-human immunoglobulin reagent is the reporter molecule that is conjugated to it. These reporter molecules include enzymes or fluorochromes and, exceptionally, radioactive markers. These reporter systems differ in assay sensitivity. Even higher assay sensitivities can be obtained by conjugation of, for instance, biotin and subsequent incubation with streptavidin conjugated with any type of reporter molecule. In general, these highly sensitive approaches are not required for the detection of human autoantibodies.

11.4 Clinical interpretation

The goal of a diagnostic test is to distinguish between individuals with and without a particular disease. Several confounding factors may hamper the correct interpretation of test results. The variability of the test should be small compared with the reference interval or range of normal. Thus, the test has to be accurate and precise. Bias can occur due to variation in the studied subject, instrument, or observer. The applicability of a test rests on its comparison with the "gold standard", which discriminates between individuals who certainly have and those who do not have the disease. Several parameters are in use that determine the value of a test result. The most commonly used parameters are sensitivity and specificity, which both, in the gold standard, by definition are 100%. Sensitivity is defined as the probability of a positive test result in a patient with the disease under investigation. Specificity is the probability of a negative test result in a patient without the disease under investigation. Whether a test result is positive or negative is dependent on the cut-off point of the assay. In order to pinpoint the cut-off point that results in optimal sensitivity and specificity, a receiver operating characteristic curve can be generated by plotting sensitivity versus specificity. Overall, the best cut-off maximizes the sum of sensitivity and specificity. However, depending on whether test results are used to detect or exclude a disease, for monitoring exacerbations of a disease, or for population screening, different cut-off points may be optimal.

It is of great practical concern to know the predictive value of positive and negative test results — that is, the proportion of those with a positive test who actually have the disease and the proportion of those with a negative test who actually do not have the disease, respectively. These values strongly depend on the true prevalence of the disease under study. Likelihood ratios, in contrast, indicate the proportion of individuals with and without the disorder at a given level of a diagnostic test. Since the likelihood ratios are calculated as a ratio of probabilities, they are not influenced by disease prevalence. Furthermore, likelihood ratios can be used in a Bayesian context to generate a post-test probability of disease. Finally, it is important to realize that the variability of the reported values for test systems can differ because variable numbers of healthy controls and/or relevant disease controls are included in the different studies. Therefore, values given in the literature or by the manufacturer of commercial kits should be interpreted in this context, and it should be recommended that all laboratories determine their own test characteristics.

Two other test parameters that are important for interpretation of results are the intra- and interassay variation. These parameters give information on the reproducibility and reliability of the results. The intra-assay variation is determined by running multiple preparations (five or more) from the same test sample in the same assay. The intra-assay variation can be calculated as the ratio of the standard deviation and the mean and is expressed as a percentage after multiplying the ratio by 100. The interassay variation is determined by running the same test sample in multiple, consecutive assays (five or more). The formula for calculating the interassay variation is similar to the one for calculating the intra-assay variation. Preferentially, these variations are determined in samples with low, medium, and high values. In general, the interassay variation is higher than the intra-assay variation. Therefore, in the case of high interassay variation, it is recommended that consecutive follow-up samples be run in the same assay in order to obtain reliable changes in autoantibody titres.

11.5 Human immunoglobulins

11.5.1 Autoimmune disease and human immunoglobulin levels

If a patient is suspected to suffer from a certain autoimmune disease, tests on immunoglobulin levels may give an indication that such a patient has a dysregulated immune system. In general, all immunoglobulin isotypes and subclasses can be detected in the human circulation. Since antibody production is the consequence of immune stimulation, it is evident that immunoglobulin levels increase during childhood and reach relatively stable levels during adulthood. Chronic immune stimulation, as is the case in autoimmune diseases, may result in further elevation of immunoglobulin levels (i.e. hypergammaglobulinaemia). These increases in immunoglobulins may even be isotype specific. For instance, hyper-IgG levels are observed in systemic lupus erythematosus and autoimmune hepatitis, whereas hyper-IgM levels are characteristic of primary biliary cholangitis. However, not only increased antibody concentrations are associated with autoimmune diseases; antibody deficiencies may also be associated with an increased prevalence of autoimmune diseases. This is particularly evident in the case of selective IgA deficiency, which is observed in 5–10% of patients with coeliac disease, whereas the prevalence of IgA deficiency in the healthy population is only 1:800. For these reasons, several autoimmune diseases have a diagnostic indication for evaluating the immunoglobulin levels in the circulation. Furthermore, antibody quantification may also give a clue to the skewing of the immune system towards type 1 or type 2 cytokine production — i.e. pro- and anti-inflammatory cytokines, respectively. In particular, IgG subclasses and IgE responses are helpful in this respect: production of IgG1 and IgG3 is associated with type 1 cytokine responses, whereas production of IgG4 and IgE is associated with type 2 cytokine responses. This distinction is probably most apparent in the detection of anticardiolipin antibodies. These antibodies are a hallmark of the antiphospholipid syndrome; in particular, the IgG2 and IgG4 subclasses are associated with clinical manifestation of antiphospholipid syndrome. Anticardiolipin antibodies of the IgG1 and IgG3 subclasses, in contrast, are induced by infections and appear not to be involved in the immunopathogenesis of antiphospholipid syndrome. Moreover, elevated IgG4 and IgE levels are induced upon contact with several environmental factors, such as mercury and gold salts.

11.5.2 Quantification of human immunoglobulins

Many different immunoassays can be used for the quantification of immunoglobulin isotypes and subclasses, varying from ELISA/ FEIA and radial immunodiffusion (RID) to nephelometry/turbidimetry (Rose et al., 2002). The immunoglobulin isotypes IgA, IgG, and IgM in particular are present in relatively high concentrations in the circulation (0.5–20 g/l). These isotypes are often quantified by nephelometry/turbidimetry. Since the concentrations of IgD and IgE are much lower (IgD: 0.04 g/l; IgE: 3×10^{-5} g/l), more sensitive assay methods are required for the detection of these latter two isotypes.

Nephelometry and turbidimetry are based on the formation of immune complexes in solution and the subsequent effect on scattering of incident light. The basic principles of light scattering by particles are beyond the scope of this discussion. The formation of immune complexes is accomplished by the addition of an optimized dilution of specific antiserum to a dilute antigen solution, resulting in more or less equivalent presence of antigen and antibody. As already stated, immune complex formation is prevented in situations of antigen excess or antibody excess. The newly formed immune complexes will scatter light from an incident light beam. In the case of nephelometry, increased side scattering at an angle to the incident light beam is determined, whereas in the case of turbidimetry, the loss in light intensity passing straight forward through the solution, due to side scattering, is measured. Some automates combine both detection principles for calculating antigen concentrations. As mentioned above, these techniques are very suitable for quantifying the immunoglobulin isotypes IgA, IgG, and IgM. The IgG subclasses, in particular IgG3 and IgG4, are present in the circulation in relatively low concentrations. They can be quantified by nephelometry/turbidimetry if the immune complex formation is enhanced. This is achieved by coupling the specific antiserum to, for instance, latex particles. In any case, quantitative results are obtained by relating the signal of the test sample to calibrators that have assigned values for the antigen of interest.

The RID or Mancini assay is also based on the formation of immune complexes. This occurs in an agarose matrix containing the specific antiserum. The antigen is applied into a small hole in the matrix and disperses through this matrix due to diffusion. As soon as equivalent concentrations of antigen and antibody are reached, the molecules will precipitate, revealing a precipitin ring. There is a linear relationship between the antigen concentration and the squares of the ring diameters (end-point method) or between the log of the antigen concentration and the ring diameters (timed-diffusion method). The use of appropriate calibrators enables quantification of results. This technique is often applied for the detection of IgG subclasses and IgD concentrations.

Finally, the extremely low IgE concentration in the circulation requires very sensitive detection methods — i.e. ELISA/FEIA, RIA, or modifications of these methods. Basically, these techniques are similar to those described for the detection of autoantibodies. In the case of ELISA/FEIA, it concerns a capture technique where the IgE molecule is first captured by an anti-IgE monoclonal antibody and subsequently recognized by an enzyme/fluorochrome-conjugated anti-IgE monoclonal antibody.

11.6 Testing in the diagnosis of delayed-type chemical hypersensitivity

When a patient suffers from a certain autoimmune disease and one suspects the person to be exposed to a certain environmental factor, few possibilities exist to prove exposure. Several in vitro or in vivo tests, such as skin tests, serological tests, and the lymphocyte transformation test (LTT), can be performed to demonstrate a sensitization to a certain chemical (Choquet-Kastylevsky et al., 2001; Pichler, 2003).

Skin testing is based on the application of chemical solutions on the epidermis, with (scratch-patch test) or without (patch test) scarification of the epidermis. The occurrence of a typical type IV hypersensitivity reaction — i.e. erythema, vesiculation, and evidence of cellular infiltrate — 48–96 h after application is typical for a positive reaction. A drawback of this approach is that the metabolism of the chemical, leading to the generation of a reactive metabolite, and the presentation of the chemical to the immune system may be different according to the route of entry.

In vitro testing of delayed-type chemical hypersensitivity is based on the detection of chemical-specific IgG antibodies and/or T cells. Chemical-specific IgG antibodies are detected in solid-phase assays where the chemical is bound to various carriers, such as nitrocellulose or sepharose. These methods are controversial and are not recommended for the routine diagnosis of chemical hypersensitivity. Chemical-specific T cell responses are measured in the so-called LTT. This test reveals a sensitization of T cells by an enhanced proliferative response of peripheral blood mononuclear cells to a certain chemical. Generally, lymphocyte transformation is measured by [^{3}H]thymidine incorporation into DNA, but alternative, flow cytometry-based methods are available as well. Although this test can be a useful tool for clinical diagnosis, a positive LTT can only signal a previous contact with the respective chemical and is not specific for delayed-type hypersensitivity. Furthermore, in vitro testing precludes the generation of reactive metabolites, which may contain the actually involved antigen.

Altogether, accurate and reliable diagnostic tests for the evaluation of adverse chemical reactions remain problematic. At the present time, none of these tests has been properly validated as a specific and sensitive diagnostic tool of delayed-type chemical hypersensitivity. Moreover, these tests only enable immune reactivity to the chemical itself: in cases where the chemical elicits an immune reaction to autologous antigens, conventional methods for the diagnosis of autoimmune diseases, as discussed in the first part of this chapter, are more appropriate. Table 16 lists a broad panel of laboratory tests (general and immunological) to enable detection of a variety of abnormalities associated with induction of autoimmunity that may occur after environmental chemical exposure. Obviously, this screening panel should be done in conjunction with clinical evaluation, since positive results in laboratory testing do not make a diagnosis or predict the subsequent development of autoimmune disease. Further, more specific testing should be done to aid in the diagnosis of possible autoimmune disease.

11.7 Conclusions

Exposure to chemicals may have a strong impact on the immune system: chemicals or their metabolites may induce a delayed-type hypersensitivity reaction to the chemical or may even break tolerance due to conjugation with autoantigens and revealing neo-epitopes. Additionally, chemicals may induce changes in the balance between type 1 and type 2 immune responses. There exist a great variety of methods for monitoring these potential chemical-mediated effects (van Loveren et al., 2001). In contrast to the diagnostic test systems for autoantibody detection, the tests available for measuring immunity to chemicals that may cause delayed-type hypersensitivity reactions are only poorly validated for clinical purposes. Furthermore, these tests assess only immune reactivity to the chemical itself and do not measure autoimmunity.

Table 16. Laboratory tests for the assessment of abnormalities associated with induction of autoimmunity related to environmental chemical exposure

Type of test	Examples
General laboratory tests	*These tests will provide basic information about health abnormalities.*
	• Complete blood count (white and red blood cell counts, differential leukocyte counts, thrombocyte counts, haemoglobin concentration, haematocrit, red cell indices) will provide information on haematological status and inflammatory conditions.
	• Urinalysis (glucose, protein, haemoglobin by dipstick; if positive, specimen should be centrifuged and the pellet examined for red blood cells and casts) should be done to detect kidney dysfunction and/or diabetes.
	• Clinical chemistry (ALT and AST as markers of liver damage, CPK for muscle damage, creatinine for kidney dysfunction). C-reactive protein will point at an acute-phase response (inflammation).
	• T3/T4 or TSH will indicate thyroid dysfunction.
Immunological laboratory tests	*These tests will provide more specific information about immune dysregulation and autoimmune reactions.*
	• Immunoglobulin levels (IgG, IgA, IgM) should be used for detection of polyclonal stimulation. For example, polyclonal elevations of IgG levels can be a characteristic of systemic lupus erythematosus or Sjögren syndrome. IgE and/or subclasses of IgG should be determined as an indication of changes in the Th1/Th2 balance.
	• Autoantibodies:
	1. Antinuclear antibodies (by IIF). If antinuclear antibodies by IIF are positive, specificity of the antinuclear antibodies should be determined. Antinuclear antibody specificities associated with the development of systemic autoimmune diseases are: autoantibodies against double-stranded DNA, nucleosomes, histones, Ro/SS-A, La/SS-B, U1-RNP, Sm, DNA-Topoisomerase I (Scl-70), centromere protein, and Jo-1.
	2. ANCA (by ELISA for MPO-ANCA and PR3-ANCA or by IIF on normal neutrophils). ANCA are markers for the small-vessel vasculitides, such as Wegener granulomatosis, microscopic polyangiitis, and Churg-Strauss syndrome.

Table 16 (Contd)

Type of test	Examples
Immunological laboratory tests (contd)	3. Rheumatoid factor (by ELISA or, if ELISA testing is not available, by particle agglutination). Rheumatoid factor refers primarily to the IgM antibody that binds aggregated IgG as its antigen. Rheumatoid factor is associated with rheumatoid arthritis.
	4. Organ-specific antibodies, such as antithyroid (peroxidase) for detection of thyroid-specific autoimmunity. Other organ-specific autoantibodies may also be selected if organ-specific autoimmune reactions are expected.
	5. Interpretation of the tests for autoantibodies will depend on the class and titre of the antibody and the age and sex of the test subject. Autoantibodies can be found in normal, healthy individuals, especially elderly females.

ALT, alanine aminotransferase; AST, aspartate aminotransferase; CPK, creatine phosphokinase

12. RISK ASSESSMENT

12.1 Introduction

The risk assessment process involves the characterization of the potential adverse health effects in humans resulting from extrinsic factors such as exposures to environmental chemicals or therapeutics and/or lifestyle choices. The first step of risk assessment for any potential adverse effects, including autoimmune disease, is problem formulation. This represents a process that establishes a conceptual model for the risk assessment. During problem formulation, the adequacy of scientific data, data gaps, policy and public health issues, and factors to define the feasibility, scope, and objectives for the risk assessment are identified. This allows for early identification of important factors to be considered in developing a scientifically sound risk assessment. The key questions that the risk assessment is seeking to answer should be identified during this planning and scoping process, and a rationale for the focus of the assessment on specific toxic effects or susceptible populations should be included. Problem formulation is based upon a clear articulation and understanding of several key elements, including the objective, the overall scope, exposure considerations, and considerations of biological effects (Daston et al., 2004).

As described in a highly referenced document (NRC, 1983), important components of this process include hazard identification, assessment of exposure and dose–response relationships, and characterization of the risk. Uncertainty factors are built into the risk assessment process to account for variations in individual susceptibility, extrapolation of data from studies in laboratory animals to humans (i.e. interspecies variation in toxicokinetics), and extrapolation from high-dose to low-dose exposures. In the case of the association between exposure to chemicals and drugs and autoimmunity or autoimmune diseases, much of the information needed to evaluate risk in the context of the traditional United States National Research Council paradigm is not available. The following represents a discussion of issues in chemical-induced autoimmunity relevant to the use of existing data and data needs in risk assessment.

12.2 Hazard identification of chemical-induced autoimmune disease (animal models)

Validated models or strategies to assess or identify chemical or physical factors that induce autoimmune diseases are not available (see also chapter 10). Despite the fact that methods (e.g. detection of autoantibodies, histopathology) exist that could be used in a general 28-day toxicity study, potential autoimmunogenicity is usually missed. Nevertheless, any sign of inflammation in any of the animals in a 28-day study should be regarded as an alert of hazard. A chemical that produces elevated autoantibodies in experimental animals or exacerbates autoimmune disease in autoimmune-prone animals (i.e. increases severity of disease or lessens time to occurrence) is also of concern because of its potential to cause autoimmunity in humans. This is because the molecular and cellular events responsible for autoimmune disease are similar in experimental animals and humans. However, at this time, it is not possible to determine the predictive value of these models. The assumption that, for chemical-induced autoimmunity, humans are at least as sensitive as animals is a conservative estimate of sensitivity.

Because of its very complex etiology, hazard assessment of autoimmunogenic potential may require a tiered approach based on a toolbox of methods. Proposed hazard identification methods include the popliteal lymph node assay as well as oral or systemic exposure models with inbred "autoimmune-prone" animals or particularly sensitive strains, such as the Brown Norway rat. The popliteal lymph node assay (in one of its variations, but in particular in combination with an immunologically relevant readout parameter) is being considered as a first-tier model, but is limited to identifying a compound's potential to sensitize the immune system. Since sensitization is considered crucial in the induction of autoimmune disease, the potential to induce sensitization should be considered a hazard. Although frequently used in experimental settings and as a screening assay, the test is not formally validated. Supporting its potential as a first-tier assay, the popliteal lymph node assay allows screening of a set of structurally related compounds so as to select the least sensitizing, which is relevant in particular in case of drug evaluations.

12.3 Exposure assessment (animal models)

The determination and evaluation of the dose–response relationship are critical steps in the hazard characterization. A dose–response relationship is an important criterion in demonstrating chemical-induced autoimmunity. The shape of the dose–response curve and the effective dose range, if attainable, should be examined, along with consideration of the exposure (route, timing, and duration), toxicokinetics, and other issues that might affect comparisons with human exposure scenarios. The interpretation of dose–response data should identify doses associated with adverse effects (autoimmune disease), as well as doses associated with no adverse effects, to determine the most sensitive end-point(s) or other critical effect(s) occurring at the lowest-observable-adverse-effect level and no-observable-adverse-effect level or benchmark dose associated with the effect(s). Assessment of dose–response relationships of autoimmunogenic chemicals in experimental studies can be complicated by dose-dependent tolerance induction and transience of the autoimmune effects. For instance, mercury-induced autoimmune glomerulonephritis in Brown Norway rats is transient and resolves spontaneously and cannot be induced again in the same animal. In addition, low-dose pretreatment of animals with mercury(II) chloride or penicillamine prevents development of adverse immunity. Tolerance indicates that no adverse effects are observed in a "non-stimulated" immune system (e.g. immunoregulatory processes), and an additional risk factor (e.g. microbial interaction) might be required to circumvent tolerance. In contrast, the fact that low-dose tolerance occurs with certain chemicals suggests that a threshold exists.

Relevant route of exposure models are not usually used in current rodent models for studying chemical-induced autoimmunity, and more relevant exposure routes, such as inhalation, dermal, or oral, will be needed to assess dose–response relationships.

12.4 Mode of action

Structure–activity relationship analysis has proven to be useful in evaluating carcinogenicity of a chemical and is considered as a part of weight of evidence by providing valuable information on chemicals or metabolites that initiate carcinogenesis. Increasing efforts to understand the basic immunological and pharmacological processes responsible for chemical-induced autoimmune diseases have provided a conceptual framework that may help identify potential agents that can produce autoimmune response (Luster et al., 1999). Chemicals affecting these known processes could be at increased potential for inducing autoimmune reactions. For example, laboratory studies have shown that thymolytic chemicals (such as cyclosporin) can induce autoimmunity when given neonatally by altering normal patterns of autoreactive T cell deletion, a process that occurs in the thymus early in life. Chemicals that form protein adducts or damage tissue in such a way as to allow expression of cryptic determinants (e.g. halothane) would provide novel host antigens that could be recognized by T cells. Common features associated with many drugs that induce autoimmune diseases include their ability to serve as myeloperoxidase substrates (e.g. procainamide) and/or cause changes in methylation (e.g. hydralazine). The underlying biology for the latter associations is less clear but may involve formation of the specific antigenic epitopes responsible for the autoimmune response. With regard to the association with myeloperoxidase substrates, it has been suggested that many of the chemicals require metabolism in proximity to immune cells in order to be antigenic; immune cells such as monocytes contain high levels of myeloperoxidase. Agents that have adjuvant activity (e.g. mercury(II) chloride), biologicals that stimulate MHC class II molecule expression (e.g. interferons), or certain cytokines, all of which can shift the balance of Th1 and Th2 cells, which may allow exacerbation of pre-existing autoimmune disease, should also be considered. Also of potential concern are endocrine disruptors, as hormonal influences, particularly sex steroids, appear to play a role in many autoimmune diseases.

Toxicity and dose–response to an exogenous chemical are dependent upon the concentration of the toxicant at the site(s) of action (e.g. the target organ). The disposition of a chemical in an organism is dependent upon the processes of absorption, distribution, metabolism, and excretion, defined as toxicokinetic data. Qualitative and quantitative information on each of these processes would be useful in risk assessment. For autoimmune diseases, toxicokinetic data may be helpful in identifying the potential organ systems that are likely to be involved or the responsible metabolite.

12.5 Epidemiological issues

Epidemiological studies, when available, represent the "gold standard" for use in risk assessment. There are special issues in designing and standardizing epidemiological studies for general risk assessment that also apply for chemical-induced autoimmune disease. A goal of this research is to be able to estimate the "attributable risk" — that is, the proportion or number of new cases of a disease that could be prevented if a given exposure is reduced or eliminated. Randomized trials of environmental exposures are generally not feasible or ethical. Epidemiological studies use methodologies developed for observational research to reduce the potential role of confounding, selection bias, and misclassification of exposure and of disease that may bias the estimates of disease association, increase the imprecision or uncertainty of the estimates, or limit the ability to apply the results to the general population. Prospective studies in which exposure assessment is determined prior to disease onset avoid the potential problem of a differential misclassification of exposure based on disease status. For both prospective and retrospective designs, however, the adequacy of exposure assessment, in terms of both sensitivity and specificity, is extremely important and has been demonstrated to affect not just the precision, but the magnitude and direction of observed associations between exposures and autoimmune diseases (Parks et al., 2004a). In addition, there are some unique challenges in epidemiological studies for risk assessment in chemical-induced autoimmunity. For example, although the estimated prevalence of all autoimmune diseases is not rare (3–5% of the population), the incidence of specific autoimmune diseases (more than 60 are suspected) is relatively low, and extremely large populations are needed to have sufficient power to identify significant increased risk. Furthermore, there are no population-based disease registries for most autoimmune diagnoses, and the diagnosis can be difficult to ascertain accurately.

In general, autoimmune diseases persist for the life of the patient. They are often marked, however, by remission and exacerbation. Exceptions are seen in autoimmune conditions caused by drugs. For example, most cases of a lupus-like illness caused by procainamide or hydralazine usually resolve when the drug is discontinued. Some autoimmune diseases precipitated by an infection, such as post-infection autoimmune thrombocytopenia and Guillain-Barré syndrome, remit after the infection resolves, whereas others, exemplified by rheumatic fever, recur with streptococcal repeated infection. Several forms of autoimmune disease, such as Hashimoto thyroiditis and Graves disease, may arise several weeks after delivery. Characteristically, these forms of postpartum autoimmune diseases clear spontaneously after several months and, thus, may be difficult to capture in retrospective studies.

12.6 Susceptibility factors

Identification of high-risk populations is an important issue in risk assessment. As described in detail elsewhere in this document, a variety of intrinsic factors (i.e. genetic polymorphisms, sex, life stage, and hormone status) affect susceptibility to individual autoimmune diseases (see chapter 6 for details). While there is variability in the extent of female predominance and no strong association between degree of female predominance and type of disease or age at onset, sex and/or hormonal status clearly play a role in disease susceptibility. Although a majority of autoimmune diseases are less common in children and adolescents, the relative influence of early-life exposures to environmental chemicals or infectious agents on the incidence and severity of disease later in life is largely unexplored. When insufficient evidence exists pertaining to susceptibility, the assumption of equality is generally used.

Studies have shown that genetic predisposition plays an important role in susceptibility in the development of autoimmune diseases. The genetic basis for these differences is likely due to functional polymorphisms contained within multiple genes, each of which, by modulating corresponding protein expression, influences disease susceptibility. In this respect, associations have been found between the occurrence of autoimmune disease and the presence of certain MHC alleles as well as polymorphism in genes responsible for cytokines and inflammatory mediators, such as TNFα, to name a few. With the advent of genetic screening assays and their application in population-based epidemiological studies, it may be possible in the near future to establish quantitatively the increased risk associated with these factors that can be applied to the risk assessment.

Two types of extrinsic factors may influence disease susceptibility: those under the conscious control of the individual, such as lifestyle choices (e.g. cigarette smoking or consumption of ethanol), and those over which the individual has limited control, such as exposure to infectious agents or environmental agents. Our lack of understanding regarding the contribution of these individual exposures to the risk of autoimmune disease in genetically susceptible individuals and the potential for cumulative interactions of many of these components is a significant challenge for the risk assessment process.

12.7 Burden of autoimmune disease

The management of the risk process also includes cost–benefit analyses. Thus, in addition to the prevalence of disease, consideration of the burden of autoimmune disease should include mortality risk and the impact of morbidity (direct costs of health-care utilization and indirect costs from effects of employment, overall quality of life, and burden on non-paid caregivers). Many autoimmune diseases (e.g. multiple sclerosis, rheumatoid arthritis, systemic lupus erythematosus) are characterized by periods of remission and relapse, which complicates both the ability to care for patients and the ability to accurately assess the impact of disease. The annual per-patient direct costs of hospitalization, outpatient services, and medications in rheumatoid arthritis have been estimated as approximately 2000 euros, with a range of approximately 5- to 10-fold. Substantial variability is seen across studies and countries (Rat & Boissier, 2004; Rosery et al., 2005). In a Canadian study of multiple sclerosis, the average cost associated with remission (i.e. costs of health-care utilization) was increased from 7596 to 33 206 Canadian dollars across levels of disease severity, and the average cost of relapse (i.e. inability to work) was 1367 Canadian dollars (Grima et al., 2000). There are few studies pertaining to costs of many of the other autoimmune diseases. The development of new therapeutic agents has led to a substantial increase in medication costs for rheumatoid arthritis and other diseases (Rubio-Terres & Dominguez-Gil Hurle, 2005; Sorensen & Andersen, 2005).

Because of the chronic nature of these diseases, and because these diseases are currently not "cured" but rather "treated", the indirect costs associated with long-term disability are substantial.

The impact on employment is of particular concern in the diseases that most often affect young and middle-aged adults. Studies on several diseases have reported that a large percentage (30% or more) of patients are unable to work, and this figure increases with disease duration (Woolf & Pfleger, 2003; Lacaille, 2005; Alarcon et al., 2006). Furthermore, the indirect costs associated with job or productivity loss may be greater than the direct costs associated with health-care utilization (Phillips, 2004; Rat & Boissier, 2004; Hulsemann et al., 2006).

In conclusion, much of the information needed to address the risk of chemical-induced autoimmune diseases is not available.

13. CONCLUSIONS AND RECOMMENDATIONS

13.1 Conclusions

1. Autoimmune diseases include a wide variety of illnesses targeting many sites in the body. They form an important health problem, affecting at least 5% of the population. Furthermore, autoimmune mechanisms play a role in many other diseases; hence, more than these 5% will encounter autoimmune-associated health effects.

2. Autoimmunity and autoimmune diseases are consequences of multifactorial phenomena. In addition to intrinsic factors, exogenous factors include infections, dietary factors, and physical and chemical agents.

3. There is growing evidence that a wide array of environmental agents and therapeutics produce autoimmune-like diseases or exacerbate pre-existing autoimmune diseases.

4. The interaction of intrinsic and environmental factors and their consequences for autoimmune disease are poorly understood.

5. Drug-induced autoimmune diseases, autoimmune-like disorders, and hypersensitivity reactions are a major concern and have caused the withdrawal of drugs from the market or restriction of their use.

6. There is inadequate information on the prevalence of the various diseases, particularly in countries other than Europe or North America. Consequently, the current figures on prevalence may actually be underestimated.

7. There is epidemiological evidence of increasing incidence and prevalence of certain autoimmune diseases in highly industrialized countries, which cannot be attributed to better diagnostics alone.

8. The utility of the available methods for clinical measurement of immune responses has not been validated for the identification of chemical-induced autoimmunity.

9. The number of animal models of autoimmunity is extensive. These models represent a variety of systemic and organ-specific diseases and are mostly used to explore etiology and therapeutic possibilities for certain autoimmune diseases. However, for the purpose of safety evaluation, a general strategy to identify and predict the autoimmunogenic potential of a wide range of chemicals is lacking.

10. The utility of the traditional risk assessment paradigm for autoimmunity associated with environmental agents is currently limited.

13.2 Recommendations

There is an urgent need for:

1. public health authorities, health professionals, and government agencies to be made better aware of the increasing burden of autoimmune disease due to exposure to physical and chemical agents.

2. better estimates of human and economic costs to individuals and society of autoimmune diseases.

3. devising standard strategies for the clinical investigation and diagnosis of autoimmune diseases and applying them internationally to examine causes and incidences of autoimmune disorders.

4. more epidemiological information with respect to incidence and prevalence of autoimmune diseases and well designed studies evaluating associations with environmental exposure.

5. identifying causes of increased incidences of certain autoimmune diseases.

6. developing predictive testing methods to identify the ability of chemicals to induce autoimmunity. Such strategies may include

Conclusions and Recommendations

a step-by-step approach, i.e. identification of the ability to stimulate the immune system, followed by examination in suitable animal models using relevant routes of exposure and measurement of disease outcome.

7. identifying mechanisms of how environmental agents induce autoimmunity or autoimmune diseases.

8. additional information on the use of autoantibodies or other factors as biomarkers of exposure and disease.

9. surveillance strategies to provide screening and alerting systems for autoimmune disorders associated with physical and chemical agents. Current post-marketing surveillance strategies in place for medicines, pesticides, and other chemicals should be extended to provide information on autoimmune disease associated with their use.

10. more emphasis placed on studies involving perinatal exposure to chemicals in view of the sensitivity of the developing immune system to immunotoxic injury.

TERMINOLOGY

Acquired immunity. A state of protection against pathogen-induced injury, with rapid immune elimination of pathogenic invaders; due to previous immunization or vaccination.

Addison disease. Adrenocortical hypofunction characterized by hypotension, weight loss, anorexia, and weakness. The most common form is the idiopathic Addison disease, mediated by autoimmune mechanisms. Autoantibodies specific to the adrenal cortex are specific diagnostic markers of this form. 21-Hydroxylase, a cytochrome P450 steroidogenic enzyme, is one of the major targets of adrenal autoantibodies in idiopathic Addison disease as well as in Addison disease in the context of autoimmune polyglandular syndromes (➡ polyendocrinopathies, autoimmune). Hypofunction or failure of the adrenal gland may also be a manifestation of ➡ antiphospholipid syndrome due to thrombosis of the blood vessels of the adrenal glands.

Adhesion molecules. Molecules, belonging mainly to the immunoglobulin or integrin superfamily of molecules (e.g. LFA-1, ICAM-1), expressed on the membrane of various cells of the immune system. Interactions with each other as receptors and corresponding ligands facilitate cooperation (cross-talk) of cells, signal transduction, and information transfer between cells.

Adjuvant. A material that enhances immune response to substances in a non-antigen-specific manner.

Allogenic. Term describing genetically different phenotypes in different (non-inbred) individuals of the same species.

Alopecia. Loss of hair, often associated with autoimmune disease (e.g. autoimmune thyroid diseases, ➡ pernicious anaemia, ➡ Addison disease, ➡ diabetes mellitus type 1, ➡ systemic lupus erythematosus). Although a specific autoimmune response could not be found up to now, autoimmunity probably plays a role in a subset of this disease.

Alveolitis. Inflammation of the alveoli of the lung. May be a manifestation of systemic autoimmune diseases.

Anaemia. A reduction in number or mass of circulating red blood cells that may cause hypoxia in organs or tissues by the reduction in the oxygen-carrying capacity (reduction in haemoglobin concentration) of blood. Anaemia is caused either by decreased production or by increased destruction of red blood cells. Immune-mediated forms of anaemia caused by decreased production of red blood cells are autoimmune myelopathies including aplastic anaemia, pure red cell aplasia induced by autoantibodies against erythropoietin, and ➡ pernicious anaemia caused by autoantibody-mediated vitamin B_{12} deficiency (autoantibodies against gastric intrinsic factor lead to decreased absorption of vitamin B_{12}). Autoantibodies against structures of red blood cells are a main cause of acquired decreased production of red blood cells. See also: ➡ autoimmune haemolytic anaemia.

ANCA-associated vasculitides. Group of autoimmune systemic vasculitides associated with ➡ antineutrophil cytoplasmic autoantibodies: ➡ Wegener granulomatosis, ➡ microscopic polyangiitis, Churg-Strauss syndrome.

Anergy. Lack of immune responsiveness (usually defined as lack of response to common recall antigens). The failure of B or T cells to proliferate in response to defined autoantigens (➡ clonal anergy) is a primary mechanism of ➡ self-tolerance.

Animal models of autoimmunity. Used for investigations of factors and mechanisms involved in the induction and progression of pathological autoimmunity and disease development with the aim of improvement of diagnosis, prophylaxis, and therapy of human autoimmune diseases. However, most experimentally induced or spontaneously occurring animal models usually differ in some aspects from human autoimmunity. Nevertheless, important insights into the pathogenesis of autoimmune diseases can be obtained using animal models, e.g. by immunization, exposure to viruses or ➡ xenobiotics, thymectomy, manipulation of the ➡ idiotypic network, or genetic engineering (transgenic or knockout animals).

Antibody. An ➡ immunoglobulin produced by activated B cells and plasma cells after exposure to an ➡ antigen with specificity for the inducing antigen.

Antibody-dependent cell-mediated cytotoxicity (ADCC). Lysis of various target cells coated with antibody by ➡ Fc receptor-bearing killer cells, including large granular lymphocytes (➡ natural killer cells), ➡ neutrophils, eosinophils, and mononuclear phagocytes.

Antigen. Any compound recognized by antigen receptor-bearing lymphocytes. Antigens induce immune responses or tolerance. Antigens inducing immune responses only with the help of T cells are T cell-dependent antigens, while those that do not need T cell help are T cell-independent antigens. All ➡ immunogens are antigens, but not all antigens are necessarily immunogens.

Antigen-presenting cells. Cells expressing MHC gene products (➡ MHC class I gene products, ➡ MHC class II gene products) with the capacity to process and present antigen. ➡ Macrophages, ➡ dendritic cells, ➡ B lymphocytes, and ➡ Langerhans' cells are termed professional or constitutive antigen-presenting cells. However, other cells (such as endothelial cells) can acquire the ability to present antigen in certain pathological conditions.

Antigen processing and presentation. Protein antigens are processed (cleaved by enzymes) in various compartments of ➡ antigen-presenting cells. The immunogenic peptides interact with the binding sites of MHC class II products (exogenous antigens) or with those in MHC class I products (endogenous antigens, including viruses). The processed antigen–MHC complex is recognized by the antigen receptor complex of ➡ T lymphocytes.

Antigenic determinant. A single antigenic site (➡ epitope) usually exposed on the surface of a complex antigen. Epitopes are recognized by antigen receptors on T or B cells (T cell epitopes or B cell epitopes).

Antimitochondrial antibodies (AMA). Autoantibodies producing a mitochondrial staining on cryostat sections of various tissues and on tumour cell monolayers. According to the fluorescence pattern, different subtypes can be differentiated. Antimitochondrial antibodies of the subtype 2 (AMA-M2) are directed against antigens of three related 2-oxo acid dehydrogenase complexes (e.g. the E2 subunit of the pyruvate dehydrogenase complex,

PDC-E2) localized to the inner mitochondrial membrane. AMA-M2 is a specific marker of ➡ primary biliary cirrhosis.

Antineutrophil cytoplasmic autoantibodies (ANCA). Autoantibodies directed against cytoplasmic antigens of neutrophils and monocytes. ANCA are routinely detected by indirect immunofluorescence with three different patterns: cANCA (granular cytoplasmic), pANCA (perinuclear), and xANCA or aANCA (atypical). They are diagnostic markers for systemic necrotizing vasculitides (e.g. ➡ Wegener granulomatosis, ➡ microscopic polyangiitis) and ➡ inflammatory bowel diseases. See also: ➡ myeloperoxidase and ➡ proteinase 3.

Antinuclear antibodies (ANA). Non-organ-specific autoantibodies directed against various nuclear antigens, including chromatin antigens (e.g. single- or double-stranded DNA, nucleosomes, histone proteins), centromere antigens (e.g. CENP-B protein), nucleolar antigens (e.g. ➡ fibrillarin, PM-Scl proteins, RNA polymerases), splicing proteins (e.g. Sm and U1-RNP proteins), and other conserved nuclear proteins (e.g. Ro/SS-A, La/SS-B, DNA topoisomerase I). Antinuclear antibodies are frequently observed in patients with autoimmune systemic rheumatic diseases (also called connective tissue diseases), especially in patients with ➡ systemic lupus erythematosus, ➡ systemic sclerosis (scleroderma), ➡ mixed connective tissue disease, and ➡ Sjögren syndrome and in patients with ➡ autoimmune hepatitis type 1.

Antinuclear factor (ANF). Former term for ➡ antinuclear antibody.

Antiphospholipid antibodies (aPL). Autoantibodies directed against neutral or negatively charged phospholipids including anticardiolipin antibodies (aCl) and lupus anticoagulant. They are diagnostic markers of the ➡ antiphospholipid syndrome, although they are also found in patients with other (autoimmune) diseases and infections.

Antiphospholipid syndrome (APS). One of the most common autoimmune diseases, characterized by thrombosis, recurrent spontaneous abortions, and the presence of ➡ antiphospholipid antibodies. Antiphospholipd syndrome may occur as an isolated disease (primary APS) or in combination with another autoimmune disease, especially ➡ systemic lupus erythematosus (secondary APS).

Apoptosis. Programmed cell death, a physiological process whereby useless and potentially harmful cells are rapidly eliminated without tissue inflammation or damage. Apoptosis plays an important role in embryogenesis and normal tissue homeostasis, but it is also involved in the development of malignancy and autoimmunity. The dysfunction of an apoptotic pathway (e.g. defects in certain pro- and anti-apoptotic molecules), defective clearance of apoptotic cells, and abnormalities in the mechanisms of clearance, processing, and presentation of autoantigens may play an important role in the development of autoimmune diseases. See also: ➡ Fas and Fas ligand, ➡ autoimmune lymphoproliferative syndrome, ➡ Bcl-2.

Atherosclerosis. A type of arteriosclerosis that is characterized by atheroma formation. It is a multifactorial process leading to the accumulation of lipids within the vessel wall, associated with mononuclear cell infiltration and smooth muscle proliferation. Autoimmune-mediated inflammation may play an important role in accelerated atherosclerosis in autoimmune rheumatic diseases.

Autoantibodies. Immunoglobulins (➡ antibodies) that are directed against the organism's own antigens (➡ autoantigens). They circulate in the serum but may also be detectable in other body fluids or bound in target tissue structures. Autoantibodies may occur as a part of the natural immunoglobulin repertoire (➡ natural autoantibodies) or are induced by different mechanisms (non-natural or pathological autoantibodies). A number of non-natural autoantibodies are diagnostic markers of defined autoimmune diseases, regardless of their pathogenic activity. They may be directed against conserved non-organ-specific autoantigens (e.g. ➡ antinuclear antibodies), organ-specific extracellular autoantigens (e.g. autoantibodies to ➡ glomerular basement membrane), organ-specific cellular antigens (e.g. ➡ islet cell antibodies), or cell-specific autoantigens of circulating cells (e.g. ➡ antineutrophil cytoplasmic autoantibodies).

Autoantigens. Self-antigens of the organism, which may be targets of autoimmune responses by autoreactive B cells (see: ➡ autoantibodies) or T cells, including proteins (e.g. enzymes, structural proteins), glycoproteins (e.g. β_2-glycoprotein I), nucleic acids (e.g. double-stranded DNA), phospholipids (e.g. cardiolipin), and glycosphingolipids (e.g. gangliosides).

Autoimmune diseases. Disorders that are characterized by (i) the production of autoantibodies or immune effector cells that are autoreactive to self-peptides and (ii) pathological changes (e.g. tissue infiltration, damage, and/or dysfunction) that resulted from these immune responses against self-antigens (➤ autoantigens).

Autoimmune haemolytic anaemia (AIHA). Acquired haemolytic anaemia mediated by autoantibodies against antigens on the organism's own red cell membrane. Autoimmune haemolytic anaemia may be idiopathic, secondary to lymphoproliferative, autoimmune (e.g. ➤ systemic lupus erythematosus), or chronic inflammatory disorders, postinfectious or drug-induced. See also: ➤ anaemia, ➤ cold autoantibody type, ➤ warm autoantibody type, ➤ drug-induced immune haemolytic anaemia.

Autoimmune hepatitis (AIH). Chronic autoimmune-mediated hepatic inflammation characterized by antinuclear (ANA), smooth muscle (SMA)/anti-F-actin, liver–kidney microsomal (LKM), and soluble liver antigen (SLA) antibodies. Autoimmune hepatitis constitutes 10–20% of all cases of chronic hepatitis. It may be idiopathic (AIH type 1, 2, and 3), part of autoimmune polyendocrine syndrome type 1 (APECED hepatitis), or drug-induced. See also: ➤ liver–kidney microsomal antibodies, ➤ liver-specific antigens.

Autoimmune lymphoproliferative syndrome (ALPS). Also known as Canale-Smith syndrome. Characterized by lymphadenopathy, hepatosplenomegaly, autoimmune cytopenias, and hypergammaglobulinaemia. Associated with defects in the Fas–FasL apoptosis signalling pathway due to mutations in the ➤ Fas gene, the FasL gene, or other genes coding for factors of this pathway.

Autoimmune regulator (AIRE). An important DNA binding protein involved in immunoregulation (probably in the establishment and maintenance of tolerance). AIRE is expressed mostly in cells of lymphoid tissues. In the thymus, AIRE is expressed in two types of antigen-presenting cells that are central in the negative selection of self-reactive T cells. The absence of a functional AIRE protein (caused by mutations in both copies of the AIRE-1 gene) results in the APECED syndrome, also known as autoimmune polyglandular syndrome type 1. See also: ➡ polyendocrinopathies, autoimmune.

Autoimmunity. Inappropriate reaction of the immune system against the organism's own antigens (➡ autoantigens) that may be either destructive or non-destructive. Destructive autoimmunity is associated with the development of ➡ autoimmune diseases.

Bcl-2. Human oncoprotein that plays a role in tissue development and maintenance by preventing ➡ apoptosis of specific cell types. Animal models suggest that failure to induce normal levels of apoptosis due to overexpression of Bcl-2 may contribute to the development of lymphoproliferative disorders and acceleration of autoimmunity. The role in human autoimmunity is not clear at this time.

B lymphocytes (B cells). Bone marrow-derived lymphocytes, expressing an antigen–receptor complex composed of membrane-bound ➡ immunoglobulin (mIg) and associated molecular chains. B cell receptors interact with ➡ epitopes directly (no MHC restriction). Activated B lymphocytes produce ➡ antibody and are efficient ➡ antigen-presenting cells. They are the precursors of plasma cells.

Bullous skin diseases, autoimmune. Characterized by intraepidermal or subepidermal blisters (e.g. pemphigus vulgaris, bullous pemphigoid) and highly specific ➡ autoantibodies against components of the desmosome or hemidesmosome (e.g. desmoglein 3, BP180). May be idiopathic or paraneoplastic (caused by various lymphoproliferative malignancies).

Cardiolipin. Main target of ➡ antiphospholipid antibodies.

Carrier. An immunogenic macromolecule (usually protein) to which a ➡ hapten is attached, allowing the hapten to be immunogenic.

CD. A molecular marker on a cell surface that may be used operationally to define phenotype, origin, and activation state of the cell.

CD3. A molecule composed of five polypeptide chains associated with the heterodimer ➡ T cell receptor (TCR), forming the T cell receptor complex (TCR/CD3); CD3 transduces the activating signals when antigen binds to the TCR.

CD4. A cell surface antigen belonging to the ➡ immunoglobulin superfamily of molecules. Marker of T helper cells. As an adhesion molecule, it interacts with the non-polymorphic part of ➡ MHC class II gene product.

$CD4^+CD25^+$ T cells. Subtype of regulatory $CD4^+$ T cells with potential role in the regulation of the immune homeostasis. Seems to be important in preventing the development of ➡ autoimmune diseases (depletion leads to the spontaneous development of various autoimmune diseases in genetically susceptible animals; transfer prevents the development of organ-specific autoimmunity).

$CD5^+$ B lymphocytes. Lymphocytes of type B1-a, which are predominant in fetal lymphoid organs and in neonatal cord blood. In adults, these cells range from 2% to 6% of total mononuclear cells in peripheral blood. They utilize an immunoglobulin variable gene repertoire different from that of $CD5^-$ B cells and produce ➡ natural autoantibodies. The expansion of autoreactive B1-a cells has been reported in peripheral blood of patients with autoimmune diseases (e.g. ➡ rheumatoid arthritis, ➡ Sjögren syndrome, ➡ antiphospholipid syndrome). In rheumatoid arthritis, these cells can account for up to 60% of circulating B cells and may produce ➡ rheumatoid factor. The pathological relevance of these observations is unclear, however.

CD8. A cell surface molecule belonging to the ➡ immunoglobulin superfamily of molecules found, among others, on cytotoxic T cells.

$CD8^+$ T suppressor cells. Regulatory T cells that inhibit the proliferation of antigen-specific T cells. Three different subpopulations have been functionally identified in humans. Functional alterations were shown to be associated with the relapse of autoimmune diseases.

CD16. Low-affinity Fcγ receptor (FcγRIII) expressed mainly on ➡ natural killer cells, granulocytes, and ➡ macrophages, mediating ➡ antibody-dependent cell-mediated cytotoxicity.

CD23. Low-affinity Fcε receptor induced by IL-4 and expressed on activated B cells and ➡ macrophages.

CD25. Alpha-chain of the ➡ interleukin 2 receptor.

CD40 ligand (CD40L). Essential molecule for normal switching signalling through binding to CD40 on B cells. The interaction of CD40L and CD40 is also critical for optimal T cell function. See also: ➡ hyper IgM syndrome.

Cell-mediated or cellular response. A specific immune response in which ➡ T lymphocytes mediate the effects, either through the release of ➡ cytokines or through cytotoxicity.

Chemokines. Large family of small secreted proteins (8–15 kilodaltons) that control the trafficking of leukocyte subpopulations, induce leukocyte activation, and control ➡ lymphocyte differentiation and effector function. May play an important role in the pathogenesis of autoimmune diseases, because the migration and accumulation of leukocytes in the target organs are critical steps for this.

Clonal anergy. State of specific functional unresponsiveness. Failure of B or T cells to proliferate in response to antigen by downregulation of the antigen receptor complex and/or cytokine receptors and costimulatory molecules. Primary mechanism involved in the induction and maintenance of ➡ self-tolerance.

Clonal deletion. Elimination (e.g. by ➡ apoptosis, receptor editing) of self-reacting B or T cells during their maturation in central or peripheral lymphoid tissues. Primary mechanism involved in the induction and maintenance of ➡ self-tolerance.

Clonal indifference (ignorance). Failure of B or T cells expressing anti-self-receptors to interact with antigen (e.g. by low valency, low concentration, or sequestration of antigens; low receptor avidity; lack of costimulatory molecules). Primary mechanism involved in the induction and maintenance of ➡ self-tolerance.

Coeliac disease. Also known as gluten-sensitive enteropathy (GSE). A lifelong intolerance to a protein fraction of grain (e.g. gluten of wheat), leading to intestinal villous atrophy and crypt hyperplasia and characterized by specific autoimmune responses against tissue transglutaminase.

Cold autoantibody type. Autoantibodies that react optimally at low temperatures (0–5 °C) with surface antigens of red blood cells. They mediate ➡ autoimmune haemolytic anaemia by either cold agglutinins (cold haemagglutinin disease) or cold haemolysins (paroxysmal cold haemoglobinuria).

Complement system. A group of serum proteins with the capacity to interact with each other when activated. The chain reaction of the activated complement components results in formation of a lytic complex and several biologically active peptides of low molecular weight (anaphylatoxins). The system can be activated by antigen–antibody complexes (classical pathway) and by other components, e.g. bacteria (alternative pathway). As an effector mechanism of the humoral immune response, the activated complement system facilitates opsonization, phagocytosis, and lysis of cellular antigens. Some defects in components of complement are associated with autoimmune diseases (see ➡ complement deficiency).

Complement deficiency. Congenital deficiencies in the various components of the ➡ complement system. Rheumatic disorders (mainly ➡ systemic lupus erythematosus) are associated with deficiencies of the early components of the classical pathway. More than 30% of individuals with C2 deficiency and nearly 80% with either C3 or C4 deficiency have an autoimmune manifestation.

Connective tissue diseases. Systemic autoimmune rheumatic diseases, including ➡ systemic lupus erythematosus, ➡ Sjögren syndrome, ➡ systemic sclerosis (scleroderma), autoimmune ➡ myositis (polymyositis, dermatomyositis), ➡ mixed connective tissue disease, and other overlapping syndromes.

Crohn disease. An ongoing disorder that causes inflammation of the digestive tract, also referred to as the gastrointestinal tract. Crohn disease can affect any area of the gastrointestinal tract, from the mouth to the anus, but it most commonly affects the lower part of the small intestine, called the ileum.

Cross-reactivity. The ability of an antibody or a T cell specific for one antigen to react with a second antigen; a measure of relatedness between two antigenic substances and/or polyspecificity of the antibody molecule (e.g. some rheumatoid factors) or of the T cell receptor.

Cryoglobulinaemic vasculitis. Cutaneous or systemic vasculitis caused by frigolabile proteins (➡ cryoglobulins, cryofibrinogen) that leads to increased viscosity, protein precipitation or gelatinification, complement activation, and endothelial cell damage, especially in the cold. Frequently associated with chronic hepatitis C or B infection, but can also be induced by other infections and malignancies.

Cryoglobulins. Precipitating ➡ immunoglobulins, forming insoluble aggregates at temperatures below body temperature. Many cryoglobulins function as ➡ autoantibodies (e.g. ➡ rheumatoid factor). Cryoglobulins are found in lymphoproliferative diseases, a number of autoimmune diseases, as well as chronic infections. They can lead to vasculitic and secondary thrombotic manifestations (➡ cryoglobulinaemic vasculitis, glomerulonephritis).

Cytokines. Group of substances (biologically active peptides), mainly synthesized by lymphocytes (lymphokines) or monocytes/macrophages (monokines), that modulate the function of cells in immunological reactions; cytokines include ➡ interleukins. Some cytokines (pleotrophic cytokines) have a broad spectrum of biological actions, including neuromodulation, growth factor activity, and proinflammatory activity.

Cytotoxic T lymphocyte (CTL). A subpopulation of T cells with the capacity to lyse target cells displaying a determinant in association with MHC gene products, recognized by its antigen receptor complex (TCR/CD3).

Defensin. A family of potent antibiotics made within the body by ➡ neutrophils and ➡ macrophages. The defensins play important roles against invading microbes. They act against bacteria, fungi, and viruses by binding to their membranes and increasing membrane permeability. On a chemical level, the defensins are small peptides unusually rich in the amino acid cysteine (Cys). The human defensins are classified into the α-defensins and β-defensins on the basis of their sequence homology and their Cys residues.

Dendritic cell (DC). A cell type characterized by extended cytoplasmic protrusions and a high expression of ➡ adhesion molecules and ➡ MHC class II gene products effecting ➡ antigen presentation to specific ➡ lymphocytes. Dendritic cells also play a crucial role in the establishment of both central and peripheral ➡ self-tolerance. See also: ➡ Langerhans' cells.

Dermatitis. Inflammatory skin disease showing redness, swelling, infiltration, scaling, and sometimes vesicles and blisters.

Desensitization. Generally transient state of specific non-reactivity in previously sensitized individual, resulting from repeated antigen exposures.

Diabetes mellitus, insulin-dependent (IDDM). Former term for ➡ diabetes mellitus type 1.

Diabetes mellitus type 1 (T1D). Autoimmune form of diabetes mellitus caused by immune-mediated destruction of insulin-producing beta cells in the pancreas with irreversible loss of insulin production. ➡ Islet cell autoantibodies and autoantibodies directed against ➡ glutamic acid decarboxylase, insulin, and the IA2-antigen are diagnostic markers for T1D as well as risk markers for the development of this disease.

Double-stranded DNA (dsDNA). Main target of ➡ autoantibodies in patients with ➡ systemic lupus erythematosus. DsDNA autoantibody is a diagnostic marker and classification criterion of this disease.

D-Penicillamine. A drug that is able to induce a variety of autoantibodies and autoimmune diseases (e.g. ➡ myasthenia gravis, polymyositis). Disease usually remits within one year after the medication is stopped.

Drug-induced lupus (DIL). A lupus-like disorder induced by various medications that is mainly characterized by the occurrence of arthralgia, myalgia, pleuritis, erythema, fever, and ➡ antinuclear antibody production. The clinical symptoms disappear within a few days to weeks after withdrawal of the causative drug, and the associated autoimmune phenomena disappear within the course of a year. Classical lupus-inducing drugs are procainamide, hydralazine, and quinidine.

Drug-induced immune haemolytic anaemia. Anaemia caused by drug-mediated immune haemolysis of red blood cells through different antibody-mediated mechanisms: (i) drug adsorption mechanism (antibody directed against the drug bound to red blood cell surface antigen), (ii) ternary (immune) complex mechanism (antibody forms a trimolecular complex with the drug and red blood cell membrane antigen), and (iii) true autoantibody-mediated mechanism (drug-induced antibodies bind red blood cells in the absence of the drug).

Eczema. A ➡ dermatitis characterized by non-contagious inflammation of skin with typical clinical (itch, erythema, papules, seropapules, vesicles, squames, crusts, lichenification) and dermato-histological (spongiosis, acanthosis, parakeratosis, lymphocytic infiltration) findings. Often due to sensitization.

Endocytosis. The uptake by a cell of a substance from the environment by invagination of its plasma membrane; it includes both phagocytosis mediated by receptors and pinocytosis.

Enzyme-linked immunosorbent assay (ELISA). An assay in which an enzyme is linked to an antibody and a labelled substance is used to measure the activity of bound enzyme and, hence, the amount of bound antibody. With a fixed amount of immobilized antigen, the amount of labelled antibody bound decreases as the concentration of unlabelled antigen is increased, allowing quantification of unlabelled antigen (competitive ELISA). With a fixed amount of one immobilized antibody, the binding of a second, labelled antibody increases as the concentration of antigen increases, allowing quantification of antigen (sandwich ELISA). ELISAs are used for the specific determination of ➡ autoantibodies.

Epidemiology. The study of the distribution and determinants of health-related states or events in specified populations, and the application of this knowledge to manage health problems.

Epitope. Antigenic determinant, a structure of biological molecules that mediate specific recognition by the immune system.

Epitope spreading. Increase in the number of epitopes targeted by autoantibodies and/or T cells. May be on the same autoantigen (intramolecular epitope spreading) and/or on other autoantigens (intermolecular epitope spreading). Characteristic sign of progression of autoimmune disease from initial activation to a chronic state.

Experimental allergic encephalomyelitis (EAE). Autoimmune demyelinating disease induced in genetically susceptible mice, rats, or marmosets by immunization with myelin proteins or peptides. Animal model for ➡ multiple sclerosis.

Experimental autoimmune thyroiditis (EAT). Autoimmune thyroiditis experimentally induced in several strains of mice and rats by immunization with thyroglobulin or by neonatal thymectomy.

Fas. A so-called "death receptor", an inducer of extrinsic apoptosis signalling pathway, and also has a role in many other normal and pathological processes — for example, in cancer. It is a differentiation antigen (synonyms: APO-1, CD95) expressed in a variety of cell lines, including myeloid and lymphoblastoid cell lines. The primary role is to regulate peripheral immune responses, which is achieved by triggering ➡ apoptosis. Mutations of Fas or its ligand (FasL) are associated with peripheral lymphoid tissue expansion and autoimmune diseases. See also: ➡ autoimmune lymphoproliferative syndrome.

Fc receptors. Receptors expressed on a wide range of cells, interacting with the Fc portion of ➡ immunoglobulins belonging to various isotypes. Membrane-bound Fc receptors mediate different effector functions (endocytosis, ➡ antibody-dependent cell-mediated cytotoxicity) and induce mediator release. Both the membrane-bound and soluble forms of Fc receptors regulate antibody production of B cells.

Fibrillarin. A component of a nucleolar small nuclear ribonucleoprotein, functioning in vivo in ribosomal RNA processing.

FOXP3. Transcription repressor that is specifically expressed in $CD4^+CD25^+$ T cells. Mutations in the FOXP3 gene may lead to an autoimmune syndrome called ➡ IPEX (immunodysregulation–polyendocrinopathy–enteropathy–X-linked).

Gangliosides. Components of all vertebrate cell membranes. Glycolipids that are expressed at high densities in peripheral nervous tissues. Targets of autoantibodies in autoimmune ➡ peripheral neuropathies (e.g. anti-GM1, -GQ1b, -GD1b). Induced by infection, ➡ natural autoantibodies cross-reacting with gangliosides may become pathogenic after affinity maturation and class switching.

Gastritis, autoimmune. Autoimmune-mediated destruction of the gastric mucosa that may result in the development of ➡ pernicious anaemia. Autoimmune gastritis is associated with autoantibodies to H^+/K^+-ATPase of gastric parietal cells as well as autoantibodies to the intrinsic factor produced by these cells.

Gliadin. A protein that is found in wheat and some other grains, including oats, rye, barley, and millet. People with ➡ coeliac disease are sensitive to gliadin in the diet and produce antibodies to gliadin as well as autoantibodies to ➡ tissue transglutaminase.

Glomerular basement membrane (GBM). Target of autoantibodies in patients with ➡ Goodpasture disease. The autoantigenic ➡ epitope is a peptide on the α3 chain of type IV collagen, which is also found in renal tubular and alveolar basement membrane.

Glomerulonephropathy. Disease of the glomeruli, which may show either thickening of the ➡ glomerular basement membrane due to the accretion of proteins or a minimal change glomerulopathy, in which there is functional damage but little structural change by light microscopy.

Glutamic acid decarboxylase (GAD). Main autoantigen in ➡ diabetes mellitus type 1 and stiff-person syndrome (a neurological autoimmune disease). Localized in pancreatic beta cells and GABA-ergic neurons.

Goodpasture disease/syndrome. An autoimmune pulmonary–renal syndrome characterized by pulmonary haemorrhage, glomerulonephritis, and production of autoantibody to ➡ glomerular basement membrane; anti-GBM disease.

Graves disease. Hyperthyroidism associated with diffuse hyperplastic goitre resulting from production of a ➡ thyroid-stimulating hormone receptor binding autoantibody.

Hapten. A non-immunogenic compound of low molecular weight that becomes immunogenic after conjugation with a carrier protein or cell and in this form induces immune responses. Antibodies, but not T cells, can bind the hapten alone in the absence of carrier.

Hashimoto thyroiditis. Goitrous form of diffuse autoimmune thyroiditis. See also: ➡ thyroiditis, autoimmune.

Helper T lymphocyte. A functional subpopulation of T cells (expressing CD4 antigen) that helps to generate cytotoxic T cells and cooperate with B cells in the production of an antibody response. Helper T cells recognize antigen in association with ➡ MHC class II gene products. Depending on their capacity to produce various ➡ cytokines, one can functionally differentiate ➡ Th1 (IL-2 and IFN gamma producing) and ➡ Th2 (IL-3, IL-4, and IL-6 producing) cells.

Heparin-induced thrombocytopenia (HIT). Most frequent antibody-mediated drug-induced thrombocytopenia. Occurs in 1–2% of patients treated with heparin intravenously for longer than four days. Mediated by antibodies to complexes formed between heparin and the endogenous platelet factor 4 (PF4).

Hepatitis, chronic. See: ➡ autoimmune hepatitis.

Human leukocyte antigen (HLA). The major human histocompatibility complex situated on chromosome 6. Human HLA-A, -B, and -C (resembling mouse H2k, d, and l) are MHC class I molecules, whereas HLA-DP, -DQ, and -DR (resembling mouse I-A and I-E) are MHC class II molecules.

Humoral immune response. An immune response in which specific antibodies induce the effector functions (such as phagocytosis and activation of the ➡ complement system).

Hypergammaglobulinaemia. Increase of gammaglobulins in the blood by paraproteinaemia or increased production of ➡ immunoglobulins.

Hyper IgM syndrome (HIGM). Primary T cell defect due to mutations in the CD40 ligand. Characterized by recurrent (opportunistic) infections and very low levels of IgG and IgA. Autoimmune manifestations (e.g. cytopenia, arthritis, sclerosing cholangitis) are often seen.

Hyperreactivity. An abnormally increased response to a stimulus.

Hypersensitivity. Abnormally increased immunologically mediated response to a stimulus. Sometimes used loosely for any increased response.

Hypersusceptibility. Condition where adverse effects are induced in an individual under exposure conditions that result in no effects in the great majority of the population or a condition where an individual exhibits exaggerated effects in comparison with the great majority of those showing some adverse effects.

Hyperthyroidism. Hyperactivity of the thyroid gland. Autoimmunity is the most common cause of hyperthyroidism, accounting for 60–80% of cases. See also: ➡ Graves disease.

Hypothyroidism. Hypofunction (insufficiency) of the thyroid gland. Autoimmunity is the most common cause of hypothyroidism in iodine-sufficient countries. See also: ➡ thyroiditis, autoimmune; Hashimoto thyroiditis; primary myxoedema.

Idiopathic. A term that describes a "primary" symptom or disease in which no underlying cause or associated disorder could be found. In most cases, autoimmune processes are involved in the pathogenesis (e.g. ➡ idiopathic thrombocytopenic purpura, idiopathic ➡ Addison disease).

Idiopathic thrombocytopenic purpura (ITP). Autoantibody-mediated thrombocytopenia (autoimmune thrombocytopenic purpura).

Idiotype. Unique, genetically controlled determinants present on ➡ immunoglobulin variable domains and that determine the antibody specificity.

Idiotypic network. Feedback inhibition of ongoing B or T cell responses by a network of (anti-idiotype–idiotype) interactions. Secondary mechanism involved in the induction and maintenance of ➡ self-tolerance.

Immune complexes (IC). Antigen–antibody complexes formed every time ➡ antibody meets ➡ antigen. May become pathogenic by triggering a variety of inflammatory processes if not removed effectively from circulation or if formed in situ. Immune complexes play a role in vasculitic manifestations of autoimmune diseases (e.g. lupus nephritis).

Immune deviation. A regulatory mechanism of the preferential activation of one arm (cellular versus humoral; see also ➡ Th1 and ➡ Th2 cells) of the adaptive immune system at the expense of the other. Although not a form of true tolerance, this regulatory mechanism may be involved in the induction and maintenance of ➡ self-tolerance.

Immunodeficiency. Defects in one or more components of the immune system, resulting in inability to eliminate or neutralize non-autoantigens. Congenital or primary immunodeficiencies are genetic or due to developmental disorders (such as congenital thymic aplasia). Acquired or secondary immunodeficiencies develop as a consequence of malnutrition, malignancies, immunosuppressive compounds, radiation, or infection of immunocompetent T cells with human immunodeficiency virus (HIV). Defects of the nonspecific defence system may also result in immunodeficiency. Immunodeficiency and autoimmune phenomena may occur concomitantly in the same individual. Many immunodeficiency syndromes are associated with autoimmune diseases. Immune dysregulation, persistent antigen stimulation, recurrent tissue damage, and defective clearance of immune complexes are pathogenic factors that may lead to autoimmunity in immunodeficient individuals. See also: ➡ complement deficiency, ➡ selective IgA deficiency, ➡ hyper IgM syndrome.

Immunogen. A substance capable of eliciting a specific immune response manifested by the formation of specific ➡ antibodies and/or specifically committed ➡ lymphocytes. To induce an antibody response, an immunogen must possess structurally and functionally distinct determinants for activation of B cells and T cells.

Immunoglobulin (Ig). Immunity-conferring portion of the plasma or serum gammaglobulins. Various isotypes (classes and subclasses) of immunoglobulins have a common core structure of two identical light (L) and two identical heavy (H) polypeptide chains, which contain repeating homologous units folded in common globular motifs (Ig domains). The amino acid sequences of the N-terminal domains are variable (V domains), in contrast to the more conserved constant regions (C domains). The V domains contain the complementarity-determining regions forming the antigen-binding sites, whereas the C domains trigger several effector functions of the immune system. See also: ➡ antibody.

Immunoglobulin gene superfamily. Genes encoding proteins containing one or more immunoglobulin domains (homology units) that are homologous to either Ig V or C domains. Cell surface and soluble molecules mediating recognition, adhesion, or binding functions in and outside the immune system, derived from the same precursor, belong to this family of molecules (e.g. ➡ immunoglobulin, ➡ T cell receptor, ➡ MHC class I and class II, ➡ CD4, ➡ CD8, FcγR).

Incidence (epidemiological). The number of new cases of disease in a defined population during a specified period of time.

Indirect immunofluorescence. Screening method for the presence of non-organ- and organ-specific autoantibodies. Tumour cell monolayer (e.g. Hep-2 cells for analysing ➡ antinuclear antibodies), cytocentrifuged cells (e.g. neutrophil granulocytes for analysing ➡ antineutrophil cytoplasmic autoantibodies), or organ cryostat sections (e.g. liver and kidney for analysing ➡ liver–kidney microsomal antibodies, pancreas for analysing ➡ islet cell antibodies) are used as targets.

Infertility, autoimmune. Caused by sperm antibodies, autoimmune ovarian inflammation (oophoritis), or autoimmune orchitis. May be part of ➡ polyendocrinopathies.

Inflammatory bowel diseases. Chronic, relapsing, and tissue-destructive ➡ idiopathic intestinal inflammation probably as a result of inappropriate responses to luminal antigens (e.g. food breakdown products, bacterial products, or ➡ autoantigens). ➡ Autoantibodies against proteins of neutrophil granulocytes, pancreatic acinus, intestinal goblet, and colonic epithelial cells are detectable. Subtypes that differ in clinical histology and serology are ➡ Crohn disease and ➡ ulcerative colitis. Crohn disease is immunologically characterized by antibody to *Saccharomyces cerevisiae* and ➡ Th1 cell-dominated responses.

Interclonal competition. Favouring of foreign-specific ➡ lymphocytes at the expense of self-specific lymphocytes. Secondary mechanism involved in the induction and maintenance of ➡ self-tolerance.

Interleukin. Immunoregulatory proteins, also designated as lymphokines, monokines, or ➡ cytokines. General features are low molecular weight (<80 000 daltons) and frequently glycosylated; regulate immune cell function and inflammation by binding to specific cell surface receptors; transient and local production; act in paracrine, autocrine, or endocrine manner, with stimulatory or blocking effect on growth/differentiation; very potent, function at picomolar concentrations. Interleukins represent an extensive series of mediators with a wide range of overlapping functions. Other mediators in this series are *c*-kit ligand, interferons, tumour necrosis factor, transforming growth factor, and a family of low relative molecular mass mediators called ➡ chemokines.

Intolerance. Non-immunologically mediated adverse reactions. In food intolerances, these may be due to pharmacological properties of food constituents, metabolic disorders, or responses of unknown etiology.

IPEX. X-linked syndrome characterized by immunodysregulation, polyendocrinopathy (➡ diabetes mellitus type 1, ➡ thyroiditis), haemolytic anaemia, ➡ thrombocytopenia, ➡ dermatitis, and enteropathy, caused by mutations in ➡ FOXP3.

Iron. Vital metal for the proliferation of all cells including those of the immune system. May be involved in the induction of autoimmunity by influencing the antigen presentation (catalysing the production of cryptic ➡ epitopes of ➡ autoantigens).

Islet cell antibodies (ICA). Autoantibodies reacting with endocrine (pancreatic islet) cells and detectable by ➡ indirect immunofluorescence on pancreas cryostat sections. Diagnostic marker of ➡ diabetes mellitus type 1.

Kidney diseases, autoimmune. May be due to immunological reaction to renal antigens (➡ glomerular basal membrane, ➡ Goodpasture disease/syndrome) or part of systemic autoimmune disease (e.g. ➡ systemic lupus erythematosus, ➡ ANCA-associated vasculitides).

Lambert-Eaton myasthenic syndrome (LEMS). Paraneoplastic neurological disorder associated with small-cell lung cancer and caused by autoantibodies against voltage-gated calcium channels.

Langerhans' cells. Bone marrow-derived epidermal cells with a dendritic morphology, expressing CD1 marker in humans and containing the cytoplasmic organelle called the Birbeck granule. They express MHC class II antigen and are capable of antigen presentation. See also: ➡ dendritic cells.

Leukocytopenia. Amount of leukocytes below normal values. Characteristic feature of systemic autoimmune diseases (e.g. Felty syndrome, ➡ systemic lupus erythematosus, ➡ Sjögren syndrome, ➡ mixed connective tissue disease).

Leukocytosis. Abnormal increase in the number of white blood cells.

Liver disease, autoimmune. Diseases caused by autoimmune-mediated inflammation and/or fibrosis: ➡ autoimmune hepatitis, ➡ primary biliary cirrhosis, and ➡ primary sclerosing cholangitis.

Liver–kidney microsomal antibodies (LKM). Autoantibodies directed against cytochrome P450 and uridine diphosphate (UDP)-glucuronosyltransferase (UGT) antigens typically found in patients with immune-mediated hepatitis: LKM-1 antibodies (cytochrome P4502D6) in patients with ➡ autoimmune hepatitis type 2 (AIH-2) and autoimmunity associated with hepatitis C; LKM-2 (cytochrome P4502C9) in patients with drug-induced hepatitis caused by tienilic acid; and LKM-3 (UGT-1) in patients with chronic hepatitis D and AIH-2.

Liver-specific antigens. Some of these become targets of autoantibodies. Liver microsomal antibodies reacting with cytochrome P4501A2 are found in patients with drug-induced hepatitis due to dihydralazine or in ➡ autoimmune hepatitis as part of autoimmune polyendocrine syndrome type 1. Autoantibodies against soluble liver or liver–pancreas antigen are found in patients with autoimmune hepatitis. Autoantibodies against asialoglycoprotein receptor are frequently found in autoimmune liver diseases, but also in viral-induced and other liver inflammation.

Long-acting thyroid stimulator (LATS). Former term for TSH-R stimulating autoantibodies. See also: ➡ thyroid-stimulating hormone receptor.

Lymphocytopenia. Amount of ➡ lymphocytes below normal values. Characteristic feature of systemic autoimmune diseases (e.g. ➡ systemic lupus erythematosus, ➡ Sjögren syndrome, ➡ mixed connective tissue disease).

Lymphocyte. Bone marrow-derived cell with little cytoplasm, with the ability to migrate and exchange between the circulation and tissues, to home to sites of antigen exposure, and to be held back at these sites. The only cells that specifically recognize and respond to antigens (mainly with the help of accessory cells). Lymphocytes consist of various subsets differing in their function and products (e.g. ➡ B lymphocytes, ➡ helper T lymphocytes, ➡ cytotoxic T lymphocytes, ➡ regulatory T cells).

Macrophage. Mononuclear cells derived from monocytes residing in tissues. Activated by different stimuli, they may appear in various forms, such as epitheloid cells and multinucleate giant cells. Macrophages found in different organs and connective tissues have been named according to the specific locations, e.g. as microglia, alveolar macrophages, or Kupffer cells. Macrophages may function as ➡ antigen-presenting cells, effector cells of cell-mediated immunity, and phagocytes eliminating opsonized antigens.

Major histocompatibility complex (MHC). A cluster of genes encoding cell surface antigens that are polymorphic within a species and have a crucial function in signalling between lymphocytes and cells expressing antigen and in recognition of self.

MHC class I gene products. Antigens encoded by the MHC class I genes are expressed on all nucleated cells. They present antigen-derived peptides of endogenous origin.

MHC class II gene products. Antigens encoded by the MHC class II genes are expressed on antigen-presenting cells. They present antigen-derived peptides of endogenous origin.

Microscopic polyangiitis (MPA). ANCA-associated necrotizing, pauci immune vasculitis of the small vessels (capillaries, venules, arterioles) frequently associated with rapidly progressive glomerulonephritis and/or haemorrhagic alveolitis as well as autoantibodies against ➡ myeloperoxidase.

Mitogen. A substance that causes cells to synthesize DNA and proliferate without acting as an ➡ antigen.

Mixed connective tissue disease (MCTD). Systemic autoimmune disease with features of ➡ systemic lupus erythematosus, ➡ systemic sclerosis, and dermatomyositis/polymyositis and high-titred autoantibodies against U1-RNP specific proteins. See also: ➡ myositis, autoimmune.

Molecular mimicry. Existence of a cross-reactive epitope between microbial proteins and ➡ autoantigens. Suggested as one cause of initiating pathological autoimmunity.

Monocyte. Bone marrow-derived mononuclear phagocytic leukocyte, with bean-shaped nucleus and fine granular cytoplasm containing lysosomes, phagocytic vacuoles, and cytoskeletal filaments. Once transported to tissues, monocytes develop into macrophages.

Multiple sclerosis. Autoimmune disorder characterized by destruction of myelin in the central nervous system.

Muscle diseases, autoimmune. Autoimmune diseases associated with profound weakness due to immunological injury of the myofibre (➡ myositis, autoimmune) or affecting the neuromuscular junction (➡ myasthenia gravis, acquired, ➡ Lambert-Eaton myasthenic syndrome).

Myasthenia gravis, acquired. The most well understood autoimmune disease. Muscle weakness usually affecting ocular and oropharyngeal muscles due to an autoimmune attack against the neuromuscular junction (e.g. nicotinic acetylcholine receptor). May be ➡ idiopathic, paraneoplastic (thymic tumour), or drug-induced (D-penicillamine).

Myeloperoxidase (MPO). This enzyme of azurophilic granules of ➡ neutrophils is the major target of pANCA (see ➡ antineutrophil cytoplasmic autoantibodies). MPO autoantibodies are diagnostic markers for ➡ microscopic polyangiitis, rapidly progressive glomerulonephritis, and ➡ Goodpasture disease/syndrome. They are also found in patients exposed to silica or drugs (e.g. hydralazine, propylthiouracil, D-penicillamine) as well as in some patients with ➡ Wegener granulomatosis and other autoimmune diseases.

Myositis, autoimmune. Rare systemic inflammatory myopathies, including primary polymyositis, primary dermatomyositis, myositis associated with malignancy, childhood dermatomyositis, and myositis with multisystem autoimmune disease (e.g. ➡ mixed connective tissue disease, ➡ systemic sclerosis). Autoantibodies against aminoacyl-tRNA synthetases (e.g. anti-Jo-1), signal recognition particle (e.g. anti-SRP54), nuclear helicase (anti-Mi-2), tRNA and tRNA–protein complexes (e.g. anti-Mas), and translation factor (anti-KJ) have been described as myositis specific.

Natural autoantibodies (NAA). Part of the naturally occurring repertoire of polyreactive antibodies that bind to autoantigens with low affinity. They are mainly of IgM isotype and produced by ➡ $CD5^+$ B lymphocytes. Natural antibodies and their producing cells may have a physiological role in the following processes: (i) first line of protection against external invaders, (ii) elimination of degraded autoantigens and senescent cells, and (iii) tolerization of T cells by presenting autoantigens, thereby in protecting from development of pathological autoimmunity. In contrast, natural autoantibodies may become pathogenic in clonal B cell disorders, e.g. monoclonal anti-I antibodies in cold agglutinin disease cause ➡ autoimmune haemolytic anaemia.

Natural killer (NK) cell. A subset of ➡ lymphocytes found in blood and some lymphoid tissues, derived from the bone marrow and appearing as large granular lymphocytes. NK cells possess the capacity to kill certain tumour cells or virus-infected normal cells. The killing is not induced by specific antigen and is not restricted by MHC molecules.

Natural resistance-associated macrophage protein (NRAMP1). Iron transporter that plays a critical role in macrophage activation and differentiation. Allele 3 of the NRAMP1 promoter is associated with autoimmune disorders (e.g. ➡ rheumatoid arthritis, juvenile rheumatoid arthritis, ➡ diabetes mellitus type 1, ➡ multiple sclerosis).

Nephritis, autoimmune. Inflammation of the kidney (proteinuria and nephritic urinary sediment) due to immunological reaction to renal antigens (anti-glomerular basement membrane disease, ➡ Goodpasture disease/syndrome; autoimmune tubulo-interstitial nephritis with antibody to tubular basement membrane) or as part of systemic autoimmune diseases independent of renal autoantigens (lupus nephritis in ➡ systemic lupus erythematosus, interstitial nephritis in ➡ Sjögren syndrome, nephritis in ➡ ANCA-associated vasculitis, cryoglobulinaemic vasculitis or hypocomplementaemic urticarial vasculitis syndrome).

Nephropathy. Disease of the kidney that may involve either or both the glomeruli (specialized structures where blood is filtered) and the renal tubules (connected structures where the composition of the filtrate is greatly modified in accordance with the physiological needs of the body).

Nephrotic syndrome. A clinical disease in which damage to glomeruli has caused leaky filtration, resulting in major loss of protein from the body.

Neuropathies, autoimmune. Autoimmune diseases of the nervous system are a major concern in neurological practice. More and more neuropathies are described as autoimmune or possibly autoimmune in nature. Little is known about ➡ xenobiotics in the pathogenesis, but infections may play an important role in the initiation of some diseases. Autoimmune neuropathies may be manifested at the neuromuscular junction, as central nervous system diseases (e.g. ➡ multiple sclerosis, ➡ paraneoplastic neurological syndromes, stiff-person syndrome, as well as manifestations of systemic autoimmune diseases), and diseases of the peripheral nerves (e.g. various forms of acute and chronic demyelinating neuropathies). See also: ➡ muscle diseases, autoimmune.

Neutrophil (polymorphonuclear leukocyte). Granular leukocytes having a nucleus with three to five lobes and fine cytoplasmic granules stainable by neutral dyes. The cells have properties of chemotaxis, adherence to immune complexes, and phagocytosis. The cells are involved in a variety of inflammatory processes, including late-phase allergic reactions.

Oncogenes. Genes that can potentially induce neoplastic transformation. See also: ➡ proto-oncogenes.

Opsonization. Coating of antigens with antibody and/or complement components. The interaction of opsonized complexes with Fc or complement receptors facilitates their uptake by the receptor-bearing phagocytic cells.

Oral tolerance. Orally induced and immune-mediated non-responsiveness.

Ouchterlony technique. Double-radial immunodiffusion for the detection of precipitating autoantibodies against "extractable nuclear antigens". Method of high diagnostic specificity but low sensitivity for diagnosis of autoimmune rheumatic diseases.

Paraneoplastic autoimmune syndromes. Autoimmune diseases that are caused by tumour-induced perturbations of the immune system with damaging effects on various organ systems (e.g. cancer-associated retinopathy, ➡ paraneoplastic neurological syndromes, paraneoplastic cutaneous syndromes). In most cases, autoantibodies generated by antitumour immunity are responsible for the tissue injury.

Paraneoplastic neurological syndromes. Group of neurological disorders mainly caused by cancer-induced immune mechanisms. Any part of the nervous system may be affected. In most cases, the neurological symptoms (e.g. different forms of encephalitis, cerebellar degeneration, stiff-person syndrome, sensory neuronopathy, myasthenic syndromes, ➤ peripheral neuropathies) precede the diagnosis of cancer. Autoantibodies against neuromuscular junction (e.g. against proteins of acetylcholine receptor, calcium and potassium channels), Purkinje cells (e.g. anti-Yo), and antineuronuclear antibodies (e.g. anti-Hu, anti-Ri) are highly specific for these syndromes.

Peripheral neuropathies, autoimmune. Acute or chronic inflammatory neuropathies leading to demyelination and axonal damage of nerves and nerve roots associated with high-titred autoantibodies against ➤ gangliosides (e.g. Guillain-Barré syndrome, Miller-Fisher syndrome, acute sensory ataxic neuropathy).

Pernicious anaemia. End stage of 10–15% of ➤ autoimmune gastritis due to vitamin B_{12} malabsorption caused by depletion of gastric parietal cells and autoantibodies against intrinsic factor. Associated with a variety of autoimmune endocrine diseases (e.g. ➤ Hashimoto thyroiditis, ➤ Addison disease) and autoimmune myasthenic syndromes.

Photosensitivity. Skin reddening due to an abnormal reaction to sunlight. A characteristic symptom of systemic autoimmune diseases (e.g. ➤ systemic lupus erythematosus, ➤ mixed connective tissue disease), cutaneous and ➤ subacute cutaneous lupus erythematosus.

Plasma cell. A terminally differentiated B lymphocyte with little or no capacity for mitotic division that can synthesize and secrete antibody. Plasma cells have eccentric nuclei, abundant cytoplasm, and distinct perinuclear haloes. The cytoplasm contains dense rough endoplasmic reticulum and a large Golgi complex.

Polyendocrinopathies, autoimmune. Autoimmune diseases affecting multiple endocrine organs. (i) The autoimmune polyglandular syndrome type 1 is characterized by mucocutaneous candidiasis in association with endocrine manifestation (also called APECED syndrome: autoimmune polyendocrinopathy–candidiasis–ectodermal–dystrophy), while (ii) the autoimmune polyglandular syndrome type 2 exhibits any combination of adrenal insufficiency (see: ➡ Addison disease), ➡ diabetes mellitus type 1, lymphocytic thyroiditis (see: ➡ thyroiditis, autoimmune), hypoparathyroidism, and gonadal failure. In both types, organ-specific autoantibodies against a variety of endocrine glands are detectable. See also: ➡ autoimmune regulator (AIRE).

Prevalence (epidemiology). The number of cases of disease occurring in a given population at a designated time.

Primary biliary cirrhosis (PBC). Autoimmune liver disease that results in the destruction of bile ducts, leading to fibrosis and cirrhosis. Primary biliary cirrhosis-specific are ➡ antimitochondrial antibodies directed against proteins of the pyruvate dehydrogenase complex (mainly the E2 subunit).

Primary myxoedema. Atrophic form of diffuse autoimmune thyroiditis. See also: ➡ thyroiditis, autoimmune.

Primary sclerosing cholangitis (PSC). Chronic, non-bacterial inflammatory narrowing of the bile ducts. Often associated with ulcerative colitis.

Prolactin. A versatile hormone that is involved in the regulation of proliferation and differentiation of a variety of cells in the immune system. May play a role in the pathogenesis and clinical expression of autoimmune diseases (e.g. ➡ systemic lupus erythematosus).

Proteinase 3 (PR3). This multifunctional enzyme of azurophilic granules of neutrophils and monocytes is the major target of cANCA (see: ➡ antineutrophil cytoplasmic autoantibodies). PR3 autoantibodies are diagnostic markers for ➡ Wegener granulomatosis and involved in the pathogenesis of this disease. They are also found in patients with other autoimmune systemic vasculitic diseases.

Proteinuria. Condition in which urine contains an abnormal amount of protein. Main symptom of ➡ nephritis.

Proto-oncogenes. Genes that may be involved in neoplastic transformation. The products of proto-oncogenes are important regulators of biological processes (e.g. growth factors, growth factor receptors, protein kinases, signal transducers, nuclear phosphoproteins, transcription factors). Mutations or aberrant expression of some proto-oncogenes may be involved in the pathogenesis of autoimmune diseases. See also: ➡ Bcl-2.

Rate (epidemiology). The frequency with which an event occurs in a defined population.

Raynaud phenomenon. Vasospastic condition characterized by acral circulatory disorders affecting the hands and feet. The symptoms can be triggered by cold, dampness, or emotional stress. Characteristic feature of systemic autoimmune diseases. Occurs in all or virtually all patients with ➡ systemic sclerosis, ➡ mixed connective tissue disease, and polymyositis/scleroderma overlap syndrome.

Regulatory T (Treg) cells. Cells that control the maintenance of normal immune homeostasis. They are involved in controlling (anergizing or counter-regulating) autoreactive cells that escaped from thymic negative selection. See also: ➡ $CD8^+$ T suppressor cells, ➡ $CD4^+CD25^+$ cells.

Rheumatoid arthritis (RA). An episodic inflammatory systemic disease with autoimmune pathogenetic mechanisms. It primarily affects the joints, causing symmetrical lesions and severe damage to the affected joints. Rheumatoid arthritis is the most common form of inflammatory joint disease (prevalence about 0.5–1%).

Rheumatoid factor (RF). Autoantibodies directed against the Fc region of altered IgG. Although detectable in various diseases, rheumatoid factor is used as a classification criterion of ➡ rheumatoid arthritis.

Selective IgA deficiency (SIgAD). The most common form of primary immunodeficiency. Autoimmunity is the most prevalent manifestation of this deficiency. Individuals with SIgAD have an increased risk of developing systemic (e.g. ➡ systemic lupus erythematosus, ➡ rheumatoid arthritis) and organ-specific (e.g. ➡ coeliac disease) autoimmune disorders.

Self-antigens. See ➡ autoantigens.

Self-tolerance. Specific immunological unresponsiveness to a defined ➡ autoantigen. Primary (➡ clonal deletion, ➡ anergy, ➡ clonal indifference) and secondary or regulatory (➡ interclonal competition, ➡ suppression, ➡ immune deviation, ➡ vetoing, feedback regulation by the ➡ idiotypic network) mechanisms are involved in the induction and maintenance of self-tolerance. Breaking self-tolerance may lead to pathological autoimmunity and development of ➡ autoimmune disease.

Sex hormones. Affect the immune system directly (e.g. by modulating the activity of $CD4^+$ cells and ➡ cytokine production and in turn by influencing B cell function and by affecting ➡ apoptosis of ➡ lymphocytes) or indirectly (e.g. by acting on a wide range of target tissues) and may thereby be involved in the development of pathological autoimmunity.

Sjögren syndrome. Chronic inflammatory autoimmune disease of the exocrine glands of unknown etiology. Its primary symptoms are keratoconjunctivitis sicca and xerostomia. Two types of Sjögren syndrome are distinguished: a primary (isolated) type and a secondary type associated with another underlying autoimmune disease (e.g. ➡ rheumatoid arthritis, ➡ systemic lupus erythematosus, ➡ systemic sclerosis, ➡ primary biliary cirrhosis, ➡ autoimmune hepatitis, ➡ multiple sclerosis, ➡ thyroiditis, autoimmune, etc.). Ro/SS-A and La/SS-B autoantibodies are used as classification criteria.

Spontaneous autoimmune thyroiditis (SAT). Autoimmune thyroiditis (➡ thyroiditis, autoimmune) that develops spontaneously (without any apparent cause or manipulation) in certain strains of mice and rats (e.g. NOD mice, BB and BUF rats) as well as in other animals (e.g. OS chickens, marmoset monkeys, beagles).

Stem cell. Pluripotent cells, representing 0.01% of bone marrow cells, having the capacity for self-renewal and committed to differentiate along particular lineages, e.g. erythroid, megakaryocytic, granulocytic, monocytic, and lymphocytic. Cytokines stimulate the proliferation and maturation of distinct precursors.

Subacute cutaneous lupus erythematosus (SCLE). A chronic remitting form of dermatitis characterized by severe photosensitivity and Ro/SS-A and La/SS-B autoantibodies.

Suppression. Dominant immunological tolerance, a phenomenon that plays an active role in regulating T and B cell responses to both foreign antigens and autoantigens (➡ suppressor T lymphocyte). The downregulation of responses to autoantigens is a major regulatory mechanism involved in the induction and maintenance of ➡ self-tolerance.

Suppressor T lymphocyte. A subpopulation of ➡ T lymphocytes that inhibits the activation phase of immune responses. They are $CD8^+$, and their growth and differentiation may be regulated by $CD4^+$ cells.

Systemic lupus erythematosus (SLE). A chronic, remitting-relapsing inflammatory autoimmune disease affecting multiple organ systems, such as the skin, joints, serosal membranes, kidneys, blood cells, and central nervous system. The disease is very heterogeneous in clinical expression and serological factors. Autoantibodies directed against nuclear components (➡ antinuclear antibodies) are typically detected. Anti-dsDNA, anti-Sm, and ➡ antiphospholipid antibodies are used as classification criteria.

Systemic sclerosis (SSc). Fibrosing disease of unclear etiology that affects multiple organ systems. The skin ("scleroderma") and blood vessels (arteries, small vessels) are most commonly affected, but involvement of the lungs and gastrointestinal tract (oesophagus) may also be observed. Anticentromer antibodies (ACA) as well as autoantibodies against DNA topoisomerase I (scl-70) and various nucleolar antigens are diagnostic and prognostic markers and often detectable years before disease manifestation. They are also detectable in quartz dust-exposed individuals.

T cell receptor (TCR). Antigen-specific receptor on T cells composed of one set of heterodimeric chains. Two types of TCR heterodimers are known (α/β and γ/δ). Functional binding for TCR requires a complex of ➡ major histocompatibility complex, antigenic peptide, and TCR.

Th0 cells. Subpopulation of ➡ helper T lymphocytes with a less restricted cytokine profile than ➡ Th1 and ➡ Th2 cells. Th0-like responses are observed in patients with ➡ rheumatoid arthritis, ➡ Sjögren syndrome, and ➡ Graves disease.

Th1 cells. Subpopulation of ➡ helper T lymphocytes producing mainly IL-2, IFN-γ, and TNF-β, thereby responsible for phagocyte-dependent host responses. Th1-dominated responses are seen in autoimmune diseases in which cytotoxic T cells and macrophages play a major role, e.g. ➡ multiple sclerosis, ➡ diabetes mellitus type 1, ➡ Hashimoto thyroiditis, and ➡ Crohn disease. Interestingly, switching from Th1 to Th2 response can prevent Th1-mediated tissue destruction in animal models.

Th2 cells. Subpopulation of ➡ helper T lymphocytes in mice producing IL-4, IL-5, IL-6, IL-9, IL-10, and IL-13. Besides other effects, they provide optimal help for antibody responses. Th2 responses should also be regarded as an important downregulatory mechanism for exaggerated Th1 responses. Predominant Th2 cytokine profile is observed in patients with atopic disorders and graft versus host disease.

Thrombocytopenia. Abnormal decrease in the number of thrombocytes below normal values. Frequently detected in patients with autoimmune diseases (e.g. ➡ systemic lupus erythematosus, ➡ Sjögren syndrome, ➡ mixed connective tissue disease, ➡ antiphospholipid syndrome). Primary forms may be drug induced (➡ heparin-induced thrombocytopenia) or mediated by antiplatelet antibodies (➡ idiopathic thrombocytopenic purpura).

Thyroglobulin (TG). This glycoprotein secreted by thyroid follicular cells is a major autoantigen in autoimmune thyroid diseases. Thyroglobulin autoantibodies were found in patients with autoimmune thyroiditis (➡ thyroiditis, autoimmune) and ➡ Graves disease.

Thyroiditis, autoimmune. Inflammatory destruction of the thyroid gland (ranging from a mild focal thyroiditis to extensive lymphocytic infiltration and scarring) often associated with goitre and hypothyroidism. The most common types of autoimmune thyroiditis are ➡ Hashimoto disease and atrophic thyroiditis (➡ primary myxoedema). Autoantibodies directed to thyroid peroxidase and ➡ thyroglobulin are found, often at very high levels, in most of these patients. Several cell- and autoantibody-mediated mechanisms (e.g. ➡ cytotoxic T lymphocytes, complement-mediated lysis, alteration of target cell function, ➡ antibody-dependent cell-mediated cytotoxicity) contribute to the inflammatory thyroid injury. Autoimmune thyroiditis occurs spontaneously (➡ spontaneous autoimmune thyroiditis) or can be induced experimentally in animals (➡ experimental autoimmune thyroiditis).

Thyroid peroxidase (TPO). This thyroid enzyme is a major autoantigen in autoimmune thyroid diseases. Thyroid peroxidase autoantibodies were found in patients with autoimmune thyroiditis (➡ thyroiditis, autoimmune) and ➡ Graves disease.

Thyroid-stimulating hormone receptor (TSH-R). Main autoantigenic target in patients with ➡ Graves disease. Most TSH-R autoantibodies are stimulatory, acting as agonists of thyroid-stimulating hormone, but receptor-blocking antibodies were also found.

Tissue transglutaminase (tTG). Main target of autoantibodies in ➡ coeliac disease.

T lymphocytes (T cells). Thymus-dependent lymphocytes that differentiate in the thymus to express ➡ T cell receptor molecules that are specifc for complexes comprising short peptides bound to and presented by ➡ major histocompatibility complex molecules. Different subpopulations of regulatory and effector cells. See ➡ cytotoxic T lymphocytes, ➡ helper T lymphocytes, ➡ regulatory T cells, and ➡ suppressor T lymphocytes.

Tolerance. Persistent condition of specific immunological unresponsiveness, resulting from previous non-sensitizing exposure to the antigen. See also: ➡ self-tolerance.

Ulcerative colitis. A disease that causes inflammation and sores, called ulcers, in the lining of the rectum and colon. Ulcers form where inflammation has killed the cells that usually line the colon, then bleed and produce pus.

Urticaria. Transient eruption of skin characterized by erythematous or oedematous swelling (wheal) of the dermis or subcutaneous tissue.

Vasculitis. Acute or chronic inflammation of the vessel walls that can lead to necrosis, fibrosis, or thrombosis. Autoimmunity plays an important role in some vasculitides (e.g. ➡ ANCA-associated vasculitides, ➡ Goodpasture disease/syndrome, ➡ cryoglobulinaemic vasculitis).

Vetoing. Elimination (➡ apoptosis) of the self-peptide–MHC complex recognizing lymphocyte by the self-peptide presenting (veto) cell. A less important regulatory mechanism of ➡ self-tolerance.

Warm autoantibody type. Autoantibodies that react optimally at higher temperatures (37 °C) with surface antigens of red blood cells. They mediate ➡ autoimmune haemolytic anaemia.

Wegener granulomatosis (WG). Granulomatous inflammation involving the respiratory tract, and necrotizing vasculitis affecting small to medium-sized vessels (e.g. capillaries, venules, arterioles, and arteries). Necrotizing glomerulonephritis is common.

Xenobiotics. A general term for foreign compounds, but here principally means drugs and environmental pollutants that influence immune responses (immune regulation) and may lead to autoimmunity.

REFERENCES

Abedi-Valugerdi M & Möller G (2000) Contribution of H-2 and non-H-2 genes in the control of mercury-induced autoimmunity. Int Immunol, 12(10): 1425–1430.

Abel EA (1992) Diagnosis of drug-induced psoriasis. Semin Dermatol, 11(4): 269–274.

Adachi Y, Bradford BU, Gao W, Bojes HK, & Thurman RG (1994) Inactivation of Kupffer cells prevents early alcohol-induced liver injury. Hepatology, 20: 453–460.

Aida T, Kimura T, Ishikawa N, & Shinkai K (1998) Evaluation of allergenic potential of low-molecular compounds by mouse popliteal lymph node assay. J Toxicol Sci, 23(5): 425–432.

Aikoh T, Tomokuni A, Matsukii T, Hyodoh F, Ueki H, Otsuki T, & Ueki A (1998) Activation-induced cell death in human peripheral blood lymphocytes after stimulation with silicate in vitro. Int J Oncol, 12: 1355–1359.

Alarcon GS, Roseman J, Bartolucci AA, Friedman AW, Moulds JM, Goel N, Straaton KV, & Reveille JD (1998) Systemic lupus erythematosus in three ethnic groups: II. Features predictive of disease activity early in its course. LUMINA Study Group. Lupus in minority populations, nature versus nurture. Arthritis Rheum, 41(7): 1173–1180.

Alarcon GS, Bastian HM, Beasley TM, Roseman JM, Tan FK, Fessler BJ, Vila LM, McGwin G Jr, LUMINA Study Group (2006) Systemic lupus erythematosus in a multi-ethnic cohort (LUMINA): contributions of admixture and socioeconomic status to renal involvement. Lupus, 15(1): 26–31.

Albano E (2002) Free radical mechanisms in immune reactions associated with alcoholic liver disease. Free Radic Biol Med, 32: 110–114.

Albano SA, Santana-Sahagun E, & Weisman MH (2001) Cigarette smoking and rheumatoid arthritis. Semin Arthritis Rheum, 31(3): 146–159.

Albers R, Broeders A, van der Pijl A, Seinen W, & Pieters R (1997) The use of reporter antigens in the popliteal lymph node assay to assess immunomodulation by chemicals. Toxicol Appl Pharmacol, 143(1): 102–109.

Albers R, de Heer C, Bol M, Bleumink R, Seinen W, & Pieters R (1998) Selective immunomodulation by the autoimmunity-inducing xenobiotics streptozotocin and $HgCl_2$. Eur J Immunol, 28(4): 1233–1242.

Aldridge WN (1992) The toxic oil syndrome (TOS, 1981): from the disease towards a toxicological understanding of its chemical aetiology and mechanism. Toxicol Lett, 64–65: 59–70.

Alvarez-Nemegyei J, Cobarrubias-Cobos A, Escalante-Triay F, Sosa-Muñoz J, Miranda JM, & Jara LJ (1998) Bromocriptine in systemic lupus erythematosus: a double-blind, randomized, placebo-controlled study. Lupus, 7: 414–419.

References

Amino N, Izumi Y, Hidaka Y, Takeoka K, Nakata Y, Tatsumi KI, Nagata A, & Takano T (2003) No increases of blocking type anti-thyrotropin receptor antibodies during pregnancy in patients with Graves' disease. J Clin Endocrinol Metab, **88**: 5871–5874.

Anaya JM, Correa PA, Herrera M, Eskdale J, & Gallagher G (2002) Interleukin 10 (IL-10) influences autoimmune response in primary Sjögren's syndrome and is linked to IL-10 gene polymorphism. J Rheumatol, **29**: 1874–1876.

Anderton SM (2004) Post-translational modifications of self antigens: implications for autoimmunity. Curr Opin Immunol, **16**: 753–758.

Andrade F, Casciola-Rosen L, & Rosen A (2000) Apoptosis in systemic lupus erythematosus: clinical implications. Rheum Dis Clin North Am, **26**: 215–227.

Andre F, Gillon J, Andre C, Lafont S, & Jourdan G (1983) Pesticide-containing diets augment anti-sheep red blood cell nonreaginic antibody responses in mice but may prolong murine infection with *Giardia muris*. Environ Res, **32**: 145–154.

Andre M, Canon JL, Levecque P, Dermine P, Mortier C, & Leveau F (1991) Eosinophilia-myalgia syndrome associated with L-tryptophan: A case report with pulmonary manifestations and review of the literature. Acta Clin Belg, **46**: 178–182.

Angell M (1997) Antipolymer antibodies, silicone breast implants, and fibromyalgia [letter]. Lancet, **349**(9059): 1171–1172.

Angotti C (2004) Immunology of cutaneous lupus erythematosus. Clin Dermatol, **22**(2): 105–112.

Arbuckle MR, McClain MT, Rubertone MV, Scofield RH, Dennis GJ, James JA, & Harley JB (2003) Development of autoantibodies before the clinical onset of systemic lupus erythematosus. N Engl J Med, **349**(16): 1526–1533.

Arnaiz-Villena A, Vicario JL, Serrano-Rios M, Bellas C, & Mampaso F (1982) Glomerular basement-membrane antibodies and HLA-DR2 in Spanish rapeseed oil disease. N Engl J Med, **307**: 1404–1405.

Arnett FC & Moulds JM (1991) HLA class III molecules and autoimmune rheumatic diseases. Clin Exp Rheumatol, **9**: 289–296.

Arnett FC, Edworthy SM, Bloch DA, McShane DJ, Fries JF, Cooper NS, Healey LA, Kaplan SR, Liang MH, & Luthra HS (1988) The American Rheumatism Association 1987 revised criteria for the classification of rheumatoid arthritis. Arthritis Rheum, **31**: 315–324.

Arnett FC, Reveille JD, Goldstein R, Pollard KM, Leaird K, Smith EA, Leroy EC, & Fritzler MJ (1996) Autoantibodies to fibrillarin in systemic sclerosis (scleroderma). An immunogenetic, serologic, and clinical analysis. Arthritis Rheum, **39**: 1151–1160.

Arnett FC, Fritzler MJ, Ahn C, & Holian A (2000) Urinary mercury levels in patients with autoantibodies to U3-RNP (fibrillarin). J Rheumatol, **27**(2): 405–410.

Artlett CM, Smith JB, & Jimenez SA (1998) Identification of fetal DNA and cells in skin lesions from women with systemic sclerosis. N Engl J Med, **338**: 1186–1191.

Aryal BK, Khuder SA, & Schaub EA (2001) Meta-analysis of systemic sclerosis and exposure to solvents. Am J Ind Med, **40**: 271–274.

Ascherio A & Munch M (2000) Epstein-Barr virus and multiple sclerosis. Epidemiology, **11**: 220–224.

Ascherio A, Munger KL, Lennette ET, Spiegelman D, Hernán MA, Olek MJ, Hankinson SE, & Hunter DJ (2001) Epstein-Barr virus antibodies and risk of multiple sclerosis: a prospective study. JAMA, **286**: 3083–3088.

Asseman C & von Herrath M (2002) About $CD4^{pos}$ $CD25^{pos}$ regulatory cells. Autoimmun Rev, **1**: 190–197.

Aster RH (2000) Can drugs cause autoimmune thrombocytopenic purpura? Semin Hematol, **37**: 229–238.

Aten J, Bosman CB, Rozing J, Stijnen T, Hoedemaeker PJ, & Weening JJ (1988) Mercuric chloride-induced autoimmunity in the Brown Norway rat. Cellular kinetics and major histocompatibility complex antigen expression. Am J Pathol, **133**(1): 127–138.

Aten J, Veninga A, De Heer E, Rozing J, Nieuwenhuis P, Hoedemaeker PJ, & Weening JJ (1991) Susceptibility to the induction of either autoimmunity or immunosuppression by mercuric chloride is related to the major histocompatibility complex class II haplotype. Eur J Immunol, **21**(3): 611–616.

Atkinson MA & Eisenbarth GS (2001) Type 1 diabetes: new perspectives on disease pathogenesis and treatment. Lancet, **358**(9277): 221–229.

Aucoin DP (1989) Propylthiouracil-induced immune mediated disease syndrome in the cat: a novel model for a drug-induced lupus-like disease. In: Kammuller ME, Bloksma N, & Seinen W eds. Autoimmunity and toxicology: immune disregulation induced by drugs and chemicals. Amsterdam, Elsevier, pp 309–320.

Avrameas S (1991) Natural autoantibodies: from "horror autotoxicus" to "gnothi seauton". Immunol Today, **12**(5): 154–159.

Ayer LM, Edworthy SM, & Fritzler MJ (1993) Effect of procainamide and hydralazine on poly (ADP-ribosylation) in cell lines. Lupus, **2**(3): 167–172.

Bach JF (2002) The effect of infections on susceptibility to autoimmune and allergic diseases. N Engl J Med, **347**: 911–920.

Bach JF (2003) Autoimmune diseases as the loss of active "self-control". Ann N Y Acad Sci, **998**: 161–177.

Bach JF (2005) Six questions about the hygiene hypothesis. Cell Immunol, **232**(2): 158–161.

Bachmann M (2004) Novel autoimmune models: Lessons from recent transgenic and knock in animals. In: Conrad K, Bachmann M, Chan EKL, Fritzler MJ, Humbel RL, Sack U, & Shoenfeld Y eds. From animal models to human genetics. Lengerich, Pabst Science Publishers, pp 24–42.

References

Bachmann M, Tröster H, Bartsch H, & Grölz D (1996) A frame shift mutation in a hot spot of the nuclear autoantigen La/SS-B. J Autoimmun, **9**: 747–756.

Bachot N & Roujeau JC (2001) Physiopathology and treatment of severe drug eruptions. Curr Opin Allergy Clin Immunol, **1**(4): 293–298.

Bagenstose LM, Salgame P, & Monestier M (1998a) Mercury-induced autoimmunity in the absence of IL-4. Clin Exp Immunol, **114**: 9–12.

Bagenstose LM, Salgame P, & Monestier M (1998b) IL-12 down-regulates autoantibody production in mercury-induced autoimmunity. J Immunol, **160**: 1612–1617.

Bagenstose LM, Salgame P, & Monestier M (1999a) Murine mercury-induced autoimmunity: a model of chemically related autoimmunity in humans. Immunol Res, **20**(1): 67–78.

Bagenstose LM, Salgame P, & Monestier M (1999b) Cytokine regulation of a rodent model of mercury chloride-induced autoimmunity. Environ Health Perspect, **107**(Suppl 5): 807–810.

Bagenstose LM, Mentink-Kane MM, Brittingham A, Mosser DM, & Monestier M (2001) Mercury enhances susceptibility to murine leishmaniasis. Parasite Immunol, **23**(12): 633–640.

Bagenstose LM, Class R, Salgame P, & Monestier M (2002) B7-1 and B7-2 co-stimulatory molecules are required for mercury-induced autoimmunity. Clin Exp Immunol, **127**(1): 12–19.

Bagheri MM, Alagheband M, Memar OM, & Eiler DB (2002) Pemphigus foliaceus presenting as eruptive seborrheic keratosis and responding to oral gold treatment. J Drug Dermatol, **1**: 333–334.

Baird DD, Wilcox AJ, & Herbst AL (1996) Self-reported allergy, infection, and autoimmune diseases among men and women exposed in utero to diethylstilbestrol. J Clin Epidemiol, **49**: 263–266.

Balazs T (1987) Immunogenetically controlled autoimmune reactions induced by mercury, gold and D-penicillamine in laboratory animals: a review from the vantage point of premarketing safety studies. Toxicol Ind Health, **3**(3): 331–336.

Balazs T & Robinson CJ (1983) Procainamide-induced antinuclear antibodies in beagle dogs. Toxicol Appl Pharmacol, **71**(2): 299–302.

Ball JA & Young KR Jr (1998) Pulmonary manifestations of Goodpasture's syndrome. Antiglomerular basement membrane disease and related disorders. Clin Chest Med, **19**(4): 777–791.

Bardin I, Dryll A, & Debeyre N (1982) HLA system and side effects of gold and D-penicillamine teatment of rheumatoid arthritis. Ann Rheum Dis, **41**: 599–601.

Barendrecht MM, Tervaert JW, van Breda Vriesman PJ, & Damoiseaux JG (2002) Susceptibility to cyclosporin A-induced autoimmunity: strain differences in relation to autoregulatory T cells. J Autoimmun, 18(1): 39–48.

Barth H, Klein R, & Berg PA (2001) L-tryptophan contaminant "peak E" induces the release of IL-5 and IL-10 by peripheral blood mononuclear cells from patients with functional somatic syndromes. Clin Exp Immunol, 126: 186–192.

Bataller R, North KE, & Brenner DA (2003) Genetic polymorphisms and the progression of liver fibrosis: A critical appraisal. Hepatology, 37: 493–503.

Bates MN, Fawcett J, Garrett N, Cutress T, & Kjellstrom T (2004) Health effects of dental amalgam exposure: a retrospective cohort study. Int J Epidemiol, 33: 1–9.

Beaudreuil S (2005) Occupational exposure in ANCA-positive patients: a case–control study. Kidney Int, 67(5): 1961–1966.

Beech JT, Siew LK, Ghoraishian M, Stasiuk LM, Elson CJ, & Thompson SJ (1997) CD4$^+$ Th2 cells specific for mycobacterial 65-kilodalton heat shock protein protect against pristane-induced arthritis. J Immunol, 159(8): 3692–3697.

Bell SA (1996) The toxic oil syndrome: an example of an exogenously induced autoimmune reaction. Mol Biol Rep, 23: 261–263.

Bell SA, Sander C, Kuntze I, & Chatelain R (1999) The acute pathology of fatty acid anilides and linoleic diester of 3-phenylamino-1,2-propanediol in mice: possible implication as aetiologic agents for the toxic oil syndrome. Arch Toxicol, 73: 493–495.

Bell SA, Kuntze I, Caputo A, & Chatelain R (2002) Strain-dependent in vitro and in vivo effects of oleic acid anilides on splenocytes and T cells in a murine model of the toxic oil syndrome. Food Chem Toxicol, 40: 19–24.

Belluzzi A (2002) N-3 fatty acids for the treatment of inflammatory bowel diseases. Proc Nutr Soc, 61: 391–395.

Ben-Ari Z & Czaja AJ (2001) Autoimmune hepatitis and its variant syndromes. Gut, 49: 589–594.

Bennett CL, Christie P, Ramsdell F, Brunkow ME, Ferguson PJ, Whitesell L, Kelly TE, Saulsbury FT, Chance PF, & Ochs HD (2001) The immune dysregulation, polyendocrinopathy, enteropathy, X-linked syndrome (IPEX) is caused by mutations of FOXP3. Nat Genet, 27: 20–21.

Bennett ST, Lucassen AM, Gough SC, Powell EE, Undlien DE, Pritchard LE, Merriman ME, Kawaguchi Y, Dronsfield MJ, & Pociot F (1995) Susceptibility to human type 1 diabetes at IDDM2 is determined by tandem repeat variation at the insulin gene minisatellite locus. Nat Genet, 9: 284–292.

Ben-Nun A & Cohen IR (1982) Experimental autoimmune encephalomyelitis (EAE) mediated by T cell lines: process of selection of lines and characterization of the cells. J Immunol, 129(1): 303–308.

References

Berger BD, Acton RT, Koopman WJ, & Alarcon GS (1984) DR antigens and gold toxicity in white rheumatoid arthritis patients. Arthritis Rheum, 27: 601–607.

Berger T, Rubner P, Schautzer F, Egg R, Ulmer H, Mayringer I, Dilitz E, Deisenhammer F, & Reindl M (2003) Antimyelin antibodies as a predictor of clinically definite multiple sclerosis after a first demyelinating event. N Engl J Med, 349: 139–145.

Berking C, Hobbs MV, Chatelain R, Meurer M, & Bell SA (1998) Strain-dependent cytokine profile and susceptibility to oleic acid anilide in a murine model of the toxic oil syndrome. Toxicol Appl Pharmacol, 148: 222–228.

Bernard A, Roels H, Hubermont G, Buchet JP, Masson PL, & Lauwerys R (1976) Characterization of the proteinuria in cadmium-exposed workers. Int Arch Occup Environ Health, 38: 19–30.

Bernard A, Lauwerys R, Gengoux P, Mahieu P, Foidart JM, Druet P, & Weening JJ (1984) Anti-laminin antibodies in Sprague-Dawley and Brown Norway rats chronically exposed to cadmium. Toxicology, 31: 307–313.

Bernard A, Roels HR, Foidart JM, & Lauwerys RL (1987) Search for anti-laminin antibodies in the serum of workers exposed to cadmium, mercury vapour or lead. Int Arch Occup Environ Health, 59: 303–309.

Bernier J, Fournier F, Blais Y, Lombardi P, Chevalier G, & Krzystyniak K (1988) Immunotoxicity of aminocarb. I. Comparative studies of sublethal exposure to aminocarb and dieldrin in mice. Pestic Biochem Physiol, 30: 238–250.

Bernier J, Girard D, Krzystyniak K, Chevalier G, Trottier B, Nadeau D, Rola-Pleszczynski M, & Fournier M (1995) Immunotoxicity of aminocarb: III. Exposure route-dependent immunomodulation by aminocarb in mice. Toxicology, 99: 135–146.

Betterle C, Dal Pra C, Mantero F, & Zanchetta R (2002) Autoimmune adrenal insufficiency and autoimmune polyendocrine syndromes: autoantibodies, autoantigens, and their applicability in diagnosis and disease prediction. Endocrinol Rev, 23: 327–364.

Bickers DR (1987) The dermatologic manifestations of human porphyria. Ann N Y Acad Sci, 514: 261–267.

Bigazzi P (1994) Autoimmunity and heavy metals. Lupus, 3: 449–453.

Bigazzi PE (1999) Metals and kidney autoimmunity. Environ Health Perspect, 107(Suppl 5): 753–765.

Bingley PJ, Bonifacio E, Williams AJ, Genovese S, Bottazzo GF, & Gale EA (1997) Prediction of IDDM in the general population: strategies based on combinations of autoantibody markers. Diabetes, 46: 1701–1710.

Black C, Pereira S, McWhirter A, Welsh K, & Laurent R (1986) Genetic susceptibility to scleroderma-like syndrome in symptomatic and asymptomatic workers exposed to vinyl chloride. J Rheumatol, 13: 1059–1062.

Black CM, Welsh KI, Walker AE, Bernstein RM, Catoggio LJ, McGregor AR, & Jones JK (1983) Genetic susceptibility to scleroderma-like syndrome induced by vinyl chloride. Lancet, 1(8314–8315): 53–55.

Blair PB (1992) Immunologic studies of women exposed in utero to diethylstilbestrol. In: Colborn T & Clement C eds. Chemically-induced alterations in sexual and functional development: the wildlife/human connection. Princeton, New Jersey, Princeton Scientific Publishing Co., pp 289–293.

Blair PB, Noller KL, Turiel J, Forghani B, & Hagens S (1992) Disease patterns and antibody responses to viral antigens in women exposed in utero to diethylstilbestrol. In: Colborn T & Clement C eds. Chemically-induced alterations in sexual and functional development: the wildlife/human connection. Princeton, New Jersey, Princeton Scientific Publishing Co., pp 283–288.

Blank M, Krause I, Buskila D, Teitelbaum D, Kopolovic J, Afek A, Goldberg I, & Shoenfeld Y (1995) Bromocriptine immunomodulation of experimental SLE and primary antiphospholipid syndrome via induction of nonspecific T suppressor cells. Cell Immunol, **162**: 114–122.

Blauvelt A, Hwang ST, & Udey MC (2003) 11. Allergic and immunologic diseases of the skin. J Allergy Clin Immunol, **111**: S560–S570.

Blaylock BL, Hollady SD, Comment CE, Heindel JJ, & Luster MI (1992) Modulation of perinatal thymocyte surface antigen expression and inhibition of thymocyte maturation by exposure to 2,3,7,8-tetrachlorodibenzo-*p*-dioxin (TCDD). Toxicol Appl Pharmacol, **112**: 207–213.

Bloksma N, de Bakker JM, van Rooijen HJ, Punt P, Seinen W, & Kammuller ME (1994) Long-term treatment with 5,5-diphenylhydantoin reduces lymphadenopathy and anti-ssDNA autoantibodies in C57BL/6-lpr/lpr mice. Int J Immunopharmacol, **16**(3): 261–268.

Bloksma N, Kubicka-Muranyi M, Schuppe HC, Gleichmann E, & Gleichmann H (1995) Predictive immunotoxicological test systems: suitability of the popliteal lymph node assay in mice and rats. Crit Rev Toxicol, **25**(5): 369–396.

Blossom S, Pumford NR, & Gilbert KM (2004) Activation and attenuation of apoptosis of $CD4^+$ T cells following in vivo exposure to two common environmental toxicants, trichloroacetaldehyde hydrate and trichloroacetic acid. J Autoimmun, **23**: 211–220.

Bluestone JA & Tang Q (2005) How do $CD4^+CD25^+$ regulatory T cells control autoimmunity? Curr Opin Immunol, **17**: 638–642.

Boberg KM, Aadland E, Jahnsen J, Raknerud N, Stiris M, & Bell H (1998) Incidence and prevalence of primary biliary cirrhosis, primary sclerosing cholangitis, and autoimmune hepatitis in a Norwegian population. Scand J Gastroenterol, **33**(1): 99–103.

Bocquet H, Bagot M, & Roujeau JC (1996) Drug-induced pseudolymphoma and drug hypersensitivity syndrome (drug rash with eosinophilia and systemic symptoms: DRESS). Semin Cutan Med Surg, **15**: 250–257.

Bodeutsch C, de Wilde PC, Kater L, van Houwelingen JC, van den Hoogen FH, Kruize AA, Hene RJ, van de Putte LB, & Vooijs GP (1992) Quantitative immunohistologic criteria are superior to the lymphocytic focus score criterion for the diagnosis of Sjogren's syndrome. Arthritis Rheum, **35**: 1075–1087.

Bogliun G & Beghi E (2004) Incidence and clinical features of acute inflammatory polyradiculoneuropathy in Lombardy, Italy, 1996. Acta Neurol Scand, **110**(2): 100–106.

Boisseau-Garsaud AM, Garsaud P, Cales-Quist D, Helenon R, Queneherve C, & Claire RC (2000) Epidemiology of vitiligo in the French West Indies (Isle of Martinique). Int J Dermatol, **39**(1): 18–20.

Bottazzo GF, Florin-Christensen A, & Doniach D (1974) Islet-cell antibodies in diabetes mellitus with autoimmune polyendocrine deficiencies. Lancet, **2**(7892): 1279–1283.

Botto M (2001) Links between complement deficiency and apoptosis. Arthritis Res, **3**: 207–210.

Bouma G & Strober W (2003) The immunological and genetic basis of inflammatory bowel disease. Nat Rev Immunol, **3**: 521–533.

Boumpas DT, Fessler BJ, Austin HA 3rd, Balow JE, Klippel JH, & Lockshin MD (1995) Systemic lupus erythematosus: emerging concepts. Part 2: Dermatologic and joint disease, the antiphospholipid antibody syndrome, pregnancy and hormonal therapy, morbidity and mortality, and pathogenesis. Ann Intern Med, **123**: 42–53.

Bournaud C & Orgiazzi JJ (2003) Iodide excess and thyroid autoimmunity. J Endocrinol Invest, **26**(Suppl 2): 49–56.

Bovenzi M, Barbone F, Betta A, Tommasini M, & Versini W (1995) Scleroderma and occupational exposure. Scand J Work Environ Health, **21**: 289–292.

Bovenzi M, Barbone F, Pisa FE, Betta A, & Romeo L (2001) Scleroderma and occupational exposure to hand-transmitted vibration. Int Arch Occup Environ Health, **74**(8): 579–582.

Bovenzi M, Barbone F, Pisa FE, Betta A, Romeo L, Tonello A, Biasis D, & Caramaschi P (2004) A case–control study of occupational exposures and systemic sclerosis. Int Arch Occup Environ Health, **77**: 10–16.

Bowness P (2002) HLA B27 in health and disease: a double-edged sword. Rheumatology, **41**: 857–868.

Boyages SC, Bloot AM, Maberly GF, Eastman CJ, Li M, Qian QD, Liu DR, van der Gaag RD, & Drexhage HA (1989) Thyroid autoimmunity in endemic goitre caused by excessive iodine intake. Clin Endocrin (Oxf), **31**: 452–465.

Boyton RJ & Altmann DM (2002) Transgenic models of autoimmune disease. Clin Exp Immunol, **127**(1): 4–11.

Brennan P, Hajeer A, Ong KR, Worthington J, John S, Thomson W, Silman A, & Ollier B (1997) Allelic markers close to prolactin are associated with HLA-DRB1 susceptibility alleles among women with rheumatoid arthritis and systemic lupus erythematosus. Arthritis Rheum, **40**: 1383–1386.

Bridges AJ, Anderson JD, Burns DE, Kemple K, Kaplan JD, & Lorden T (1996) Autoantibodies in patients with silicone implants. Curr Top Microbiol Immunol, **210**: 277–282.

Brik R, Tenenbaum G, Blank M, Shoenfeld Y, Barzilai D, Bloch K, & Vardi P (1995) D-penicillamine-induced autoantibodies in a mouse model. Clin Exp Rheumatol, **13**(4): 483–488.

Brostoff J, Blanca M, Boulton P, & Serrano S (1982) Absence of specific IgE antibodies in toxic oil syndrome. Lancet, **1**(8266): 277.

Broughton A, Thrasher JD, & Madison R (1990) Chronic health effects and immunological alterations associated with exposure to pesticide. Comments Toxicol, **4**: 59–71.

Brouwer A, Longnecker MP, Birnbaum LS, Cogliano J, Kostyniak P, Moore J, Schantz S, & Winneke G (1999) Characterization of potential endocrine-related health effects at low-dose levels of exposure to PCBs. Environ Health Perspect, **107**(Suppl 4): 639–649.

Brown JM, Archer AJ, Pfau JC, & Holian A (2003) Silica accelerated systemic autoimmune disease in lupus-prone New Zealand mixed mice. Clin Exp Immunol, **131**(3): 415–421.

Brown LM, Gridley G, Olsen JH, Mellemkjaer L, Linet MS, & Fraumeni JF (1997) Cancer risk and mortality patterns among silicotic men in Sweden and Denmark. J Occup Environ Med, **66**: 323–333.

Brown SL (2002) Epidemiology of silicone breast implants. Epidemiology, **13**: S34–S39.

Brown SL, Pennello G, Berg WA, Soo MS, & Middleton MS (2001) Silicone gel breast implant rupture, extracapsular silicone, and health status in a population of women. J Rheumatol, **28**: 996–1003.

Brownlie BE & Wells JE (1990) The epidemiology of thyrotoxicosis in New Zealand: incidence and geographical distribution in North Canterbury, 1983–1985. Clin Endocrinol (Oxf), **33**(2): 249–259.

Bruining GJ, Molenaar JL, Grobbee DE, Hofman A, Scheffer GJ, Bruining HA, de Bruyn AM, & Valkenburg HA (1989) Ten-year follow-up study of islet-cell antibodies and childhood diabetes mellitus. Lancet, **1**(8647): 1100–1103.

Brun JG, Madland TM, & Vedeler CA (2002) Immunoglobulin G Fc-receptor (Fcγ R) IIA, IIIA, and IIIB polymorphisms related to disease severity in rheumatoid arthritis. J Rheumatol, **29**: 1135–1140.

Burns CJ, Laing TJ, Gillespie BW, Heeringa SG, Alcser KH, Mayes MD, Wasko MC, Cooper BC, Garabrant DH, & Schottenfeld D (1996) The epidemiology of scleroderma among women: assessment of risk from exposure to silicone and silica. J Rheumatol, **23**: 1904–1911.

Burns C, Burns P, & Holsapple M (2000) "Of Mice and Men" (John Steinbeck) — How do we determine the potential for immunotoxicity in humans? Ann Epidemiol, **10**(7): 471–472.

Caforio AL, Mahon NJ, Tona F, & McKenna WJ (2002) Circulating cardiac autoantibodies in dilated cardiomyopathy and myocarditis: pathogenetic and clinical significance. Eur J Heart Fail, **4**: 411–417.

Calder PC (1997) n-3 polyunsaturated fatty acids and cytokine production in health and disease. Ann Nutr Metab, **41**: 203–234.

Calemine JB, Gogal RM Jr, Lengi A, Sponenberg P, & Ahmed SA (2002) Immunomodulation by diethylstilbestrol is dose and gender related: effects on thymocyte apoptosis and mitogen-induced proliferation. Toxicology, **178**: 101–118.

Calkins BM (1989) A meta-analysis of the role of smoking in inflammatory bowel disease. Dig Dis Sci, **34**: 1841–1854.

Cam C (1958) Cases of skin porphyria related to hexachlorobenzene intoxication. Saglik Dergisi, **32**: 215–216.

Cantagrel A, Navaux F, Loubet-Lescoulié P, Nourhashemi F, Enault G, Abbal M, Constantin A, Laroche M, & Maziéres B (1999) Interleukin-1β, interleukin-1 receptor antagonist, interleukin-4, and interleukin-10 gene polymorphisms. Relationship to occurrence and severity of rheumatoid arthritis. Arthritis Rheum, **42**: 1093–1100.

Caplan A (1953) Certain unusual radiological appearances in the chest of coalminers suffering from rheumatoid arthritis. Thorax, **8**: 29–35.

Cardaba B, Enzendam J, Gallardo S, del Poza V, Izquierdo Martinez M, Martin C, Cortegano MI, Aceituno E, Rojo M, Arrieta I, Palomino P, Posada de la Paz M, & Lahoz C (1999) DR2 antigens are associated with severity of disease in toxic oil syndrome (TOS). Tissue Antigens, **55**: 110–117.

Carr L, Ruther E, Berg PA, & Lehnert H (1994) Eosinophilia-myalgia syndrome in Germany: an epidemiologic review. Mayo Clin Proc, **69**: 620–625.

Carr LG, Hartleroad JY, Liang Y, Mendenhall C, Moritz T, & Thomasson H (1995) Polymorphism at the P450IIE1 locus is not associated with alcoholic liver disease in Caucasian men. Alcohol Clin Exp Res, **19**: 182–184.

Carreno BM & Collins M (2002) The B7 family of ligands and its receptors: new pathways for costimulation and inhibition of immune responses. Annu Rev Immunol, **20**: 29–53.

Carroll MC (2004) A protective role for innate immunity in systemic lupus erythematosus. Nat Rev Immunol, **4**(10): 825–831.

Casciola-Rosen L, Wigley F, & Rosen A (1997) Scleroderma autoantigens are uniquely fragmented by metal-catalyzed oxidation reactions: implications for pathogenesis. J Exp Med, **185**: 71–79.

Castano P (1971) Chronic intoxication by cadmium experimentally induced in rabbits. A study of kidney ultrastructure. Path Microbiol, **37**: 280–301.

Castranova V, Vallyathan V, Ramsey DM, McLaurin JL, Pack D, Leonard S, Barger MW, Ma JY, Dalal NS, & Teass A (1997) Augmentation of pulmonary reactions to quartz inhalation by trace amounts of iron-containing particles. Environ Health Perspect, **105**(Suppl 5): 1319–1324.

Cerhan JR, Saag KG, Merlino LA, Mikuls TR, & Criswell LA (2003) Antioxidant micronutrients and risk of rheumatoid arthritis in a cohort of older women. Am J Epidemiol, **157**: 345–354.

Chan OT, Madaio MP, & Shlomchik MJ (1999) The central and multiple roles of B cells in lupus pathogenesis. Immunol Rev, **169**: 107–121.

Charmley P, Nepom BB, & Concannon P (1994) HLA and T cell receptor β-chain DNA polymorphisms identify a distinct subset of patients with pauciarticular-onset juvenile rheumatoid arthritis. Arthritis Rheum, **37**: 685–701.

Chen M, Hemmerich P, & Von Mikecz A (2002) Platinum-induced autoantibodies target nucleoplasmic antigens related to active transcription. Immunobiology, **206**: 474–483.

Chenuaud P, Larcher T, Rabinowitz JE, Provost N, Cherel Y, Casadevall N, Samulski RJ, & Moullier P (2004) Autoimmune anemia in macaques following erythropoietin gene therapy. Blood, **103**(9): 3303–3304.

Chernajovsky Y, Dreja H, Daly G, Annenkov A, Gould D, Adams G, Croxford JL, Baker D, Podhajcer OL, & Mageed RA (2000) Immuno- and genetic therapy in autoimmune diseases. Genes Immun, **1**(5): 295–307.

Chiang SY, Swenberg JA, Weisman WH, & Skopek TR (1997) Mutagenicity of vinyl chloride and its reactive metabolites, chloroethylene oxide and chloroacetaldehyde, in a metabolically competent human B-lymphoblastoid line. Carcinogenesis, **18**: 31–36.

Choquet-Kastylevsky G, Vial T, & Descotes J (2001) Drug allergy diagnosis in humans: possibilities and pitfalls. Toxicology, **158**: 1–10.

Christner PJ, Artlett CM, Conway RF, & Jimenez SA (2000) Increased numbers of microchimeric cells of fetal origin are associated with dermal fibrosis in mice following injection of vinyl chloride. Arthritis Rheum, **43**: 2598–2605.

Chu JL, Drappa J, Parnassa A, & Elkon KB (1993) The defect in Fas mRNA expression in MRL/lpr mice is associated with insertion of the retrotransposon, ETn. J Exp Med, **178**: 723–730.

Cines DB & Blanchette VS (2002) Immune thrombocytopenic purpura. N Engl J Med, **346**: 995–1008.

Clarkson TW (2002) The three modern faces of mercury. Environ Health Perspect, **110**(Suppl 1): 11–23.

Clarkson TW, Magos L, & Myers GJ (2003) The toxicology of mercury — current exposures and clinical manifestations. N Engl J Med, **349**: 1731–1737.

References

Clot P, Albano E, Eliasson E, Tabone M, Arico S, Israel Y, Moncada C, & Ingelman-Sundberg M (1996) Cytochrome P4502E1 hydroxyethyl radical adducts as the major antigen in autoantibody formation among alcoholics. Gastroenterology, **111**(1): 206–216.

Colosio C, Maroni M, Barcellini W, Meroni P, Alcini D, Colombi A, Cavallo D, & Foa V (1993) Toxicological and immune findings in workers exposed to pentachlorophenol (PCP). Arch Environ Health, **48**(2): 81–88.

Colosio C, Barcellini W, Maroni M, Alcini D, Bersani M, Cavallo D, Galli A, Meroni PL, Pastorelli R, Rizzardi GP, Soleo L, & Foà V (1996) Immunomodulatory effects of occupational exposure to mancozeb. Arch Environ Health, **51**(6): 445–451.

Compston A & Coles A (2002) Multiple sclerosis. Lancet, **359**(9313): 1221–1231.

Comstock GW, Burke AE, Hoffman SC, Helzlsouer KJ, Bendich A, Masi AT, Norkus EP, Malamet RL, & Gershwin ME (1997) Serum concentrations of α tocopherol, β carotene, and retinol preceding the diagnosis of rheumatoid arthritis and systemic lupus erythematosus. Ann Rheum Dis, **56**: 323–325.

Confavreux C, Hutchinson M, Hours MM, Cortinovis-Tourniaire P, & Moreau T (1998) Rate of pregnancy-related relapse in multiple sclerosis: Pregnancy in multiple sclerosis group. N Engl J Med, **339**: 285–291.

Conrad K, Melhorn J, Luthke K, Dorner T, & Frank KH (1996) Systemic lupus erythematosus after heavy exposure to quartz dust in uranium mines: clinical and serological characteristics. Lupus, **5**: 62–69.

Constant CM, Swaak AJ, Wiggers T, Wai RT, & Van Geel AN (2000) First evaluation study of the Dutch Working Party on silicone breast implants (SBI) and the silicone-related symptom complex (SRSC). Clin Rheumatol, **19**: 458–463.

Cooper GS & Stroehla BC (2003) The epidemiology of autoimmune diseases. Autoimmun Rev, **2**: 119–125.

Cooper GS, Dooley MA, Treadwell EL, St Clair EW, Parks CG, & Gilkeson GS (1998) Hormonal, environmental, and infectious risk factors for developing systemic lupus erythematosus. Arthritis Rheum, **41**: 1714–1724.

Cooper GS, Miller FW, & Pandey JP (1999) The role of genetic factors in autoimmune disease: Implications for environmental research. Environ Health Perspect, **107**(Suppl 5): 693–700.

Cooper GS, Miller FW, & Germolec DR (2002) Occupational exposure and autoimmune diseases. Int Immunopharmacol, **2**: 303–313.

Cooper GS, Parks CG, Treadwell EL, St Clair EW, Gilkeson GS, & Dooley MA (2004) Occupational risk factors for the development of systemic lupus erythematosus. J Rheum, **31**: 1928–1933.

Corbett EL, Mozzato-Chamay N, Butterworth AE, De Cock KM, Williams BG, Churchyard GJ, & Conway DJ (2002) Polymorphisms in the tumor necrosis factor-alpha gene promoter may predispose to severe silicosis in black South African miners. Am J Respir Crit Care Med, **165**: 690–693.

Corsini E, Birindelli S, Fustinoni S, De Paschale G, Mammone T, Visentin S, Galli CL, Marinovich M, & Colosio C (2005) Immunomodulatory effects of the fungicide Mancozeb in agricultural workers. Toxicol Appl Pharmacol, **208**(2): 178–185.

Costenbader KH, Kim DJ, Peerzada J, Lockman S, Nobles-Knight D, Petri M, & Karlson EW (2004) Cigarette smoking and the risk of systemic lupus erythematosus: a meta-analysis. Arthritis Rheum, **50**: 849–857.

Cotch MF, Hoffman GS, Yerg DE, Kaufman GI, Targonski P, & Kaslow RA (1996) The epidemiology of Wegener's granulomatosis: Estimates of the five-year period prevalence, annual mortality, and geographic disease distribution from population-based data sources. Arthritis Rheum, **39**(1): 87–92.

Cowie RL (1987) Silica-dust-exposed mine workers with scleroderma (systemic sclerosis). Chest, **92**: 260–262

Craig WY, Ledue TB, Johnson AM, & Ritchie RF (1999) The distribution of antinuclear antibody titers in "normal" children and adults. J Rheum, **26**: 914–919.

Crilly A, Hamilton J, Clark CJ, Jardine A, & Madhok R (2002) Analysis of transforming growth factor β1 gene polymorphisms in patients with systemic sclerosis. Ann Rheum Dis, **61**: 678–681.

Cripps DJ, Peters HA, Gocmen A, & Dogramici I (1984) Porphyria turcica due to hexachlorobenzene: a 20 to 30 year follow-up study on 204 patients. Br J Dermatol, **111**: 413–422.

Crommelin DJ, Storm G, Verrijk R, de Leede L, Jiskoot W, & Hennink WE (2003) Shifting paradigms: biopharmaceuticals versus low molecular weight drugs. Int J Pharm, **266**(1–2): 3–16.

Cuadrado JI, de Pedro-Cuesta J, Ara JR, Cemillan CA, Diaz M, Duarte J, Fernandez MD, Fernandez O, Garcia-Lopez F, Garcia-Merino A, Velasquez JM, Martinez-Matos JA, Palomo F, Pardo J, & Tobias A (2004) Public health surveillance and incidence of adulthood Guillain-Barre syndrome in Spain, 1998–1999: the view from a sentinel network of neurologists. Neurol Sci, **25**(2): 57–65.

Cuellar ML, Gluck O, Molina JF, Guttiérrez S, Garcia C, & Espinoza R (1995) Silicone breast implant-associated musculoskeletal manifestations. Clin Rheumatol, **14**: 667–672.

Cuttres TW (1997) Dental amalgam and human health, current situation — a New Zealand review. In: Mjor IA & Pakomov GN eds. Dental amalgam and alternative direct restorative materials. Geneva, World Health Organization, pp 63–67.

Cutolo M, Sulli A, Capellino S, Villaggio B, Montagna P, Seriolo B, & Straub RH (2004) Sex hormones influence on the immune system: basic and clinical aspects in autoimmunity. Lupus, **13**: 635–638.

Czernielewski A, Kiec-Swierczynska M, Gluszcz M, & Wozniak L (1979) Dermatological aspects of so called vinyl chloride monomer disease. Derm Beruf Umwelt, 27: 108–112.

Czirjak L & Kumánovics G (2002) Exposure to solvents in female patients with scleroderma. Clin Rheumatol, 21: 114–118.

Dalakas MC & Hohlfeld R (2003) Polymyositis and dermatomyositis. Lancet, 362(9388): 971–982.

D'Alfonso S, Rampi M, Bocchio D, Colombo G, Scorza-Smeraldi R, & Momigliano-Richiardi P (2000) Systemic lupus erythematosus candidate genes in the Italian population: Evidence for a significant association with interleukin-10. Arthritis Rheum, 43: 120–128.

Daly AK (1995) Molecular basis of polymorphic drug metabolism. Mol Med, 73: 539–553.

Dambinova SA, Granstrem OK, Tourov A, Salluzzo R, Castello F, & Izykenova GA (1998) Monitoring of brain spiking activity and autoantibodies to N-terminus domain of GluR1 subunit of AMPA receptors in blood serum of rats with cobalt-induced epilepsy. J Neurochem, 71: 2088–2093.

Damoiseaux JG (2002) Cyclosporin A-induced autoimmunity in the rat: central versus peripheral tolerance. Int J Immunopathol Pharmacol, 15(2): 81–87.

Damoiseaux JG, Dopp EA, & Dijkstra CD (1991) Cellular binding mechanism on rat macrophages for sialylated glycoconjugates, inhibited by the monoclonal antibody ED3. J Leukoc Biol, 49: 434–441.

Dantas DCM & Queiroz MLS (1997) Immunoglobulin E and autoantibodies in mercury-exposed workers. Immunopharmacol Immunotoxicol, 19(3): 383–392.

Darnell RB & Posner JB (2003) Paraneoplastic syndromes involving the nervous system. N Engl J Med, 349: 1543–1554.

Das P, Abraham R, & David C (2000) HLA transgenic mice as models of human autoimmune diseases. Rev Immunogenet, 2(1): 105–114.

Das YT, Bagchi M, Bagchi D, & Preuss HG (2004) Safety of 5-hydroxy-L-tryptophan. Toxicol Lett, 150: 111–122.

Daston G, Faustman E, Ginsberg G, Fenner-Crisp P, Olin S, Sonawane B, Bruckner J, Breslin W, & McLaughlin TJ (2004) A framework for assessing risks to children from exposure to environmental agents. Environ Health Perspect, 112(2): 238–256.

David CS (1997) The mystery of HLA-B27 and disease. Immunogenetics, 46: 73–77.

D'Cruz D (2000) Autoimmune diseases associated with drugs, chemicals and environmental factors. Toxicol Lett, 112/113: 421–432.

Dean GS, Tyrell-Price J, Crawley J, & Isenberg DA (2000) Cytokines and systemic lupus erythematosus. Ann Rheum Dis, 59: 243–251.

Degoul F, Sutton A, Mansouri A, Cepanec C, Degott C, Fromenty B, Beaugrand M, Valla D, & Pessayre D (2001) Homozygosity for alanine in the mitochondrial targeting sequence of superoxide dismutase and risk for severe alcoholic liver disease. Gastroenterology, **120**: 1468–1474.

De Heer C, Van Driesten G, Shuurman HJ, Rozing J, & van Loveren H (1995) No evidence for emergence of autoreactive V beta 6+ T cells in Mls-1a mice following exposure to a thymotoxic dose of 2,3,7,8-tetrachlorodibenzo-*p*-dioxin. Toxicology, **10**: 195–203.

DeHoratius RJ, Pillarisetty R, Messner RP, & Talal N (1975) Anti-nucleic acid antibodies in systemic lupus erythematosus patients and their families. Incidence and correlation with lymphocytotoxic antibodies. J Clin Invest, **56**: 1149–1154.

De Jong WH, Goldhoorn CA, Kallewaard M, Geertsma RE, van Loveren H, Bijlsma JWJ, & Schouten JSAG (2002) Study to determine the presence of antipolymer antibodies in a group of Dutch women with a silicone breast implant. Clin Exp Rheumatol, **20**(2):151–160.

De Jong WH, Kallewaard M, Goldhoorn CA, Verhoef CM, Bijlsma JWJ, Schouten JSAG, & van Loveren H (2004) Long-term exposure to silicone breast implants does not induce antipolymer antibodies. Biomaterials, **25**: 1095–1103.

Delamere JP, Jobson S, Mackintosh LP, Wells L, & Walton KW (1983) Penicillamine-induced myasthenia in rheumatoid arthritis: its clinical and genetic features. Ann Rheum Dis, **42**(5): 500–504.

del Puente A, Knowler WC, Pettitt DJ, & Bennett PH (1988) The incidence of rheumatoid arthritis is predicted by rheumatoid factor titer in a longitudinal population study. Arthritis Rheum, **31**: 1239–1244.

Deluca HF & Cantorna MT (2001) Vitamin D: its role and uses in immunology. FASEB J, **15**: 2579–2585.

Demoly P & Bousquet J (2001) Epidemiology of drug allergy. Curr Opin Allergy Clin Immunol, **1**(4): 305–310.

Deng C, Lu Q, Zhang Z, Rao T, Attwood J, Yung R, & Richardson B (2003) Hydralazine may induce autoimmunity by inhibiting extracellular signal-regulated kinase pathway signaling. Arthritis Rheum, **48**(3): 746–756.

Depta JP & Pichler WJ (2003) Cross-reactivity with drugs at the T cell level. Curr Opin Allergy Clin Immunol, **3**(4): 261–267.

Derk CT & Jimenez SA (2003) Systemic sclerosis: current views of its pathogenesis. Autoimmunol Rev, **2**: 181–191.

De Rycke L, Kruithof E, Van Damme N, Hoffman IE, Van den Bossche N, Van den Bosch F, Veys EM, & De Keyser F (2003) Antinuclear antibodies following infliximab treatment in patients with rheumatoid arthritis or spondylarthropathy. Arthritis Rheum, **48**: 1015–1023.

Descotes J (1992) The popliteal lymph node assay: a tool for studying the mechanisms of drug-induced autoimmune disorders. Toxicol Lett, **64–65**: 101–107.

Deutsch M, Tsopanou E, & Dourakis SP (2004) The autoimmune lymphoproliferative syndrome (Canale-Smith) in adulthood. Clin Rheumatol, **23**: 43–44.

De Waal EJ, Schuurman H-J, Loeber JG, van Loveren H, & Vos JG (1992) Alterations in the cortical thymic epithelium of rats after in vivo exposure to 2,3,7,8-tetrachlorodibenzo-*p*-dioxin (TCDD): an immunohistological study. Toxicol Appl Pharmacol, **115**: 80–88.

Dexter SL (1984) Zimeldine induced neuropathies. Hum Toxicol, **3**(2): 141–143.

DHHS (1993) Dental amalgam: a scientific review and recommended Public Health Service strategy for research, education and regulation. Final report of the Subcommittee on Risk Management of the Committee to Co-ordinate Environmental Health and Related Progams. Washington, DC, United States Department of Health and Human Services, Public Health Service.

Dianzani U, Bragardo M, DiFranco D, Alliaudi C, Scagni P, Buonfiglio D, Redoglia V, Bonissoni S, Correra A, Dianzani I, & Ramenghi U (1997) Deficiency of the Fas apoptosis pathway without gene mutations in pediatric patients with autoimmunity/lymphoproliferation. Blood, **89**: 2871–2879.

Dietrich LL, Bridges AJ, & Albertini MR (2000) Dermatomyositis after interferon alpha treatment. Med Oncol, **17**: 64–69.

Diggle GE (2001) The toxic oil syndrome: 20 years on. Int J Clin Pract, **55**: 371–375.

Dijkstra CD, Dopp EA, Vogels IM, & Van Noorden CJ (1987) Macrophages and dendritic cells in antigen-induced arthritis. An immunohistochemical study using cryostat sections of the whole knee joint of rat. Scand J Immunol, **26**: 513–523.

Dijkstra CD, Dopp EA, Huitinga I, & Damoiseaux JG (1992) Macrophages in experimental autoimmune diseases in the rat: a review. Curr Eye Res, **11**(Suppl): 75–79.

Diot E, Lesire V, Guilmot JL, Metzger MD, Pilore R, Rogier S, Stadler M, Diot P, Lemarie E, & Lasfargues G (2002) Systemic sclerosis and occupational risk factors: a case–control study. Occup Environ Med, **59**(8): 545–549.

Dodson VN, Dinman BD, Whitehouse WM, Nasr ANM, & Magnuson HJ (1971) Occupational acroosteolysis. Arch Environ Health, **22**: 83–91.

Donker AJ, Venuto RC, Vladutiu AO, Brentjens JR, & Andres GA (1984) Effects of prolonged administration of D-penicillamine or captopril in various strains of rats. Brown Norway rats treated with D-penicillamine develop autoantibodies, circulating immune complexes, and disseminated intravascular coagulation. Clin Immunol Immunopathol, **30**(1): 142–155.

Doran MF, Pond GR, Crowson CS, O'Fallon WM, & Gabriel SE (2002) Trends in incidence and mortality in rheumatoid arthritis in Rochester, Minnesota, over a forty-year period. Arthritis Rheum, **46**: 625–631.

Drappa J, Vaishnaw AK, Sullivan KA, Chu JL, & Elkon KB (1996) Fas gene mutations in the Canale-Smith syndrome, an inherited lymphoproliferative disorder associated with autoimmunity. N Engl J Med, **335**: 1643–1649.

Drossaers-Bakker KW, Zwinderman AH, van Zeben D, Breedveld FC, & Hazes JM (2002) Pregnancy and oral contraceptive use do not significantly influence outcome in long term rheumatoid arthritis. Ann Rheum Dis, **61**: 405–408.

Dubey D, Kuhn J, Vial MC, Druet P, & Bellon B (1993) Anti-interleukin-2 receptor monoclonal antibody therapy supports a role for Th1 like cells in $HgCl_2$-induced autoimmunity in rats. Scand J Immunol, **37**(4): 406–412.

Dubois EL & Strain L (1972) Failure of procainamide to induce a systemic lupus erythematosus-like disease in animals. Toxicol Appl Pharmacol, **21**(2): 253–259.

Dwosh E, Guimond C, Duquette P, & Sadovnick AD (2003) The interaction of MS and pregnancy: a critical review. Int MS J, **10**: 38–42.

Dyment DA, Ebers GC, & Sadovnick AD (2004) Genetics of multiple sclerosis. Lancet Neurol, **3**(2): 104–110.

Edberg JE, Langefeld CD, Wu J, Moser KL, Kaufman KM, Kelly J, Bansal V, Brown WM, Salmon JE, Rich SS, Harley JB, & Kimberly RP (2002) Genetic linkage and association of Fcγ receptor IIIA (CD16A) on chromosome 1q23 with human systemic lupus erythematosus. Arthritis Rheum, **46**: 2132–2140.

Edlavitch SA (1997) Antipolymer antibodies, silicone breast implants, and fibromyalgia [letter]. Lancet, **349**(9059): 1170.

Edworthy SM, Martin L, Barr SG, Birdsell DC, Brant RF, & Fritzler MJ (1998) A clinical study of the relationship between silicone breast implants and connective tissue disease. J Rheumatol, **25**: 254–260.

Elenkov IJ, Papanicolaou DA, Wilder RL, & Chrousos GP (1996) Modulatory effects of glucocorticoids and catecholamines on human interleukin-12 and interleukin-10 production: clinical implications. Proc Assoc Am Physicians, **108**: 374–381.

Elenkov IJ, Wilder RL, Bakalov VK, Link AA, Dimitrov MA, Fisher S, Crane M, Kanik KS, & Chrousos GP (2001) IL-12, TNF-alpha, and hormonal changes during late pregnancy and early postpartum: implications for autoimmune disease activity during these times. J Clin Endocrinol Metab, **86**: 4933–4938.

Emery P & Panayi GS (1989) Autoimmune reactions to D-penicillamine. In: Kammuller ME, Bloksma N, & Seinen W eds. Autoimmunity and toxicology: immune disregulation induced by drugs and chemicals. Amsterdam, Elsevier, pp 167–182.

Emslie-Smith AM, Engel A, Duffy J, & Bowles CA (1991) Eosinophilia myalgia syndrome: I. Immunocytochemical evidence for a T-cell mediated immune effector response. Ann Neurol, **29**: 524–528.

Eneström S & Hultman P (1995) Does amalgam affect the immune system? A controversial issue. Int Arch Allergy Immunol, **106**: 180–203.

Englert H, Small-McMahon J, Davis K, O'Connor H, Chambers P, & Brooks P (2000) Male systemic sclerosis and occupational silica exposure — a population-based study. Aust NZ J Med, **30**: 215–220.

Enzer I, Dunn G, Jacobsson L, Bennett PH, Knowler WC, & Silman A (2002) An epidemiologic study of trends in prevalence of rheumatoid factor for seropositivity in Pima Indians: evidence of a decline due to both secular and birth-cohort influences. Arthritis Rheum, **46**: 1729–1734.

Etzioni A (2003) Immune deficiency and autoimmunity. Autoimmunity Rev, **2**: 364–369.

Evans HL, Taioli E, Toniolo P, & El-Fawal HAN (1994) Serum autoantibody to nervous proteins: Isotypes in workers exposed to cadmium and nickel. Toxicologist, **14**: 291.

Everson MP & Blackburn WD Jr (1997) Antipolymer antibodies, silicone breast implants, and fibromyalgia [letter]. Lancet, **349**(9059): 1171.

Evron E, Brautbar C, Becker S, Fenakel G, Abend Y, Sthoeger Z, Cohen P, & Geltner D (1995) Correlation between gold-induced enterocolitis and the presence of the HLA-DRB1*0404 allele. Arthritis Rheum, **38**: 755–759.

Ezendam J (2004) Mechanisms of hexachlorobenzene-induced adverse immune effects [thesis]. Utrecht, Utrecht University.

Ezendam J, Hassing I, Bleumink R, Vos JG, & Pieters R (2004a) Hexachlorobenzene-induced immunopathology in Brown Norway rats is partly mediated by T cells. Toxicol Sci, **78**: 88–95.

Ezendam J, Staedtler F, Pennings J, Vandebriel RJ, Pieters R, Harleman JH, & Vos JG (2004b) Toxicogenomics of subchronic hexachlorobenzene exposure in Brown Norway rats. Environ Health Perspect, **112**(7): 782–791.

Fabris P, Floreani A, Tositti G, Vergani D, De Lalla F, & Betterle C (2003) Type 1 diabetes mellitus in patients with chronic hepatitis C before and after interferon therapy. Aliment Pharmacol Ther, **18**(6): 549–558.

Fagius J, Osterman PO, Siden A, & Wiholm BE (1985) Guillain-Barre syndrome following zimeldine treatment. J Neurol Neurosurg Psychiatry, **48**(1): 65–69.

Fairweather D, Kaya Z, Shellam GR, Lawson CM, & Rose NR (2001) From infection to autoimmunity. J Autoimmunol, **16**: 175–186.

Farrell RJ & Kelly CP (2002) Celiac sprue. N Engl J Med, **346**: 180–188.

Farrell RJ & Peppercorn MA (2002) Ulcerative colitis. Lancet, **359**(9303): 331–340.

Feghali-Bostwick C, Medsger TA Jr, & Wright TM (2003) Analysis of systemic sclerosis in twins reveals low concordance for disease and high concordance for the presence of antinuclear antibodies. Arthritis Rheum, **48**: 1956–1963.

Feld JJ & Heathcote EJ (2003) Epidemiology of autoimmune liver disease. J Gastroenterol Hepatol, **18**(10): 1118–1128.

Fellermann K, Wehkamp J, Herrlinger KR, & Stange EF (2003) Crohn's disease: a defensin deficiency syndrome? Eur J Gastroenterol Hepatol, 15: 627–634.

Ferucci ED, Templin DW, & Lanier AP (2005) Rheumatoid arthritis in American Indians and Alaska Natives: a review of the literature. Semin Arthritis Rheum, 34: 662–667.

Field AC, Caccavelli L, Fillion J, Kuhn J, Mandet C, Druet P, & Bellon B (2000) Neonatal induction of tolerance to T(h)2-mediated autoimmunity in rats. Int Immunol, 12(10): 1467–1477.

Field AC, Caccavelli L, Bloch MF, & Bellon B (2003) Regulatory $CD8^+$ T cells control neonatal tolerance to a Th2-mediated autoimmunity. J Immunol, 170(5): 2508–2515.

Field T & Bridges AJ (1996) Clinical and laboratory features of patients with scleroderma and silicone implants. Curr Top Microbiol Immunol, 210: 283–290.

Fife MS, Fisher SA, John S, Worthington J, Shah CJ, Ollier WER, Panayi GS, Lewis CM, & Lanchbury JS (2000) Multipoint linkage analysis of a candidate gene locus in rheumatoid arthritis demonstrates significant evidence of linkage and association with the corticotropin-releasing hormone genomic region. Arthritis Rheum, 43: 1673–1678.

Filaci G & Suciu-Foca N (2002) $CD8^+$ T suppressor cells are back to the game: are they players in autoimmunity? Autoimmunity Rev, 1: 279–283.

Firestein GS (2003) Evolving concepts of rheumatoid arthritis. Nature (Lond), 423: 356–361.

Firestein GS, Echeverri F, Yeo M, Zvaifler NJ, & Green DR (1997) Somatic mutations in the p53 tumor suppressor gene in rheumatoid arthritis synovium. Proc Natl Acad Sci U S A, 94: 10895–10900.

Fisher GH, Rosenberg FJ, Straus SE, Dale JK, Middleton LA, Lin AY, Strober W, Leonardo MJ, & Puck JM (1995) Dominant interfering Fas gene mutations impair apoptosis in a human autoimmune lymphoproliferative syndrome. Cell, 81: 935–946.

Flassbeck D, Pfleiderer B, Klemens P, Heumann KG, Eltze E, & Hirner AV (2003) Determination of siloxanes, silicon, and platinum in tissues of women with silicone gel-filled implants. Anal Bioanal Chem, 375: 356–362.

Flescher E & Talal N (1991) Do viruses contribute to the development of Sjögren's syndrome? Am J Med, 90: 283–285.

Flockhart DA, Clauw DJ, Buchert Sale E, Hewett J, & Woosley R (1994) Pharmacogenetic characteristics of the eosinophilia-myalgia syndrome. Clin Pharmacol Ther, 56: 398–405.

Folwaczny C, Glas J, & Török HP (2003) Crohn's disease: an immunodeficiency? Eur J Gastroenterol Hepatol, 15: 621–626.

Ford CD, Johnson GH, & Smith WG (1983) Natural killer cells in in utero diethylstilbestrol-exposed patients. Gynecol Oncol, 16: 400–404.

Forsberg JG (2000) Neonatal estrogen treatment and its consequences for thymus development, serum level of autoantibodies to cardiolipin, and the delayed-type hypersensitivity response. J Toxicol Environ Health A, **60**: 185–213.

Fortin PR, Lew RA, Liang MH, Wright EA, Beckett LA, Chalmers TC, & Sperling RI (1995) Validation of a meta-analysis: the effects of fish oil in rheumatoid arthritis. J Clin Epidemiol, **48**: 1379–1390.

Fournie GJ, Mas M, Cautain B, Savignac M, Subra JF, Pelletier L, Saoudi A, Lagrange D, Calise M, & Druet P (2001) Induction of autoimmunity through bystander effects. Lessons from immunological disorders induced by heavy metals. J Autoimmun, **16**: 319–326.

Fox RI, Luppi M, Pisa P, & Kang HL (1992) Potential role of Epstein-Barr virus in Sjögren's syndrome and rheumatoid arthritis. J Rheumatol, **19**: 18–24.

Fraser PA, Ding WZ, Mohseni M, Treadwell EL, Dooley MA, St Clair EW, Gilkeson GS, & Cooper GS (2003) Glutathione S-transferase M null homozygosity and risk of systemic lupus erythematosus associated with sun exposure: a possible gene–environmental interaction for autoimmunity. J Rheumatol, **30**: 276–282.

Frenkel K, Karkoszka J, Cohen B, Baranski B, Jakubowski M, Cosma G, Taioli E, & Toniolo P (1994) Occupational exposures to Cd, Ni, and Cr modulate titers of anti-oxidized DNA base autoantibodies. Environ Health Perspect, **102**(Suppl 3): 221–229.

Friedetzky A, Grau V, Wieckenberg M, Lewen A, Gemsa D, & Garn H (2002) Long term iNOS expression in thoracic lymph nodes of silicotic rats. Immunobiology, **205**(3): 219–230.

Friedman SL (1999) Stellate cell activation in alcoholic fibrosis — an overview. Alcohol Clin Exp Res, **23**(5): 904–910.

Friis S, Mellemkjaer L, McLaughlin JK, Breiting V, Kjaer SK, Blot W, & Olson JH (1997) Connective tissue disease and other rheumatic conditions following breast implants in Denmark. Ann Plast Surg, **39**: 1–8.

Fritzler MJ, Pauls JD, Kinsella TD, & Bowen TJ (1985) Antinuclear, anticytoplasmic, and anti-Sjogren's syndrome antigen A (SS-A/Ro) antibodies in female blood donors. Clin Immunol Immunopathol, **36**: 120–128.

Froicu M, Weaver V, Wynn TA, McDowell MA, Welsh JE, & Cantorna MT (2003) A crucial role for the vitamin D receptor in experimental inflammatory bowel diseases. Mol Endocrinol, **17**: 2386–2392.

Fronczak CM, Baron AE, Chase HP, Ross C, Brady HL, Hoffman M, Eisenbarth GS, Rewers M, & Norris JM (2003) In utero dietary exposures and risk of islet autoimmunity in children. Diabetes Care, **26**: 3237–3242.

Fryzek JP, Signorello LB, Hakelius L, Lipworth L, McLaughlin JK, Blot WJ, & Nyren O (2001) Local complications and subsequent symptom reporting among women with cosmetic breast implants. Plast Reconstr Surg, **107**(1): 214–221.

Gabriel SE, O'Fallon WM, Kurland LT, Beard CM, Woods JE, & Melton LJ (1994) Risk of connective-tissue diseases and other disorders after breast implantation. N Engl J Med, **330**: 1697–1702.

Gadoth N (2003) Multiple sclerosis in children. Brain Dev, **25**(4): 229–232.

Gallardo S, del Pozo V, Cardaba B, de Andres B, Martin-Orozco E, Fernandez JC, Tramon P, Posada de la Paz M, Abaitua Borda I, Palomino P, & Lahoz C (1994) Immunological basis of toxic oil syndrome (TOS). Toxicology, **93**: 289–299.

Gallardo S, Cardaba B, del Poza V, Belen DA, Cortegano MI, Jurado A, Tramon P, Palomino P, & Lahoz C (1997) Study of apoptosis in human lymphocytes by toxic substances implicated in toxic oil syndrome. Toxicology, **118**: 71–82.

Garabrant DH, Lacey JV Jr, Laing TJ, Gillespie BW, Mayes MD, Cooper BC, & Schottenfeld D (2003) Scleroderma and solvent exposure among women. Am J Epidemiol, **157**: 493–500.

Garchon HJ (2003) Genetics of autoimmune myasthenia gravis, a model for antibody-mediated autoimmunity in man. J Autoimmun, **21**: 105–110.

Garn H, Friedetzky A, Kirchner A, Jager R, & Gemsa D (2000) Experimental silicosis: a shift to a preferential IFN-gamma-based Th1 response in thoracic lymph nodes. Am J Physiol Lung Cell Mol Physiol, **278**(6): L1221–1230.

Gatenby PA (1991) The role of complement in the aetiopathogenesis of systemic lupus erythematosus. Autoimmunity, **11**(1): 61–66.

Gaubitz M, Jackisch C, Domschke W, Heindel W, & Pfleiderer B (2002) Silicone breast implants: correlation between implant ruptures, magnetic resonance spectroscopically estimated silicone presence in the liver, antibody status and clinical symptoms. Rheumatology, **41**: 129–135.

Gehrs BC & Friedberg RC (2002) Autoimmune hemolytic anemia. Am J Hematol, **69**: 258–271.

Geier MR & Geier DA (2003) Neurodevelopmental disorders after thimerosal-containing vaccines: a brief communication. Exp Biol Med, **228**: 660–664.

Gelpi E, Posada de la Paz M, Terracini B, Abaitua I, Gomez de la Camara A, Kilbourne EM, Lahoz C, Nemery B, Philen RM, Soldevilla L, & Tarkowski S (2002) The Spanish toxic oil syndrome 20 years after its onset: a multidisciplinary review of scientific knowledge. Environ Health Perspect, **110**: 457–464.

Gerszten PC (1999) A formal risk assessment of silicone breast implants. Biomaterials, **20**: 1063–1069.

Gherardi RK, Coquet M, Cherin P, Belec L, Moretto P, Dreyfus PA, Pelissier JF, Chariot P, & Authier FJ (2001) Macrophagic myofasciitis lesions assess long-term persistence of vaccine-derived aluminium hydroxide in muscle. Brain, **124**: 1821–1831.

Gherardi RK & Authier FJ (2003) Aluminum inclusion macrophagic myofasciitis: a recently identified condition. Immunol Allergy Clin North Am, **23**(4): 699–712.

Ghio AJ, Kennedy TP, Schapira RM, Crumbliss AL, & Hoisal JR (1990) Hypothesis: is lung disease after silicate inhalation caused by oxidant generation? Lancet, **336**(8721): 967–969.

Ghosh S, Shand A, & Ferguson A (2000) Ulcerative colitis. Brit Med J, **320**: 1119–1123.

Gilbert KM, Whitlow AB, & Pumford NR (2004) Environmental contaminant and disinfection by-product trichloroacetaldehyde stimulates T cells in vitro. Int Immunopharmacol, **4**: 25–36.

Gleichmann H (1981) Studies on the mechanism of drug sensitization: T-cell-dependent popliteal lymph node reaction to diphenylhydantoin. Clin Immunol Immunopathol, **18**(2): 203–211.

Gocmen A, Peters HA, Cripps DJ, Morris CR, & Dogramaci I (1986) Porphyria turcica: hexachlorobenzene-induced porphyria. In: Morris C & Cabral JR eds. Hexachlorobenzene: Proceedings of an international symposium. Lyon, International Agency for Research on Cancer, pp 567–573 (IARC Scientific Publications No. 77).

Goebel C, Griem P, Sachs B, Bloksma N, & Gleichmann E (1996) The popliteal lymph node assay in mice: screening of drugs and other chemicals for immunotoxic hazard. Inflamm Res, **45**(Suppl 2): S85–S90.

Goebel C, Vogel C, Wulferink M, Mittmann S, Sachs B, Schraa S, Abel J, Degen G, Uetrecht J, & Gleichmann E (1999) Procainamide, a drug causing lupus, induces prostaglandin H synthase-2 and formation of T cell-sensitizing drug metabolites in mouse macrophages. Chem Res Toxicol, **12**(6): 488–500.

Gomez de la Camara A, Abaitua Borda I, & Posada de la Paz M (1997) Toxicologists versus toxicological disasters: toxic oil syndrome, clinical aspects. Berlin/Heidelberg, Springer Verlag.

González S, Martínez-Borra J, López-Vásquez A, García-Fernández S, Torre-Alonso JC, & López-Larrea C (2002) MICA rather than MICB, TNFA, or HLA-DRB1 is associated with susceptibility to psoriatic arthritis. J Rheumatol, **29**: 973–978.

González-Escribano NF, Morales J, García-Lozano JR, Castillo MJ, Sánchez-Roman J, Núnez-Roldán A, & Sanchez B (1995) TAP polymorphism in patients with Behcet's disease. Ann Rheum Dis, **54**: 386–388.

Gonzalez-Gay MA, Garcia-Porrua C, Guerrero J, Rodriguez-Ledo P, & Llorca J (2003) The epidemiology of the primary systemic vasculitides in northwest Spain: implications of the Chapel Hill Consensus Conference definitions. Arthritis Rheum, **49**(3): 388–393.

Goodin DS (2004) Relationship between multiple sclerosis exacerbations and stress. Psychosom Med, **66**: 287–289.

Gorrie MJ, Qasim FJ, Whittle CJ, Gillespie KM, Szeto CC, Nicoletti F, Bolton EM, Bradley JA, & Mathieson PW (2000) Exogenous type-1 cytokines modulate mercury-induced hyper-IgE in the rat. Clin Exp Immunol, **121**: 17–22.

Goter-Robinson CJ, Balasz T, & Egorov IK (1986) Mercuric chloride, gold sodium thiomalate, and D-penicillamine induced antinuclear antibodies in mice. Toxicol Appl Pharmacol, **86**: 159–169.

Goverman J (1999) Tolerance and autoimmunity in TCR transgenic mice specific for myelin basic protein. Immunol Rev, **169**: 147–159.

Graham RR, Ortmann WA, Langefeld CD, Jawaheer D, Selby SA, Rodine PR, Baechler EC, Rohlf KE, Shark KB, Espe KJ, Green LE, Nair RP, Stuart PE, Elder JT, King RA, Moser KL, Gaffney PM, Bugawan TL, Erlich HA, Rich SS, Gregersen PK, & Behrens TW (2002) Visualizing human leukocyte antigen class II risk haplotypes in human systemic lupus erythematosus. Am J Hum Genet, **71**: 543–553.

Gran JT, Husby G, & Thorsby E (1983) HLA-DR antigens and gold toxicity. Ann Rheum Dis, **41**: 63–71.

Granum B, Gardner PI, Groeng E, Leikvold R, Namork E, & Lovik M (2001) Fine particles of widely different composition have an adjuvant effect on the production of allergen-specific antibodies. Toxicol Lett, **118**: 171–181.

Green DR, Droin N, & Pinkoski M (2003) Activation-induced cell death in T cells. Immunol Rev, **193**: 70–81.

Greenberg GN & Dement JM (1994) Exposure assessment and gender differences. J Occup Environ Med, **36**: 907–912.

Gregersen PK, Silver J, & Winchester RJ (1987) The shared epitope hypothesis: an approach to understanding the molecular genetics of susceptibility to rheumatoid arthritis. Arthritis Rheum, **30**: 1205–1213.

Gregorini G, Ferioli A, Donato F, Tira P, Morassi L, Tardanico R, Lancini L, & Maiorca R (1993) Association between silica exposure and necrotizing crescentic glomerulonephritis with p-ANCA and anti-MPO antibodies: a hospital-based case–control study. Adv Exp Med Biol, **336**: 435–440.

Gregorini G, Tira P, Frizza J, D'Haese PC, Elseviers MM, Nuyts G, Maiorca R, & De Broe ME (1997) ANCA-associated diseases and silica exposure. Clin Rev Allergy Immunol, **15**: 21–40.

Greinacher A, Eichler P, Lubenow N, & Kiefel V (2001) Drug-induced and drug-dependent immune thrombocytopenias. Rev Clin Exp Hematol, **5**(3): 166–200, 311–312.

Griem P, Panthel K, Kalbacher H, & Gleichmann E (1996) Alteration of a model antigen by Au(III) leads to T cell sensitization to cryptic peptides. Eur J Immunol, **26**(2): 279–287.

Griem P, Wulferink M, Sachs B, González JB, & Gleichmann E (1998) Allergic and autoimmune reactions to xenobiotics: how do they arise? Immunol Today, **19**: 133–141.

Griffin JM, Gilbert KM, Lamps LW, & Pumford NR (2000a) CD4(+) T-cell activation and induction of autoimmune hepatitis following trichloroethylene treatment in MRL +/+ mice. Toxicol Sci, **57**: 345–352.

Griffin JM, Gilbert KM, & Pumford NR (2000b) Inhibition of CYP2E1 reverses $CD4^+$ T-cell alterations in trichloroethylene-treated MRL+/+ mice. Toxicol Sci, **54**: 384–389.

Grima DT, Torrance GW, Francis G, Rice G, Rosner AJ, & Lafortune L (2000) Cost and health related quality of life consequences of multiple sclerosis. Mult Scler, **6**: 91–98.

Grodzicky T & Elkon KB (2002) Apoptosis: a case where too much or too little can lead to autoimmunity. Mt Sinai J Med, **69**: 208–219.

Grove J, Daly AK, Bassendine MF, & Day CP (1997) Association of a tumor necrosis factor promoter polymorphism with susceptibility to alcoholic steatohepatitis. Hepatology, **26**: 143–146.

Grove J, Brown AS, Daly AK, Bassendine MF, James OF, & Day CP (1998) The Rsal polymorphism of CYP2E1 and susceptibility to alcoholic liver disease in Caucasians: effect on age of presentation and dependence on alcohol dehydrogenase genotype. Pharmacogenetics, **8**(4): 335–342.

Grove J, Daly AK, Bassendine MF, Gilvarry E, & Day CP (2000) Interleukin 10 promoter region polymorphisms and susceptibility to advanced alcoholic liver disease. Gut, **46**: 540–545.

Guo XM & Rhodes J (1990) An essential role for constitutive Schiff base-forming ligands in antigen presentation to murine T cell clones. J Immunol, **144**: 2883–2890.

Gutierrez MA, Garcia ME, Rodriguez JA, Rivero S, & Jacobelli S (1998) Hypothalamic–pituitary–adrenal axis function and prolactin secretion in systemic lupus erythematosus. Lupus, **7**: 404–408.

Gutting BW, Schomaker SJ, Kaplan AH, & Amacher DE (1999) A comparison of the direct and reporter antigen popliteal lymph node assay for the detection of immunomodulation by low molecular weight compounds. Toxicol Sci, **51**(1): 71–79.

Gutting BW, Updyke LW, & Amacher DE (2002a) Investigating the TNP-OVA and direct popliteal lymph node assays for the detection of immunostimulation by drugs associated with anaphylaxis in humans. J Appl Toxicol, **22**(3): 177–183.

Gutting BW, Updyke LW, & Amacher DE (2002b) BALB/c mice orally pretreated with diclofenac have augmented and accelerated PLNA responses to diclofenac. Toxicology, **172**(3): 217–230.

Hajeer AH, Worthington J, Silman AJ, & Ollier WER (1996) Association of tumor necrosis factor microsatellite polymorphisms with HLA-DRB1*04-bearing haplotypes in rheumatoid arthritis patients. Arthritis Rheum, **39**: 1109–1114.

Hakala M, Silvennoinen-Kassinen S, Ikäheimo I, Isosomppi J, & Tilikainen A (1997) HLA markers in a community based rheumatoid arthritis series. Ann Med, **29**: 291–296.

Hall A, Kane M, Roure C, & Meheus A (1999) Multiple sclerosis and hepatitis B vaccine? Vaccine, **17**: 2473–2475.

Hall AJ, Yee LJ, & Thomas SL (2002) Life course epidemiology and infectious diseases. Int J Epidemiol, **31**(2): 300–301.

Hall GM, Daniels M, Huskisson EC, & Spector TD (1994) A randomized controlled trial of the effect of hormone replacement therapy on disease activity in postmenopausal rheumatoid arthritis. Ann Rheum Dis, **53**: 112–116.

Hammarstrom L, Vorechovsky I, & Webster D (2000) Selective IgA deficiency (SIgAD) and common variable immunodeficiency (CVID). Clin Exp Immunol, **120**(2): 225–231.

Han Z, Boyle DL, Shi Y, Green DR, & Firestein GS (1999) Dominant-negative p53 mutations in rheumatoid arthritis. Arthritis Rheum, **42**: 1088–1092.

Hanley GA, Schiffenbauer J, & Sobel ES (1998) Resistance to $HgCl_2$-induced autoimmunity in haplotype-heterozygous mice is an intrinsic property of B cells. J Immunol, **161**: 1778–1785.

Hard GC (2000) Short-term adverse effects in humans of ingested mineral oils, their additives, and possible contaminants — a review. Hum Exp Toxicol, **19**: 158–172.

Hard GC (2002) A search for an animal model of the Spanish toxic oil syndrome. Food Chem Toxicol, **40**: 1551–1567.

Hari CK, Raza SA, & Clayton MI (1998) Hydralazine-induced lupus and vocal fold paralysis. J Laryngol Otol, **112**(9): 875–877.

Harness J & McCombe PA (2001) The effects of pregnancy on myelin basic protein-induced experimental autoimmune encephalomyelitis in Lewis rats: Suppression of clinical disease, modulation of cytokine expression in the spinal cord inflammatory infiltrate and suppression of lymphocyte proliferation by pregnancy sera. Am J Reprod Immunol, **46**: 405–412.

Harness J, Cavanagh A, Morton H, & McCombe P (2003) A protective effect of early pregnancy factor on experimental autoimmune encephalomyelitis induced in Lewis rats by inoculation with myelin basic protein. J Neurol Sci, **216**: 33–41.

Harrison BJ (2002) Influence of cigarette smoking on disease outcome in rheumatoid arthritis. Curr Opin Rheumatol, **14**: 93–97.

Haustein UF & Ziegler V (1985) Environmentally induced systemic sclerosis-like disorders. Int J Dermatol, **24**: 147–151.

Havarinasab S, Lambertsson L, Qvarnstrom J, & Hultman P (2004) Dose–response study of thimerosal induced murine systemic autoimmunity. Toxicol Appl Pharmacol, **194**: 169–179.

Hawkins BR, Dawkins RL, Burger HG, MacKay IR, Cheah PS, Whittingham S, Patel Y, & Welborn TA (1980) Diagnostic significance of thyroid microsomal antibodies in randomly selected population. Lancet, **2**(8203): 1057–1059.

He XS, Ansari AA, & Gershwin ME (2001) Xenobiotic considerations for the development of autoimmune liver diseases: bad genes and bad luck. Rev Environ Health, **16**: 191–201.

References

Heldt C, Listing J, Sözeri O, Bläsing F, Frishbutter S, & Müller B (2003) Differential expression of HLA class II genes associated with disease susceptibility and progression in rheumatoid arthritis. Arthritis Rheum, **48**: 2779–2787.

Heliovaara M, Aho K, Knekt P, Impivaara O, Reunanen A, & Aromaa A (2000) Coffee consumption, rheumatoid factor, and the risk of rheumatoid arthritis. Ann Rheum Dis, **59**: 631–635.

Hennekens CH, Lee IM, Cook NR, Hebert PR, Karlson EW, LaMotte F, Manson JE, & Buring JE (1996) Self-reported breast implants and connective-tissue diseases in female health professionals. A retrospective cohort study. J Am Med Assoc, **275**: 616–621.

Henry J, Miller MM, & Pontarotti P (1999) Structure and evolution of the extended B7 family. Immunol Today, **20**(6): 285–288.

Hernán MA, Hohol MJ, Olek MJ, Spiegelman D, & Ascherio A (2000) Oral contraceptives and the incidence of multiple sclerosis. Neurology, **55**: 848–854.

Hernán MA, Oleky MJ, & Ascherio A (2001) Cigarette smoking and incidence of multiple sclerosis. Am J Epidemiol, **154**: 69–74.

Herold KC, Vezys V, Sun Q, Viktora D, Seung E, Reiner S, & Brown DR (1996) Regulation of cytokine production during development of autoimmune diabetes induced with multiple low doses of streptozotocin. J Immunol, **156**(9): 3521–3527.

Hertzman PA, Blevins WL, Mayer J, Greenfield B, Ting M, & Gleich GJ (1990) Association of the eosinophilia-myalgia syndrome with the ingestion of tryptophan. N Engl J Med, **322**: 869–873.

Hertzman PA, Clauw DJ, Kaufman LD, Varga J, Silver RM, Thacker HL, Mease P, Espinoza LR, & Pincus T (1995) The eosinophilia myalgia syndrome: status of 205 patients and results of treatment two years after onset. Ann Intern Med, **122**: 851–855.

Hill RH, Caudill SP, Philen RM, Bailey SL, Flanders WD, Driskell WJ, Kamb ML, Needham LL, & Sampson EJ (1993) Contaminants in L-tryptophan associated with eosinophilia myalgia syndrome. Arch Environ Contam Toxicol, **25**: 134–142.

Hirsch F, Couderc J, Sapin C, Fournie G, & Druet P (1982) Polyclonal effect of $HgCl_2$ in the rat, its possible role in an experimental autoimmune disease. Eur J Immunol, **12**(7): 620–625.

Hirsch F, Kuhn J, Ventura M, Vial MC, Fournie G, & Druet P (1986) Autoimmunity induced by $HgCl_2$ in Brown-Norway rats. I. Production of monoclonal antibodies. J Immunol, **136**(9): 3272–3276.

Hitraya EG, Jimenez SA, Ludwicka A, Silver RM, & Varga J (1997) Increased activity of the α1(I) procollagen promoter in skin fibroblasts from patients with chronic eosinophilia-myalgia syndrome. Int J Biochem Cell Biol, **29**: 135–141.

Hochberg MC & Perlmutter DL (1996) The association of augmentation mammoplasty with connective tissue disease, including systemic sclerosis (scleroderma): a meta-analysis. Curr Top Microbiol Immunol, **210**: 411–417.

Hochberg MC & Petri M (1993) Clinical features of systemic lupus erythematosus. Curr Opin Rheumatol, **5**: 575–586.

Hochberg MC, Perlmutter DL, Medsger TA Jr, Nguyen K, Steen V, Weisman MH, White B, & Wigley FM (1996) Lack of association between augmentation mammoplasty and systemic sclerosis (scleroderma). Arthritis Rheum, **39**: 1125–1131.

Hoebe K, Janssen E, & Beutler B (2004) The interface between innate and adaptive immunity. Nat Immunol, **5**(10): 971–974.

Hoek RM, Ruuls SR, Murphy CA, Wright GJ, Goddard R, Zurawski SM, Blom B, Homola ME, Streit WJ, Brown MH, Barclay AN, & Sedgwick JD (2000) Downregulation of the macrophage lineage through interaction with OX2 (CD200). Science, **290**: 1768–1771.

Hogan SL, Satterly KK, Dooley MA, Nachman PH, Jennette JC, & Falk RJ (2001) Silica exposure in anti-neutrophil cytoplasmic autoantibody-associated glomerulonephritis and lupus nephritis. J Am Soc Nephrol, **12**: 134–142.

Holladay SD (1999) Prenatal immunotoxicant exposure and postnatal autoimmune disease. Environ Health Perspect, **107**(Suppl 5): 687–691.

Hollowell JG, Staehling NW, Flanders WD, Hannon WH, Gunter EW, Spencer CA, & Braverman LE (2002) Serum TSH, T(4), and thyroid antibodies in the United States population (1988 to 1994): National Health and Nutrition Examination Survey (NHANES III). J Clin Endocrinol Metab, **87**: 489–499.

Holmdahl R, Andersson EC, Andersen CB, Svejgaard A, & Fugger L (1999) Transgenic mouse models of rheumatoid arthritis. Immunol Rev, **169**: 161–173.

Holmich LR, Friis S, Fryzek JP, Vejborg IM, Conrad C, Sletting S, Kjoller K, McLaughlin JK, & Olsen JH (2003) Incidence of silicone breast implant rupture. Arch Surg, **138**: 801–806.

Hopkinson ND, Doherty M, & Powell RJ (1993) The prevalence and incidence of systemic lupus erythematosus in Nottingham, UK, 1989–1990. Br J Rheumatol, **32**: 110–115.

Horiuchi T, Nishizaka H, Yasunaga S, Higuchi M, Tsukamoto H, Hayashi H, & Nagasawa K (1999) Association of Fas/Apo-1 gene polymorphism with systemic lupus erythematosus in Japanese. Rheumatology (Oxford), **38**: 516–520.

Horseman ND & Yu-Lee LY (1994) Transcriptional regulation by the helix bundle peptide hormones: growth hormone, prolactin, and hematopoietic cytokines. Endocrinol Rev, **15**: 627–649.

Hrubec Z & Omenn GS (1981) Evidence of genetic predisposition to alcoholic cirrhosis and psychosis: twin concordances for alcoholism and its biological end points by zygosity among male veterans. Alcohol Clin Exp Res, **5**: 207–215.

Huang SH, Hubbs AF, Stanley CF, Vallyathan V, Schnabel PC, Rojanasakul Y, Ma JK, Banks DE, & Weissman DN (2001) Immunoglobulin responses to experimental silicosis. Toxicol Sci, **59**: 108–117.

Hudson CA, Cao L, Kasten-Jolly J, Kirkwood JN, & Lawrence DA (2003) Susceptibility of lupus-prone NZM mouse strains to lead exacerbation of systemic lupus erythematosus symptoms. J Toxicol Environ Health, **A23**: 895–918.

Huizinga TW, van der Linder MW, Deneys-Laporte V, & Breedveld FC (1999) Interleukin-10 as an explanation for pregnancy-induced flare in systemic lupus erythematosus. Rheumatology, **38**: 496–498.

Hulsemann JL, Ruof J, Zeidler H, & Mittendorf T (2006) Costs in rheumatology: results and lessons learned from the "Hannover Costing Study". Rheumatol Int, **26**(8): 704–711 [Epub 1 November 2005].

Hultman P & Enestrom S (1992) Dose–response studies in murine mercury-induced autoimmunity and immune-complex disease. Toxicol Appl Pharmacol, **113**(2): 199–208.

Hultman P & Nielsen JB (2001) The effect of dose, gender, and non-H-2 genes in murine mercury-induced autoimmunity. J Autoimmun, **17**: 27–37.

Hultman P, Johansson U, Turley SJ, Lindh U, Enestrom S, & Pollard KM (1994) Adverse immunological effects and autoimmunity induced by dental amalgam and alloy in mice. FASEB J, **8**: 1183–1190.

Hultman P, Turley SJ, Enestrom S, Lindh U, & Pollard KM (1996) Murine genotype influences the specificity, magnitude and persistence of murine mercury-induced autoimmunity. J Autoimmun, **9**: 139.

Hunter I, Greene SA, MacDonald TM, & Morris AD (2000) Prevalence and aetiology of hypothyroidism in the young. Arch Dis Child, **83**(3): 207–210.

Hunziker H (1978) Gold induced autoimmunohemolytic anemia. Praxis, **67**: 702–704.

Hurtenbach U, Gleichmann H, Nagata N, & Gleichmann E (1987) Immunity to D-penicillamine: genetic, cellular, and chemical requirements for induction of popliteal lymph node enlargement in the mouse. J Immunol, **139**(2): 411–416.

Hviid A, Stellfield M, Wohlfahrt J, & Melbye M (2004) Childhood vaccination and type 1 diabetes. N Engl J Med, **350**: 1398–1404.

Hypponen E (2004) Micronutrients and the risk of type 1 diabetes: vitamin D, vitamin E, and nicotinamide. Nutr Rev, **62**: 340–347.

Hypponen E, Laara E, Reunanen A, Jarvelin MR, & Virtanen SM (2001) Intake of vitamin D and risk of type 1 diabetes: a birth-cohort study. Lancet, **358**(9292): 1500–1503.

Hyrich KL, Silman AJ, Watson KD, & Symmons DPM (2004) Anti-tumour necrosis factor α therapy in rheumatoid arthritis: an update on safety. Ann Rheum Dis, **63**: 1538–1543.

Iannello S, Camuto M, Cantarella S, Cavaleri A, Ferriero P, Leanza A, Milazzo P, & Belfiore F (2002) Rheumatoid syndrome associated with lung interstitial disorder in a dental technician exposed to ceramic silica dust. A case report and critical literature review. Clin Rheumatol, **21**(1): 76–81.

Imai S, Tezuka H, & Fujita K (2001) A factor of inducing IgE from a filarial parasite prevents insulin-dependent diabetes mellitus in nonobese diabetic mice. Biochem Biophys Res Commun, **286**(5): 1051–1058.

IPCS (1996) Principles and methods for assessing direct immunotoxicity associated with exposure to chemicals. Geneva, World Health Organization, International Programme on Chemical Safety (Environmental Health Criteria 180).

IPCS (1999) Principles and methods for assessing allergic hypersensitization associated with exposure to chemicals. Geneva, World Health Organization, International Programme on Chemical Safety (Environmental Health Criteria 212).

Iwasaki A & Medzhitov R (2004) Toll-like receptor control of the adaptive immune responses. Nat Immunol, **5**(10): 987–995.

Iyer R, Hamilton RE, Li L, & Holian A (1996) Silica-induced apoptosis mediated via scavenger receptor in human alveolar macrophages. Toxicol Appl Pharmacol, **141**: 84–92.

Izumi Y, Tanaka S, Hidaka Y, Shimaoka Y, Tatsumi KI, Takano T, Kaneko A, Oku K, & Amino N (2003) Relation between post-partum liver dysfunction and anti-cytochrome 2D6 antibodies. Am J Reprod Immunol, **50**: 355–362.

Jacobson DL, Gange SJ, Rose NR, & Graham NM (1997) Epidemiology and estimated population burden of selected autoimmune diseases in the United States. Clin Immunol Immunopathol, **84**(3): 223–243.

James JA, Kaufman KM, Farris AD, Taylor-Albert E, Lehman TJ, & Harley JB (1997) An increased prevalence of Epstein-Barr virus infection in young patients suggests a possible etiology for systemic lupus erythematosus. J Clin Invest, **100**: 3019–3026.

James JA, Neas BR, Moser KL, Hall T, Bruner GR, Sestak AL, & Harley JB (2001) Systemic lupus erythematosus in adults is associated with previous Epstein-Barr virus exposure. Arthritis Rheum, **44**: 1122–1126.

Janeway CA Jr & Medzhitov R (2002) Innate immune recognition. Annu Rev Immunol, **20**: 197–216.

Janowsky EC, Kupper LL, & Hulka BS (2000) Meta-analysis of the relation between silicone breast implants and the risk of connective tissue diseases. N Engl J Med, **342**: 781–790.

Jarvelainen HA, Orpana A, Perola M, Savolainen VT, Karhunen PJ, & Lindros KO (2001) Promoter polymorphism of the CD14 endotoxin receptor gene as a risk factor for alcoholic liver disease. Hepatology, **33**: 1148–1153.

Jennings AM, Wild G, Ward JD, & Ward AM (1988) Immunological abnormalities 17 years after accidental exposure to 2,3,7,8-tetrachlorodibenzo-*p*-dioxin. Br J Ind Med, **45**: 701–704.

Jensen B, Wittrup IH, Wiik A, Bliddal H, Friis AS, McLaughlin JK, Danneskiold-Samsoe B, & Olsen JH (2004) Antipolymer antibodies in Danish fibromyalgia patients. Clin Exp Rheumatol, **22**: 227–229.

Johnson AE, Gordon C, Palmer RG, & Bacon PA (1995) The prevalence and incidence of systemic lupus erythematosus in Birmingham, England. Relationship to ethnicity and country of birth. Arthritis Rheum, **38**: 551–558.

Johnson EO, Vlachoyiannopoulos PG, Skopouli FN, Tzioufas AG, & Moustsopoulos HM (1998) Hypofunction of the stress axis in Sjogren's syndrome. J Rheumatol, **25**: 1508–1514.

Jonsson R, Haga HJ, & Gordon TP (2000) Current concepts on diagnosis, autoantibodies and therapy in Sjogren's syndrome. Scand J Rheumatol, **29**: 341–348.

Jonsson TH, Thorsteinsson J, & Valdimarsson H (1998) Does smoking stimulate rheumatoid factor production in nonrheumatic individuals? APMIS, **106**: 970–974.

Joshi BG, Dwivedi C, Powell A, & Holscher M (1981) Immune complex nephritis in rats induced by long-term oral exposure to cadmium. J Comp Pathol, **91**: 11–15.

Jung D, Berg PA, Edler L, Ehrenthal W, Fenner D, Flesch-Janys D, Huber C, Klein R, Koitka C, Lucier G, Manz A, Muttray A, Needham L, Päpke O, Pietsch M, Portier C, Patterson D, Prellwitz W, Rose DM, Thews A, & Konietzko J (1998) Immunological findings in workers formerly exposed to 2,3,7,8-tetrachlorodibenzo-p-dioxin and its congeners. Environ Health Perspect, **106**(Suppl 2): 689–695.

Kahaly G, Dienes HP, Beyer J, & Hommel G (1997) Randomized, double blind, placebo-controlled trial of low dose iodide in endemic goiter. J Clin Endocrinol Metab, **82**(12): 4049–4053.

Kahaly GJ, Dienes HP, Beyer J, & Hommel G (1998) Iodide induces thyroid autoimmunity in patients with endemic goitre: a randomised, double-blind, placebo-controlled trial. Eur J Endocrinol, **139**(3): 290–297.

Kalb B, Matell G, Pirskanen R, & Lambe M (2002) Epidemiology of myasthenia gravis: a population-based study in Stockholm, Sweden. Neuroepidemiology, **21**: 221–225.

Kamb ML, Murphy JJ, Jones JL, Caston JC, Nederlof K, Horney LF, Swygert LA, Falk H, & Kilbourne EM (1992) Eosinophilia-myalgia syndrome in L-tryptophan-exposed patients. J Am Med Assoc, **267**: 77–82.

Kammuller ME & Seinen W (1988) Structural requirements for hydantoins and 2-thiohydantoins to induce lymphoproliferative popliteal lymph node reactions in the mouse. Int J Immunopharmacol, **10**(8): 997–1010.

Kammuller ME, Bloksma N, & Seinen W (1988) Chemical-induced autoimmune reactions and Spanish toxic oil syndrome: focus on hydantoins and related compounds. Clin Toxicol, **26**: 157–174.

Kammuller ME, Bloksma N, & Seinen S (1989a) Autoimmunity and toxicology: immune disregulation induced by drugs and chemicals. In: Kammuller ME, Bloksma N, & Seinen W eds. Autoimmunity and toxicology: immune disregulation induced by drugs and chemicals. Amsterdam, Elsevier, pp 3–34.

Kammuller ME, Thomas C, De Bakker JM, Bloksma N, & Seinen W (1989b) The popliteal lymph node assay in mice to screen for the immune disregulating potential of chemicals — a preliminary study. Int J Immunopharmacol, **11**(3): 293–300.

Kanemitsu S, Ihara K, Saifddin A, Otsuka T, Takeuchi T, Nagayama J, Kuwano M, & Hara T (2002) A functional polymorphism in Fas (CD95/APO-1) gene promotor associated with systemic lupus erythematosus. J Rheumatol, **29**: 1183–1188.

Karlson EW, Hankinson SE, Liang MH, Sanchez-Guerrero J, Colditz GA, Rosenau BJ, Speizer FE, & Schur PH (1999) Association of silicone breast implants with immunologic abnormalities: a prospective study. Am J Med, **106**: 11–19.

Karvonen M, Viik-Kajander M, Moltchanova E, Libman I, LaPorte R, & Tuomilehto J (2000) Incidence of childhood type 1 diabetes worldwide. Diabetes Mondiale (DiaMond) Project Group. Diabetes Care, **78**(1): 84–88.

Katsutani N & Shionoya H (1992) Drug-specific immune responses induced by immunization with drugs in guinea pigs and mice. J Toxicol Sci, **17**(4): 169–183.

Kaufman L & Krupp L (1995) Eosinophilia-myalgia syndrome, toxic-oil syndrome, and diffuse fasciitis with eosinophilia. Curr Opin Rheumatol, **7**: 560–567.

Kaufman LD, Gruber BL, & Gregersen PK (1991) Clinical follow-up and immunogenetic studies of 32 patients with eosinophilia-myalgia syndrome. Lancet, **337**(8749): 1071–1074.

Kaufman LD, Izquierdo Martinez M, Serrano JM, & Gomez-Reino JJ (1995) 12-year followup study of epidemic Spanish toxic oil syndrome. J Rheumatol, **22**: 282–288.

Khamashta MA, Ruiz-Irastorza G, & Hughes GR (1997) Systemic lupus erythematosus flares during pregnancy. Rheum Dis Clin North Am, **23**: 15–30.

Khan MA (2000) HLA-B27 polymorphism and association with disease. J Rheumatol, **27**(5): 1110–1114.

Khan MF, Kaphalia BS, Prabhakar BS, Kanz MF, & Ansari GA (1995) Trichloroethene induced autoimmune response in female MRL +/+ mice. Toxicol Appl Pharmacol, **134**: 155–160.

Khan MF, Wu X, & Ansari GA (2001) Anti-malondialdehyde antibodies in MRL +/+ mice treated with trichloroethene and dichloroacetyl chloride: possible role of lipid peroxidation in autoimmunity. Toxicol Appl Pharmacol, **170**: 88–92.

Khani-Hanjani A, Lacaille D, Horne C, Chalmers A, Hoar DI, Balshaw R, & Keown PA (2002) Expression of QK/QR/RRRAA or DERAA motifs at the third hypervariable region of HLA-DRB1 and disease severity in rheumatoid arthritis. J Rheumatol, **29**: 1358–1365.

Khurana R & Chauhan RS (2002) Pesticide induced immune complex mediated glomerulonephritis in sheep. J Immunol Immunopathol, **4**(1–2): 40–42.

Kim HA, Kim EM, Park YC, Yu JY, Hong SK, Jeon SH, Park KL, Hur SJ, & Heo Y (2003) Immunotoxicological effects of Agent Orange exposure to the Vietnam War Korean veterans. Ind Health, **41**: 158–166.

References

Kim HJ, Jeong KS, Park SJ, Cho SW, Son HY, Kim SR, Kim SH, An MY, & Ryu SY (2003) Effect of benzo[a]pyrene, 2-bromopropane, phenol and 2,3,7,8-tetrachlorodibenzo-p-dioxin on IL-6 production in mice after single or repeated exposure. In Vivo, **17**: 269–275.

Kimber I & Dearman R (2002) Immunologic basis for autoimmunity and the potential influences of xenobiotics. Toxicol Lett, **127**: 77–81.

Kimpimaki T, Kupila A, Hamalainen AM, Kukko M, Kulmala P, Savola K, Simell T, Keskinen P, Ilonen J, Simell O, & Knip M (2001) The first signs of beta-cell autoimmunity appear in infancy in genetically susceptible children from the general population: the Finnish Type 1 Diabetes Prediction and Prevention Study. J Clin Endocrinol Metab, **86**: 4782–4788.

Kirchner J, Stein A, Viel K, & Jacobi V (1997) [Hamman-Rich syndrome in a goldsmith.] Aktuelle Radiol, **7**: 321–323 (in German).

Kjoller K, Friis S, Mellemkjaer L, McLaughlin JK, Winther JF, Lipworth L, Blot WJ, Fryzek J, & Olsen JH (2001) Connective tissue disease and other rheumatic conditions following cosmetic breast implantation in Denmark. Arch Intern Med, **161**: 973–979.

Klinkhammer C, Dohle C, & Gleichmann H (1989) T cell-dependent class II major histocompatibility complex antigen expression in vivo induced by the diabetogen streptozotocin. Immunobiology, **180**(1): 1–11.

Klockars M, Koskela R-S, Jarvinen E, Kolari PJ, & Rossi A (1987) Silica exposure and rheumatoid arthritis: a follow-up study of granite workers 1940–81. Br Med J, **294**: 997–1000.

Knekt P, Heliovaara M, Aho K, Alfthan G, Marniemi J, & Aromaa A (2000) Serum selenium, serum alpha-tocopherol, and the risk of rheumatoid arthritis. Epidemiology, **11**: 402–405.

Knowles SR, Shapiro LE, & Shear NH (1999) Anticonvulsant hypersensitivity syndrome — incidence, prevention and management. Drug Saf, **21**: 489–501.

Koller LD (1980) Immunotoxicology of heavy metals. Int J Immunopharmacol, **2**(4): 269–279.

Koller LD, Stang BV, Posada de la Paz M, & Ruiz-Mendez MV (2001) Pathology of "toxic oils" and selected metals in the MRL/lpr mouse. Toxicol Pathol, **29**(6): 630–638.

Koller LD, Stang BV, Hall JA, Posada de la Paz M, & Ruiz-Mendez MV (2002) Immunoglobulin and autoantibody responses in MRL/lpr mice treated with "toxic oils". Toxicology, **178**: 119–133.

Kono DH, Balomenos D, Park MS, & Theofilopoulos AN (2000) Development of lupus in BXSB mice is independent of IL-4. J Immunol, **164**: 38–42.

Korn JH (1997) Antipolymer antibodies, silicone breast implants, and fibromyalgia [letter]. Lancet, **349**(9059): 1171.

Kornek B & Lassmann H (2003) Neuropathology of multiple sclerosis — new concepts. Brain Res Bull, **61**: 321–326.

Korpilähde T, Heliovaara M, Kaipiainen-Seppanen O, Knekt P, & Aho K (2003) Regional differences in Finland in the prevalence of rheumatoid factor in the presence and absence of arthritis. Ann Rheum Dis, **62**: 353–355.

Kosuda LL & Bigazzi PE (1996) Chemical-induced autoimmunity. In: Smialowicz RJ & Holsapple MP eds. Experimental immunotoxicology. Boca Raton, Florida, CRC Press, pp. 419–465.

Kosuda LL, Hosseinzadeh H, Greiner DL, & Bigazzi PE (1994) Role of RT6+ T lymphocytes in mercury-induced renal autoimmunity: experimental manipulations of "susceptible" and "resistant" rats. J Toxicol Environ Health, **42**(3): 303–321.

Kosugi A, Sharrow SO, & Shearer GM (1989) Effect of cyclosporin A on lymphopoiesis. I. Absence of mature T cells in thymus and periphery of bone marrow transplanted mice treated with cyclosporin A. J Immunol, **142**(9): 3026–3032.

Kotsy MP, Hench PK, Tani P, & McMillan R (1989) Thrombocytopenia associated with aurofin therapy: evidence for a gold-dependent immunologic mechanism. Am J Hematol, **30**: 236–239.

Kozhevnikova G, Kuzmin I, Roumak V, & Karaulov A (1991) Immune alteration in South Vietnamese exposed to Agent Orange. In: Dioxin '91 — Proceedings of the 11th international symposium on chlorinated dioxins and related compounds. Research Triangle Park, North Carolina, p 117.

Kralovicova J, Hammarström L, Plebani A, Webster ADB, & Vorechovsky I (2003) Fine-scale mapping at IGAD1 and genome-wide genetic lingage analysis implicate HLA-DQ/DR as a major susceptibility locus in selective IgA deficiency and common variable immunodeficiency. J Immunol, **170**: 2765–2775.

Kretz-Rommel A & Rubin RL (1999) Persistence of autoreactive T cell drive is required to elicit anti-chromatin antibodies in a murine model of drug-induced lupus. J Immunol, **162**(2): 813–820.

Kretz-Rommel A & Rubin RL (2000) Disruption of positive selection of thymocytes causes autoimmunity. Nat Med, **6**(3): 298–305.

Kretz-Rommel A & Rubin RL (2001) Early cellular events in systemic autoimmunity driven by chromatin-reactive T cell. Cell Immunol, **208**(2): 125–136.

Kretz-Rommel A, Duncan SR, & Rubin RL (1997) Autoimmunity caused by disruption of central T cell tolerance. A murine model of drug-induced lupus. J Clin Invest, **99**(8): 1888–1896.

Kristofferson A & Nilsson BS (1989) Zimeldine: febrile reactions and peripheral neuropathy. In: Kammuller ME, Bloksma N, & Seinen W eds. Autoimmunity and toxicology: immune disregulation induced by drugs and chemicals. Amsterdam, Elsevier, pp 183–214.

References

Kubicka-Muranyi M, Griem P, Lubben B, Rottmann N, Luhrmann R, & Gleichmann E (1995) Mercuric-chloride-induced autoimmunity in mice involves up-regulated presentation by spleen cells of altered and unaltered nucleolar self antigen. Int Arch Allergy Immunol, **108**(1): 1–10.

Kubicka-Muranyi M, Kremer J, Rottmann N, Lubben B, Albers R, Bloksma N, Luhrmann R, & Gleichmann E (1996) Murine systemic autoimmune disease induced by mercuric chloride: T helper cells reacting to self proteins. Int Arch Allergy Immunol, **109**(1): 11–20.

Kühtreiber WM, Hayashi T, Dale EA, & Faustman DL (2003) Central role of defective apoptosis in autoimmunity. J Mol Endocrinol, **31**: 373–399.

Kulmala P, Savola K, Petersen JS, Vahasalo P, Karjalainen J, Lopponen T, Dyrberg T, Akerblom HK, & Knip M (1998) Prediction of insulin-dependent diabetes mellitus in siblings of children with diabetes: a population-based study. The Childhood Diabetes in Finland Study Group. J Clin Invest, **101**: 327–336.

Kuroda Y, Nacionales DC, Akaogi J, Reeves WH, & Satoh M (2004) Autoimmunity induced by adjuvant hydrocarbon oil components of vaccine. Biomed Pharmacother, **58**: 325–337.

Kurtzke JF, Beebe GW, & Norman JE Jr (1979) Epidemiology of multiple sclerosis in U.S. veterans: 1. Race, sex, and geographic distribution. Neurology, **29**: 1228–1235.

Kuwabara S (2004) Guillain-Barre syndrome: epidemiology, pathophysiology and management. Drugs, **64**: 597–610.

Lacaille D (2005) Arthritis and employment research: where are we? Where do we need to go? J Rheumatol Suppl, **72**: 42–45.

Lacey JV, Garabrant DH, Laing TJ, Gillespie BW, Mayes MD, Cooper BC, & Schottenfeld D (1999) Petroleum distillate solvents as risk factors for undifferentiated connective tissue disease (UCTD). Am J Epidemiol, **149**: 761–770.

Ladona MG, Izquierdo Martinez M, Posada de la Paz M, de la Torre R, Ampurdanes C, Segura J, & Sanz EJ (2001) Pharmacogenetic profile of xenobiotic enzyme metabolism in survivors of the Spanish toxic oil syndrome. Environ Health Perspect, **109**: 369–375.

LaGasse JM, Brantley MS, Leech NJ, Rowe RE, Monks S, Palmer JP, Nepom GT, McCulloch DK, & Hagopian WA (2002) Successful prospective prediction of type 1 diabetes in schoolchildren through multiple defined autoantibodies: an 8-year follow-up of the Washington State Diabetes Prediction Study. Diabetes Care, **25**: 505–511.

Lahoz C, del Pozo V, Gallardo S, Cardaba B, Jurado A, Cortegano MI, del Amo A, Arrieta I, & Palomino P (1997) Immunological aspects of the toxic oil syndrome. Berlin/Heidelberg, Springer Verlag.

Laing TJ, Gillespie BW, Toth MB, Mayes MD, Gallavan RH Jr, Burns CJ, Johanns JR, Cooper BC, Keroack BJ, Wasko MC, Lacey JV Jr, & Schottenfeld D (1997) Racial differences in scleroderma among women in Michigan. Arthritis Rheum, **40**(4): 734–742.

Lambré CR & Alaoui-Silimani N (1986) An enzyme immunoassay for auto-antibodies to keratin in normal human serum and in pleural fluids from patients with various malignant or non-malignant lung diseases. J Clin Lab Immunol, **20**: 171–176.

Lander ES & Schork NJ (1994) Genetic dissection of complex traits. Science, **265**: 2037–2048.

Landtblom AM, Floden U, Söderfeldt B, Wolfson C, & Axelson O (1996) Organic solvents and multiple sclerosis: a synthesis of the current evidence. Epidemiology, **7**: 429–433.

Lane SE, Watts RA, Bentham G, Innes NJ, & Scott DG (2003) Are environmental factors important in primary systemic vasculitis? A case–control study. Arthritis Rheum, **48**: 814–823.

Langer P, Tajtakova M, Fodor G, Kocan A, Bohov P, Michalek J, & Kreze A (1998) Increased thyroid volume and prevalence of thyroid disorders in an area heavily polluted by polychlorinated biphenyls. Eur J Endocrinol, **139**(4): 402–409.

Langer P, Tajtakova M, Guretzki HJ, Kocan A, Petrik J, Chovancova J, Drobna B, Jursa S, Pavuk M, Trnovec T, Sebokova E, & Klimes I (2002) High prevalence of anti-glutamic acid decarboxylase (anti-GAD) antibodies in employees at a polychlorinated biphenyl production factory. Arch Environ Health, **57**(5): 412–415.

Langer P, Kocan A, Tajtakova M, Petrik J, Chovancova J, Drobna B, Jursa S, Pavuk M, Koska J, Trnovec T, Sebokova E, & Klimes I (2003) Possible effects of polychlorinated biphenyls and organochlorinated pesticides on the thyroid after long-term exposure to heavy environmental pollution. J Occup Environ Med, **45**(5): 526–532.

Lauwerys RR, Bernard A, Roels HA, Buchet J-P, & Viau C (1984) Characterization of cadmium proteinuria in man and rat. Environ Health Perspect, **54**: 147–152.

Lawrence DA & McCabe MJ (1995) Immune modulation by toxic metals. In: Goyer RA, Klaassen CD, & Waalkes MP eds. Metal toxicology. San Diego, California, Academic Press, pp 305–337.

Lawrence DA, Mudzinski S, Rusofsky U, & Warner G (1987) Mechanisms of metal-induced immunotoxicity. In: Berlin A, Dean J, Draper MH, Smith EMB, & Spreafico F eds. Immunotoxicology. Dordrecht, Martinus-Nijhoff, pp 293–307.

Lawson BR, Baccala R, Song J, Croft M, Kono DH, & Theofilopoulos AN (2004) Deficiency of the cyclin kinase inhibitor p21 (WAF-1/CIP-1) promotes apoptosis of activated/memory T cells and inhibits spontaneous systemic autoimmunity. J Exp Med, **199**: 547–557.

Layland LE, Wulferink M, Dierkes S, & Gleichmann E (2004) Drug-induced autoantibody formation in mice: triggering by primed $CD4^+CD25^-$ T cells, prevention by primed $CD4^+CD25^+$ T cells. Eur J Immunol, **34**(1): 36–46.

Lebwohl M (2003) Psoriasis. Lancet, **361**(9364): 1197–1204.

Leffel EK, Wolf C, Poklis A, & White KL Jr (2003) Drinking water exposure to cadmium, an environmental contaminant, results in the exacerbation of autoimmune disease in the murine model. Toxicology, **188**: 233–250.

Lehmann PV, Sercarz EE, Forsthuber T, Dayan CM, & Gammon G (1993) Determinant spreading and the dynamics of the autoimmune T-cell repertoire. Immunol Today, **14**(5): 203–208.

Leiba A, Amital H, Gershwin ME, & Shoenfeld Y (2001) Diet and lupus. Lupus, **10**: 246–248.

Leiter EH (1982) Multiple low-dose streptozotocin-induced hyperglycemia and insulitis in C57BL mice: influence of inbred background, sex, and thymus. Proc Natl Acad Sci U S A, **79**(2): 630–634.

Lemire JM, Archer DC, Beck L, & Spiegelberg HL (1995) Immunosuppressive actions of 1,25-dihydroxyvitamin D3: preferential inhibition of Th1 functions. J Nutr, **125**(6): 1704S–1708S.

Levin LI, Munger KL, Rubertone MV, Peck CA, Lennette ET, Spiegelman D, & Ascherio A (2005) Temporal relationship between elevation of Epstein-Barr virus antibody titers and initial onset of neurological symptoms in multiple sclerosis. JAMA, **293**: 2496–2500.

Levine JS, Branch DW, & Rauch J (2002) The antiphospholipid syndrome. N Engl J Med, **346**: 752–763.

Levine S & Sowinski R (1980) Enhancement of allergic encephalomyelitis by particulate adjuvants inoculated long before antigen. Am J Pathol, **99**: 291–304.

Li FK, Tse KC, Lam MF, Yip TP, Lui SL, Chan GS, Chan KW, Chan EY, Choy BY, Lo WK, Chan TM, & Lai KN (2004) Incidence and outcome of antiglomerular basement membrane disease in Chinese. Nephrology (Carlton), **9**: 100–104.

Li J, Johansen C, Bronnum-Hansen H, Stenager E, Koch-Henriksen N, & Olsen J (2004) The risk of multiple sclerosis in bereaved patients: A nationwide cohort study in Denmark. Neurology, **62**: 726–729.

Ligier S & Sternberg EM (1999) Neuroendocrine host factors and inflammatory disease susceptibility. Environ Health Perspect, **107**(Suppl 5): 701–707.

Lind P, Langsteger W, Molnar M, Gallowitsch HJ, Mikosch P, & Gomez I (1998) Epidemiology of thyroid diseases in iodine sufficiency. Thyroid, **8**(12): 1179–1183.

Liu G, Schwartz JA, & Brooks SC (2000) Estrogen receptor protects p53 from deactivation by human double minute-2. Cancer Res, **60**: 1810–1814.

Liu Z (2002) Are anti-BP180 IgG1 or IgG4 autoantibodies pathogenic? J Invest Dermatol, **119**: 989–990.

Loftus EV Jr (2004) Clinical epidemiology of inflammatory bowel disease: incidence, prevalence, and environmental influences. Gastroenterology, **126**: 1504–1517.

Long SA, Van de Water J, & Gershwin ME (2002) Antimitochondrial antibodies in primary biliary cirrhosis: the role of xenobiotics. Autoimmunol Rev, **1**: 37–42.

Lorenzi M, Cagliero E, & Schmidt NJ (1985) Racial differences in incidence of juvenile-onset type 1 diabetes: epidemiologic studies in southern California. Diabetologia, **28**: 734–738.

Lovas K & Husebye ES (2002) High prevalence and increasing incidence of Addison's disease in western Norway. Clin Endocrinol (Oxf), **56**(6): 787–791.

Lundberg I, Alfredsson L, Plato N, Sverdrup B, Klareskog L, & Kleinau S (1994) Occupation, occupational exposure to chemicals and rheumatological disease. Scand J Rheumatol, **23**: 305–310.

Lundin KE, Scott H, Hansen T, Paulsen G, Halstensen TS, Fausa O, Thorsby E, & Sollid LM (1993) Gliadin-specific, HLA-DQ (alpha 1*0501, beta 1*0201) restricted T cells isolated from the small intestinal mucosa of celiac disease patients. J Exp Med, **178**: 187–196.

Luster MI, Hayes HT, Korach K, Tucker AN, Dean JH, Greenlee WF, & Boorman GA (1984) Estrogen immunosuppression is regulated through estrogenic responses in the thymus. J Immunol, **133**: 110–116.

Luster MI, Simeonova PP, Galluci R, & Matheson J (1999) Autoimmunity and risk assessment. Environ Health Perspect, **107**(Suppl 5): 679–680.

Lykissa ED, Kala SV, Hurley JB, & Lebovitz RM (1997) Release of low molecular weight silicones and platinum from silicone breast implants. Anal Chem, **69**: 4912–4916.

Lytton SD, Helander A, Zhang-Gouillon ZQ, Stokkeland K, Bordone R, Arico S, Albano E, French SW, & Ingelman-Sundberg M (1999) Autoantibodies against cytochromes P-4502E1 and P-4503A in alcoholics. Mol Pharmacol, **55**: 223–233.

MacPhee IA, Turner DR, Yagita H, & Oliveira DB (2001) CD80(B7.1) and CD86(B7.2) do not have distinct roles in setting the Th1/Th2 balance in autoimmunity in rats. Scand J Immunol, **54**(5): 486–494.

Madsen KM, Lauritsen MB, Pedersen CB, Thorsen P, Plesner AM, Andersen PH, & Mortensen PB (2003) Thimerosal and the occurrence of autism: negative ecological evidence from Danish population-based data. Pediatrics, **112**: 604–606.

Magistrelli C, Samoilova E, Agarwal RK, Banki K, Ferrante P, Vladutiu A, Phillips PE, & Perl A (1999) Polymorphic genotypes of the HRES-1 human endogenous retrovirus locus correlate with systemic lupus erythematosus and autoreactivity. Immunogenetics, **49**: 829–834.

Maharaj SVN (2004) Platinum concentration in silicone breast implant material and capsular tissue by ICP-MS. Anal Bioanal Chem, **380**: 84–89.

Maibach H (1975) Acute laryngeal obstruction presumed secondary to thimerosal (Merthiolate) delayed hypersensitivity. Contact Dermatitis, **1**: 221–222.

Maitre A, Hours M, Bonneterre V, Arnaud J, Arslan MT, Carpentier P, Bergeret A, & de Gaudemaris R (2004) Systemic sclerosis and occupational risk factors: role of solvents and cleaning products. J Rheumatol, **31**: 2395–2401.

Maksymowych WP, Suarez-Almazor M, Chou CT, & Russell AS (1995) Polymorphism in the LMP2 gene influences susceptibility to extraspinal disease in HLA-B27 positive individuals with ankylosing spondylitis. Ann Rheum Dis, **54**: 321–324.

Manger K, Repp R, Jansen M, Geisselbrecht M, Wassmuth R, Westerdaal NAC, Pfahlberg A, Manger B, & van de Winkel JGJ (2002) Fcγ receptor IIa, IIIa and IIIb polymorphisms in German patients with systemic lupus erythematosus: association with clinical symptoms. Ann Rheum Dis, **61**: 786–792.

Marchetti B, Morale MC, Testa N, Tirolo C, Caniglia S, Amor S, Dijkstra CD, & Barden N (2001) Stress, the immune system and vulnerability to degenerative disorders of the central nervous system in transgenic mice expressing glucocorticoid receptor antisense RNA. Brain Res Rev, **37**: 259–272.

Margolin L (2003) Non-L-tryptophan related eosinophilia-myalgia syndrome with hypoproteinemia and hypoalbuminemia. J Rheumatol, **30**: 628–629.

Marie I, Hatron PY, Levesque H, Hachulla E, Hellot MF, Michon-Pasturel U, Courtois H, & Devulder B (1999) Influence of age on characteristics of polymyositis and dermatomyositis in adults. Medicine (Baltimore), **78**: 139–147.

Marinovich M, Guizzetti M, Ghilardi F, Viviani B, Corsini E, & Galli CL (1997) Thyroid peroxidase as toxicity target for dithiocarbamates. Arch Toxicol, **71**(8): 508–512.

Martel P & Joly P (2001) Pemphigus: autoimmune diseases of keratinocyte's adhesion molecules. Clin Dermatol, **19**: 662–674.

Martinez A, Fernández-Arquero M, Pascual-Salcedo D, Conejero L, Alves H, Balsa A, & de la Concha EG (2000) Primary association of tumor necrosis factor-region genetic markers with susceptibility to rheumatoid arthritis. Arthritis Rheum, **43**: 1366–1370.

Martyn CN, Cruddas M, & Compston DA (1993) Symptomatic Epstein-Barr virus infection and multiple sclerosis. J Neurol Neurosurg Psychiatry, **56**: 167–168.

Masi AT & Chrousos GP (1996) Hypothalamic–pituitary–adrenal–glucocorticoid axis function in rheumatoid arthritis. J Rheumatol, **23**: 577–581.

Mason JW (2003) Myocarditis and dilated cardiomyopathy: an inflammatory link. Cardiovasc Res, **60**: 5–10.

Masson MJ & Uetrecht JP (2004) Tolerance induced by low dose D-penicillamine in the Brown Norway rat model of drug-induced autoimmunity is immune-mediated. Chem Res Toxicol, **17**(1): 82–94.

Matarese G, Sanna V, Lechler RI, Sarvetnick N, Fontana S, Zappacosta S, & La Cava A (2002) Leptin accelerates autoimmune diabetes in female NOD mice. Diabetes, **51**: 1356–1361.

Matheson D, Clarkson T, & Gelfand E (1980) Mercury toxicity (acrodynia) induced by long-term injection of gamma globulin. J Pediatr, **97**: 153–155.

Michielsen C, Zeamari S, Leusink-Muis A, Vos J, & Bloksma N (2002) The environmental pollutant hexachlorobenzene causes eosinophilic and granulomatous inflammation and in vitro airways hyperreactivity in the Brown Norway rat. Arch Toxicol, **76**: 236–247.

Miller AS 3rd, Willard V, Kline K, Tarpley S, Guillotte J, Lawler FH, & Pendell GM 3rd (1998) Absence of longitudinal changes in rheumatologic parameters after silicone breast implantation: a prospective 13-year study. Plast Reconstr Surg, **102**: 2299–2303.

Minami Y, Sasaki T, Arai Y, Kurisu Y, & Hisamichi S (2003) Diet and systemic lupus erythematosus: a 4 year prospective study of Japanese patients. J Rheumatol, **30**: 747–754.

Mirtcheva J, Pfeiffer C, De Bruijn JA, Jacquesmart F, & Gleichmann E (1989) Immunological alterations inducible by mercury compounds. III. H-2A acts as an immune response and H-2E as an immune "suppression" locus for $HgCl_2$-induced antinucleolar autoantibodies. Eur J Immunol, **19**(12): 2257–2261.

Miyaura H & Iwata M (2002) Direct and indirect inhibition of Th1 development by progesterone and glucocorticoids. J Immunol, **168**: 1087–1094.

Mohr DC, Hart SL, Julian L, Cox D, & Pelletier D (2004) Association between stressful life events and exacerbation in multiple sclerosis: a meta-analysis. Brit Med J, **328**: 731–736.

Monestier M, Novick KE, & Losman MJ (1994) D-penicillamine- and quinidine-induced antinuclear antibodies in A.SW (H-2s) mice: similarities with autoantibodies in spontaneous and heavy metal-induced autoimmunity. Eur J Immunol, **24**(3): 723–730.

Mongey AB & Hess E (2001) In vitro production of antibodies to histones in patients receiving chronic procainamide therapy. J Rheumatol, **28**(9): 1992–1998.

Monzani F, Caraccio N, Dardano A, & Ferrannini E (2004) Thyroid autoimmunity and dysfunction associated with type I interferon therapy. Clin Exp Med, **3**: 199–210.

Monzoni A, Masutti F, Saccoccio G, Bellentani S, Tiribelli C, & Giacca M (2001) Genetic determinants of ethanol-induced liver damage. Mol Med, **7**: 255–262.

Mordes JP, Desemone J, & Rossini AA (1987) The BB rat. Diabetes Metab Rev, **3**(3): 725–750.

Morelli AE & Thomson AW (2003) Dendritic cells: regulators of alloimmunity and opportunities for tolerance induction. Immunol Rev, **196**: 125–146.

Mortensen JT, Brønnum-Hansen H, & Rasmussen K (1998) Multiple sclerosis and organic solvents. Epidemiology, **9**: 168–171.

Moudgil KD & Sercarz EE (1994) The T cell repertoire against cryptic self determinants and its involvement in autoimmunity and cancer. Clin Immunol Immunopathol, **73**(3): 283–289.

Mu H, Charmley P, King MC, & Criswell LA (1996) Synergy between T cell receptor β gene polymorphism and HLA-DR4 in susceptibility to rheumatoid arthritis. Arthritis Rheum, **39**: 931–937.

Mueller PW, Paschal DC, Hammel RR, Klincewicz SL, MacNeil ML, Spierto B, & Steinberg KK (1992) Chronic renal effects in three studies of men and women occupationally exposed to cadmium. Arch Environ Contam Toxicol, **23**: 125–136.

Muller H, de Toledo FW, & Resch KL (2001) Fasting followed by vegetarian diet in patients with rheumatoid arthritis: a systematic review. Scand J Rheumatol, **30**: 1–10.

Mulloy KB (2003) Silica exposure and systemic vasculitis. Environ Health Perspect, **111**(16): 1933–1938.

Munger KL, Zhang SM, O'Reilly E, Hernán MA, Olek MJ, Willett WC, & Ascherio A (2004) Vitamin D intake and incidence of multiple sclerosis. Neurology, **62**: 60–65.

Murray J (2002) Infection as a cause of multiple sclerosis. Brit Med J, **325**: 1128.

Nagata S & Suda T (1995) Fas and Fas ligand: lpr and gld mutations. Immunol Today, **16**: 39–43.

Nagayama J, Tsuji H, Iida T, Hirakawa H, Matsueda T, & Ohki M (2001) Effects of contamination level of dioxins and related chemicals on thyroid hormone and immune response systems in patients with "Yusho". Chemosphere, **43**: 1005–1010.

Nagi AH & Khan AH (1984) Gold nephropathy in rabbits using an indigenous preparation. A morphological study. Intern Urol Nephrol, **16**: 49–59.

Nagi AH, Alexander F, & Barabas AZ (1971) Gold nephropathy in rats. Light and electron microscopic studies. Exp Mol Pathol, **15**: 354–362.

Naisbitt DJ, Gordon SF, Pirmohamed M, Burkhart C, Cribb AE, Pichler WJ, & Park BK (2001) Antigenicity and immunogenicity of sulphamethoxazole: demonstration of metabolism-dependent haptenation and T-cell proliferation in vivo. Br J Pharmacol, **133**(2): 295–305.

Nakken B, Jonsson R, & Bolstad AI (2001) Polymorphisms of the Ro52 gene associated with anti-Ro 52-kd autoantibodies in patients with primary Sjögren's syndrome. Arthritis Rheum, **44**: 638–646.

Neidhart M (1997) Bromocriptine has little direct effect on murine lymphocytes, the immunomodulatory effect being mediated by the suppression of prolactin secretion. Biomed Pharmacother, **51**: 118–125.

Neidhart M (1998) Prolactin in autoimmune diseases. Proc Soc Exp Biol Med, **217**: 408–419.

Nepom GT (1993) Immunogenetics and IDDM. Diabetes Rev, **1**: 93–103.

Nepom GT (1998) Major histocompatibility complex-directed susceptibility to rheumatoid arthritis. Adv Immunol, **68**: 315–332.

Neuberger J (1998) Halothane hepatitis. Eur J Gastroenterol Hepatol, **10**: 631–633.

Nielsen JB & Hultman P (2002) Mercury-induced autoimmunity in mice. Environ Health Perspect, **110**(Suppl 5): 877–881.

Nierkens S, van Helden P, Bol M, Bleumink R, van Kooten P, Ramdien-Murli S, Boon L, & Pieters R (2002) Selective requirement for CD40-CD154 in drug-induced type 1 versus type 2 responses to trinitrophenyl-ovalbumin. J Immunol, **168**(8): 3747–3754.

Nierkens S, Nieuwenhuijsen L, Thomas M, & Pieters R (2004) Evaluation of the use of reporter antigens in an auricular lymph node assay to assess the immunosensitizing potential of drugs. Toxicol Sci, **79**(1): 90–97.

Nierkens S, Aalbers M, Bol M, van Wijk F, Hassing I, & Pieters R (2005) Development of an oral exposure mouse model to predict drug-induced hypersensitivity reactions by using reporter antigens. Toxicol Sci, **83**(2): 273–281.

Nietert PJ, Sutherland SE, Silver RM, Pandey JP, & Dosemeci M (1999) Solvent oriented hobbies and the risk of systemic sclerosis. J Rheumatol, **26**: 2369–2372.

Nisipeanu P & Korczyn AD (1993) Psychological stress as risk factor for exacerbations in multiple sclerosis. Neurology, **43**: 1311–1312.

Noli C, Koeman JP, & Willemse T (1995) A retrospective evaluation of adverse reactions to trimethoprim-sulphonamide combinations in dogs and cats. Vet Q, **17**(4): 123–128.

Noller KL, Blair PB, O'Brien PC, & Mellon LJ (1988) Increased occurrence of auto-immune disease among women exposed in utero to diethylstilbestrol. Fertil Steril, **49**: 1080–1082.

Noone RB (1997) A review of the possible health implications of silicone breast implants. Cancer, **79**: 1747–1756.

Nowack R, Flores-Suarez LF, & van der Woude FJ (1998) New developments in pathogenesis of systemic vasculitis. Curr Opin Rheumatol, **10**: 3–11.

NRC (1983) Risk assessment in the federal government: Managing the process. Washington, DC, National Research Council, National Academy Press.

Nuriya S, Yagita H, Okumura K, & Azuma M (1996) The differential role of CD86 and CD80 co-stimulatory molecules in the induction and the effector phases of contact hypersensitivity. Int Immunol, **8**(6): 917–926.

Nuyts GD, Van Vlem E, Vos AD, Daelemans RA, Rovive G, Elseviers MM, Schurgers M, Segaert M, D'Haese PC, & De Broe ME (1995) Wegener granulomatosis is associated to exposure to silicon compounds: a case–control study. Nephrol Dialysis Trans, **10**: 1162–1165.

Nyren O, Yin L, Josefsson S, McLaughlin JK, Blot WJ, Engqvist M, Hakelius L, Boice JD, & Adami HO (1998) Risk of connective tissue disease and related disorders among women with breast implants: a nation-wide retrospective cohort study in Sweden. Br Med J, **316**: 417–422.

References

Ochel M, Vohr HW, Pfeiffer C, & Gleichmann E (1991) IL-4 is required for the IgE and IgG1 increase and IgG1 autoantibody formation in mice treated with mercuric chloride. J Immunol, **146**(9): 3006–3011.

Oen K (2000) Comparative epidemiology of the rheumatic diseases in children. Curr Opin Rheumatol, **12**(5): 410–414.

Offit PA & Hackett CA (2003) Addressing parents' concerns: Do vaccines cause allergic or autoimmune diseases? Pediatrics, **111**(3): 653–659.

Ohsawa M (1993) Nutritional and toxicological implication of trace elements in the immune response. In: Prasad AS ed. Essential and toxic elements in human health and disease: An update. Prog Clin Biol Res, **380**: 283–298.

Ohsawa M, Takahashi K, & Otsuka F (1988) Induction of anti-nuclear antibodies in mice orally exposed to cadmium at low concentrations. Clin Exp Immunol, **73**: 98–102.

Ohsawa M, Otsuka F, & Takahashi K (1990) Modulation of the immune response by trace elements. In: Tomita H ed. Trace elements in clinical medicine. Tokyo, Springer Verlag, pp 165–171.

Okada K, Sugiura T, Kuroda E, Tsuji S, & Yamashita U (2001) Phenytoin promotes Th2 type immune response in mice. Clin Exp Immunol, **124**(3): 406–413.

Oldstone MB (1987) Molecular mimicry and autoimmune disease. Cell, **50**: 819–820.

Olofsson P, Holmberg J, Pettersson U, & Holmdahl R (2003) Identification and isolation of dominant susceptibility loci for pristane-induced arthritis. J Immunol, **171**(1): 407–416.

Olsen NJ (2004) Drug-induced autoimmunity. Best Pract Res Clin Rheumatol, **18**: 677–688.

Olsson AR, Skogh T, Axelson O, & Wingren C (2004) Occupations and exposures in the work environment as determinants for rheumatoid arthritis. Occup Environ Med, **61**(3): 233–238.

Otsuki T, Sakaguchi H, Tomokuni A, Aikoh T, Matsuki T, Kawakami Y, Kuaska M, Ueki H, Kita S, & Ueki A (1998) Soluble Fas mRNA is dominantly expressed in cases with silicosis. Immunology, **94**: 258–262.

Owen CJ, Jennings CE, Imrie H, Lachaux A, Bridges NA, Cheetham TD, & Pearce SH (2003) Mutational analysis of the FOXP3 gene and evidence for genetic heterogeneity in the immunodysregulation, polyendocrinopathy, enteropathy syndrome. J Clin Endocrinol Metab, **88**: 6034–6039.

Oya H, Kawamura T, Shimizu T, Bannai M, Kawamura H, Minagawa M, Watanabe H, Hatakeyama K, & Abo T (2000) The differential effect of stress on natural killer T (NKT) and NK cell function. Clin Exp Immunol, **121**: 384–390.

Pablos JL, Santiago B, Galindo M, Carreira PE, Ballestin C, & Gomez-Reino JJ (1999) Keratinocyte apoptosis and p53 expression in cutaneous lupus and dermatomyositis. J Pathol, **188**(1): 63–68.

Padyukov L, Silva C, Stolt P, Alfredsson L, & Klareskog L (2004) A gene–environment interaction between smoking and shared epitope genes in HLA-DR provides a high risk of seropositive rheumatoid arthritis. Arthritis Rheum, **50**: 3085–3089.

Paivonsalo-Hietanen T, Tuominen J, & Saari KM (2000) Uveitis in children: population-based study in Finland. Acta Ophthalmol Scand, **78**: 84–88.

Park Y, Moon Y, & Chung HY (2003) AIRE-1 (autoimmune regulator type 1) as a regulator of the thymic induction of negative selection. Ann NY Acad Sci, **1005**: 431–435.

Parks CG, Conrad K, & Cooper GS (1999) Occupational exposure to crystalline silica and autoimmune disease. Environ Health Perspect, **107**(Suppl 5): 793–802.

Parks CG, Cooper GS, Nylander-French LA, Sanderson WT, Dement JM, Cohen PL, Dooley MA, Treadwell EL, St Clair EW, Gilkerson GS, Hoppin JA, & Savitz DA (2002) Occupational exposure to crystalline silica and risk of systemic lupus erythematosus: a population-based, case–control study in the southeastern United States. Arthritis Rheum, **46**: 1840–1850.

Parks CG, Cooper GS, Nylander-French LA, Hoppin JA, Sanderson WT, & Dement JM (2004a) Comparing methods to assess occupational silica exposure in a population-based case–control study of systemic lupus erythematosus. Epidemiology, **15**: 433–441.

Parks CG, Pandey JP, Dooley MA, Treadwell EL, St Clair EW, Gilkeson GS, Feghali-Bostwick CA, & Cooper GS (2004b) Genetic polymorphism in tumor necrosis factor (TNF)-alpha and TNF-beta in a population-based study of systemic lupus erythematosus: associations and interaction with the interleukin-1alpha-889 C/T polymorphism. Hum Immunol, **65**: 622–631.

Parks CG, Cooper GS, Hudson LL, Dooley MA, Treadwell EL, St Clair EW, Gilkeson GS, & Pandey JP (2005) Association of Epstein-Barr virus and systemic lupus erythematosus: effect modification by race, age and cytotoxic T lymphocyte-associated antigen 4 genotype. Arthritis Rheum, **52**: 1148–1159.

Paronetto F (1993) Immunologic reactions in alcoholic liver disease. Semin Liver Dis, **13**: 183–195.

Pattison DJ, Harrison RA, & Symmons DP (2004) The role of diet in susceptibility to rheumatoid arthritis: a systematic review. J Rheumatol, **31**: 1310–1319.

Pearce EN, Farwell AP, & Braverman LE (2003) Thyroiditis. N Engl J Med, **348**: 2646–2655.

Pearson CM (1956) Development of arthritis, periarthritis and periostitis in rats given adjuvants. Proc Soc Exp Biol Med, **91**(1): 95–101.

Pellegrini I, Lebrun JJ, Ali S, & Kelly PA (1992) Expression of prolactin and its receptor in human lymphoid cells. Mol Endocrinol, **6**: 1023–1031.

Pelletier L, Pasquier R, Rossert J, & Druet P (1987) $HgCl_2$ induces nonspecific immunosuppression in Lewis rats. Eur J Immunol, **17**(1): 49–54.

Pelletier L, Rossert J, Pasquier R, Villarroya H, Belair MF, Vial MC, Oriol R, & Druet P (1988) Effect of $HgCl_2$ on experimental allergic encephalomyelitis in Lewis rats. $HgCl_2$-induced down-modulation of the disease. Eur J Immunol, **18**(2): 243–247.

Pelletier L, Rossert J, Pasquier R, Vial MC, & Druet P (1990) Role of $CD8^+$ T cells in mercury-induced autoimmunity or immunosuppression in the rat. Scand J Immunol, **31**(1): 65–74.

Peltonen J, Varga J, Solberg S, Uitto J, & Jimenez S (1991) Elevated expression of the genes for transforming growth factor-beta 1 and type IV collagen in diffuse fasciitis associated with the eosinophilia-myalgia syndrome. J Invest Dermatol, **96**: 20–25.

Perkins LL, Clark BD, Klein PJ, & Cook RR (1995) A meta-analysis of breast implants and connective tissue disease. Ann Plast Surg, **35**: 561–570.

Pernis B & Paronetto F (1962) Adjuvant effects of silica (tridymite) on antibody production. Proc Soc Exp Biol Med, **110**: 390–392.

Peschken CA & Esdaile JM (2000) Systemic lupus erythematosus in North American Indians: a population based study. J Rheumatol, **27**(8): 1884–1891.

Peter JB & Shoenfeld Y (1996) Autoantibodies. Amsterdam, Elsevier Science.

Peters H, Cripps D, Gocmen A, Bryan G, Erturk E, & Morris C (1987) Turkish epidemic hexachlorobenzene porphyria: a 30-year study. Ann NY Acad Sci, **514**: 183–190.

Petri M, Howard D, & Repke J (1991) Frequency of lupus flare in pregnancy: the Hopkins Lupus Pregnancy Center experience. Arthritis Rheum, **34**: 1538–1545.

Pfau JC, Brown JM, & Holian A (2004) Silica-exposed mice generate autoantibodies to apoptotic cells. Toxicology, **195**: 167–176.

Philen R & Dicker R (2000) TOS (toxic oil syndrome) an epidemic of mass proportions in Spain, 1981. United States Department of Health and Human Services, Public Health Service, Centers for Disease Control and Prevention, National Center for Environmental Health (Case Studies in Applied Epidemiology No. 002-800; http://iier.isciii.es/ea/pdf/ea_tos1.htm; accessed 1 May 2005).

Philen RM, Posada de la Paz M, Hill RH, Schurz HH, Abaitua Borda I, Gomez de la Camara A, & Kilbourne EM (1997) Epidemiology of the toxic oil syndrome. Berlin/Heidelberg, Springer Verlag.

Phillips CJ (2004) The cost of multiple sclerosis and the cost effectiveness of disease-modifying agents in its treatment. CNS Drugs, **18**: 561–574.

Pichler WJ (2002) Modes of presentation of chemical neoantigens to the immune system. Toxicology, **181–182**: 49–54.

Pichler WJ (2003) Drug-induced autoimmunity. Curr Opin Allergy Clin Immunol, **3**: 249–253.

Pieters R & Albers R (1999) Screening tests for autoimmune-related immunotoxicity. Environ Health Perspect, **107**(Suppl 5): 673–677.

Pietsch P, Vohr H-W, Degitz K, & Gleichmann E (1989) Immunological alterations inducible by mercury compounds. II. $HgCl_2$ and gold sodium thiomalate enhance serum IgE and IgG concentrations in susceptible mouse strains. Int Arch Allergy Appl Immunol, **90**: 47–53.

Pilatte Y, Tisserand EM, Greffard A, Bignon J, & Lambré CR (1990) Anticarbohydrate autoantibodies to sialidase-treated erythrocytes and thymocytes in serum from patients with pulmonary sarcoidosis. Am J Med, **88**: 486–492.

Pillemer SR, Matteson EL, Jacobsson LT, Martens PB, Melton LJ 3rd, O'Fallon WM, & Fox PC (2001) Incidence of physician-diagnosed primary Sjogren syndrome in residents of Olmsted County, Minnesota. Mayo Clin Proc, **76**(6): 593–599.

Pittoni V & Valesini G (2002) The clearance of apoptotic cells: implications for autoimmunity. Autoimmunity Rev, **1**: 154–161.

Pociot F, Briant L, Jongeneel CV, Mølvig J, Worsaae H, Abbal M, Thomsen M, Nerup J, & Cambon-Thomsen A (1993) Association of tumor necrosis factor (TNF) and class II major histocompatibility complex alleles with the secretion of TNFα and TNFβ by human mononuclear cells: a possible link to insulin-dependent diabetes mellitus. Eur J Immunol, **23**: 224–231.

Podolsky DK (2002) Inflammatory bowel disease. N Engl J Med, **347**: 417–429.

Pollard KM & Landberg GP (2001) The in vitro proliferation of murine lymphocytes to mercuric chloride is restricted to mature T cells and is interleukin 1 dependent. Int Immunopharmacol, **1**: 581–593.

Pollard KM, Pearson DL, Hultman P, Hildebrandt B, & Kono DH (1999) Lupus-prone mice as models to study xenobiotic-induced acceleration of systemic autoimmunity. Environ Health Perspect, **107**(Suppl 5): 729–735.

Ponsonby AL, McMichael A, & van der Mei I (2002) Ultraviolet radiation and autoimmune disease: insights from epidemiological research. Toxicology, **181–182**: 71–78.

Ponsonby AL, Lucas RM, & van der Mei IA (2005) UVR, vitamin D and three autoimmune diseases — multiple sclerosis, type 1 diabetes, rheumatoid arthritis. Photochem Photobiol, **81**(6): 1267–1275.

Popovic M, Nierkens S, Pieters R, & Uetrecht J (2004) Investigating the role of 2-phenylpropenal in felbamate-induced idiosyncratic drug reactions. Chem Res Toxicol, **17**(12): 1568–1576.

Posada de la Paz M, Abaitua Borda I, Kilbourne EM, Tabuenca Oliver J, Diaz de Rojas F, & Castro Garcia M (1989) Late cases of toxic oil syndrome: Evidence that the aetiological agent persisted in oil stored for up to one year. Food Chem Toxicol, **27**: 517–521.

Posada de la Paz M, Philen RM, Abaitua Borda I, Sicilia Socias JM, Gomez de la Camara A, & Kilbourne EM (1996) Toxic oil syndrome: Traceback of the toxic oil and evidence for a point source epidemic. Food Chem Toxicol, **34**: 251–257.

Poulas K, Tsibri E, Kokla A, Papanastasiou D, Tsouloufis T, Marinou M, Tsantili P, Papapetropoulos T, & Tzartos SJ (2001) Epidemiology of seropositive myasthenia gravis in Greece. J Neurol Neurosurg Psychiatry, **71**(3): 352–356.

Povey A, Guppy MJ, Wood M, Knight C, Black CM, & Silman AJ (2001) Cytochrome P2 polymorphism and susceptibility to scleroderma following exposure to organic solvents. Arthritis Rheum, **44**: 662–665.

Powell J, Van de Water J, & Gershwin E (1999) Evidence for the role of environmental agents in the initiation or progression of autoimmune conditions. Environ Health Perspect, **107**(Suppl 5): 667–677.

Pozzilli P, Manfrini S, & Monetini L (2001) Biochemical markers of type 1 diabetes: clinical use. Scand J Clin Lab Invest, **61**(Suppl 235): 38–44.

Prentice LM, Phillips DIW, Sarsero D, Beever K, McLachlan SM, & Smith B (1990) Geographical distribution of subclinical autoimmune thyroid disease in Britain: a study using highly sensitive direct assays for autoantibodies to thyroglobulin and thyroid peroxidase. Acta Endocrinol, **123**: 493–498.

Prins JB, Herberg L, Den Bieman M, & van Zutphen LF (1991) Genetic variation within and between lines of diabetes-prone and non-diabetes-prone BB rats; allele distribution of 8 protein markers. Lab Anim, **25**(3): 207–211.

Prummel MF & Laurberg P (2003) Interferon-α and autoimmune thyroid disease. Thyroid, **13**: 547–551.

Pugliese A, Zeller M, Fernandez A, Zalcberg LJ, Bartlett RJ, Ricordi C, Pietropaolo M, Eisenbarth GS, Bennett ST, & Patel DD (1997) The insulin gene is transcribed in the human thymus and transcription levels correlate with allelic variation at the INS VNTR-IDDM2 susceptibility locus for type I diabetes. Nat Genet, **15**: 293–297.

Pugliese A, Brown D, Garza D, Murchison D, Zeller M, Redondo M, Diez J, Eisenbarth GS, Patel DD, & Ricordi C (2001) Self-antigen presenting cells expressing islet cell molecules in human thymus and peripheral lymphoid organs: phenotypic characterization and implications for immunological tolerance and type 1 diabetes. J Clin Invest, **107**: 555–564.

Qasim FJ, Thiru S, & Gillespie K (1997) Gold and D-penicillamine induce vasculitis and up-regulate mRNA for IL-4 in the Brown Norway rat: support for a role for Th2 cell activity. Clin Exp Immunol, **108**(3): 438–445.

Quddus J, Johnson KJ, Gavalchin J, Amento EP, Chrisp CE, Yung RL, & Richardson BC (1993) Treating activated CD4$^+$ T cell with either of two distinct DNA methyltransferase inhibitors, 5-azacytidine or procainamide, is sufficient to cause lupus-like disease in syngeneic mice. J Clin Invest, **92**(1): 38–53.

Queiroz MLS & Dantas DCM (1997) B lymphocytes in mercury-exposed workers. Pharmacol Toxicol, **81**: 130–133.

Queiroz MLS, Perlingeiro RCR, Dantas DCM, Annichino Bizzacchi JM, & De Capitani EM (1994) Immunoglobulin levels in workers exposed to inorganic mercury. Pharmacol Toxicol, **74**: 72–75.

Queiroz MLS, Bincoletto C, Perlingeiro RC, Quadros MR, & Souza CA (1998a) Immunoglobulin levels in workers exposed to hexachlorobenzene. Hum Exp Toxicol, **17**: 172–175.

Queiroz MLS, Quadros MR, Valadares MC, & Silveira JP (1998b) Polymorphonuclear phagocytosis and killing in workers occupationally exposed to hexachlorobenzene. Immunopharmacol Immunotoxicol, **20**: 447–454.

Quero C, Colome N, Prieto MR, Carrascal M, Posada de la Paz M, Gelpi E, & Abian J (2004) Determination of protein markers in human serum: analysis of protein expression in toxic oil syndrome studies. Proteomics, **4**: 303–315.

Ramenghi U, Bonissoni S, Migliaretti G, DeFranco S, Bottarel F, Gambaruto C, DiFranco D, Priori R, Conti F, Dianzani I, Valesini G, Merletti F, & Dianzani U (2000) Deficiency of the Fas apoptosis pathway without Fas gene mutations is a familial trait predisposing to development of autoimmune diseases and cancer. Blood, **95**: 3176–3182.

Rantapaa-Dahlqvist S, de Jong BA, Berglin E, Hallmans G, Wadell G, Stenlund H, Sundin U, & van Venrooij WJ (2003) Antibodies against cyclic citrullinated peptide and IgA rheumatoid factor predict the development of rheumatoid arthritis. Arthritis Rheum, **48**: 2741–2749.

Rat AC & Boissier MC (2004) Rheumatoid arthritis: direct and indirect costs. Joint Bone Spine, **71**: 518–524.

Raulet DH (2004) Interplay of natural killer cells and their receptors with the adaptive immune response. Nat Immunol, **5**(10): 996–1002.

Ravel G & Descotes J (2005) Popliteal lymph node assay: facts and perspectives. J Appl Toxicol, **25**(6): 451–458.

Reed T, Page WF, Viken RJ, & Christian JC (1996) Genetic predisposition to organ-specific endpoints of alcoholism. Alcohol Clin Exp Res, **20**: 1528–1533.

Regius O, Lengyel E, Borzsonyi L, & Beregi E (1988) The effect of smoking on the presence of antinuclear antibodies and on the morphology of lymphocytes in aged subjects. Z Gerontol, **21**: 161–163.

Regius O, Rajczy K, Gergely I, Borzsonyi L, Lengyel E, & Vargha P (1990) The effect of smoking on peripheral blood lymphocytes and on some immunological parameters of old age. Z Gerontol, **23**: 163–167.

Renzoni E, Lympany P, Sestini P, Pantelidis P, Wells A, Black C, Welsh K, Brunn C, Knight C, Foley P, & du Bois RM (2000) Distribution of novel polymorphisms of the interleukin-8 and CXC receptor 1 and 2 genes in systemic sclerosis and cryptogenic fibrosing alveolitis. Arthritis Rheum, **43**: 1633–1640.

Rhodes J, Chen H, Hall SR, Beesley JE, Jenkins DC, Collins P, & Zheng B (1995) Therapeutic potentiation of the immune system by costimulatory Schiff-base-forming drugs. Nature (Lond), **270**: 21433–21436.

Richardson BC (2002) Role of DNA methylation in the regulation of cell function: autoimmunity, aging, cancer. J Nutr, **132**: 2401S–2405S.

Richardson BC (2003) DNA methylation and autoimmune disease. Clin Immunol, **109**: 72–79.

Richardson BC, Scheinbart L, Strahler J, Gross L, Hanash S, & Johnson M (1990) Evidence for impaired T cell DNA methylation in systemic lupus erythematosus and rheumatoid arthritis. Arthritis Rheum, **33**: 1665–1673.

Richardson BC, Strahler JR, Pivirotto TS, Quddus J, Bayliss GE, Gross LA, O'Rourke KS, Powers D, Hanash SM, & Johnson MA (1992) Phenotypic and functional similarities between 5-azacytidine-treated T cells and T cell subset in patients with active systemic lupus erythematosus and rheumatoid arthritis. Arthritis Rheum, **35**: 647–662.

Rider LG, Artlett CM, Foster CB, Ahmed A, Neeman T, Chanock SJ, Jimenez SA, & Miller FW, for the Childhood Myositis Heterogeneity Collaborative Study Group (2000) Polymorphisms in the IL-1 receptor antagonist gene VNTR are responsible risk factors for juvenile idiopathic inflammatory myopathies. Clin Exp Immunol, **121**: 47–52.

Rieux-Laucat F, Le Deist F, Hivroz C, Roberts IAG, Debatin KM, Fischer A, & de Villarty JP (1995) Mutations in Fas associated with human lymphoproliferative syndrome and autoimmunity. Science, **268**: 1347–1349.

Rieux-Laucat F, Blachère S, Danielan S, de Villarty JP, Oleastro M, Solary E, Bader-Meunier B, Arkwright P, Pondaré C, Bernaudin F, Chapel H, Nielsen S, Berrah M, Fischer A, & Le Deist F (1999) Lymphoproliferative syndrome with autoimmunity: a possible genetic basis for dominant expression of the clinical manifestations. Blood, **94**: 2575–2582.

Riise T, Moen BE, & Kyvik KR (2002) Organic solvents and the risk of multiple sclerosis. Epidemiology, **13**: 718–720.

Riise T, Nortvedt MW, & Ascherio A (2003) Smoking is a risk factor for multiple sclerosis. Neurology, **61**: 1122–1124.

Riskind PN, Massacesi L, Doolittle TH, & Hauser SL (1991) The role of prolactin in autoimmune demyelination: suppression of experimental allergic encephalomyelitis by bromocriptine. Ann Neurol, **29**(5): 542–547.

Rivas E, Gomez-Arnaiz M, Ricoy JR, Mateos F, Simon R, Garcia-Silva MT, Martin E, Vasquez M, Ferreira A, & Cabello A (2005) Macrophage myofasciitis in childhood: a controversial entity. Pediatric Neurol, **33**(5): 350–356.

Robinson CJ, Balazs T, & Egorov IK (1986) Mercuric chloride-, gold sodium thiomalate-, and D-penicillamine-induced antinuclear antibodies in mice. Toxicol Appl Pharmacol, **86**(2): 159–169.

Rodgers KE (1997) Effects of oral administration of malathion on the course of disease in MRL-lpr mice. J Autoimmun, **10**: 367–373.

Rodgers KE & Ellefson DD (1990) Modulation of respiratory burst activity and mitogenic response of human peripheral blood mononuclear cells and murine splenocytes and peritoneal cells by malathion. Appl Toxicol, **14**: 309–317.

Rodgers KE & Xiong S (1997) Effect of acute administration of malathion by oral and dermal routes on serum histamine levels. Int J Immunopharmacol, **19**: 437–441.

Rodgers KE, Leung N, Devens B, Ware CF, & Imamura T (1986) Lack of immunosuppressive effects of acute and subacute administration of malathion on murine cellular and humoral immune responses. Pest Biochem Physiol, **25**: 358–365.

Rodriguez-Perez M, Gonzalez-Dominguez J, Mataran L, Garcia-Perez S, & Salvatierra D (1994) Association of HLA-DR5 with mucocutaneous lesions in patients with rheumatoid arthritis receiving gold sodium thiomalate. J Rheumatol, **21**: 41–43.

Romagnani S (2004) Immunologic influences on allergy and the Th1/Th2 balance. J Allergy Clin Immunol, **113**: 395–400.

Ronningen KS, Spurkland A, Tait BD, Drummond B, Lopez-Larrea C, Baranda FS, Menendez-Diaz MJ, Caillat-Zucman S, Beaurain G, Garchon HJ, Ilonen J, Reijonen H, Knip M, Boehm BO, Rosak C, Loliger C, Kuhnl P, Ottenhoff T, Contu L, Carcassi C, Savi M, Zanelli P, Neri TM, Hamaguchi K, Kimura A, Dong RP, Chikuba N, Nagataki S, Gorodezky C, Debaz H, Robles C, Coimbra HB, Martinho A, Ruas MA, Sachs JA, Garcia-Pachedo M, Biro A, Nikaein A, Dombrausky L, Gonwa T, Zmijewski C, Monos D, Kamoun M, Layrisse Z, Magli MC, Balducci P, & Thorsby E (1992) HLA class II associations in insulin-dependent diabetes mellitus among Blacks, Caucasoids, and Japanese. In: Tsuji K, Aizawa A, & Sasazuki T eds. HLA 1991 — Proceedings of the 11th international histocompatibility workshop and conference. Oxford, Oxford University Press, vol 1, pp 713–722.

Rood MJ, van Krugten MV, Zanelli E, van der Linden MW, Keijsers V, Schneuder GMT, Verduyn W, Westendorp RGJ, de Vries RRP, Breedveld FC, Verweij CL, & Huizinga TWJ (2000) TNF-308A and HLA-DR3 alleles contribute independently to susceptibility to systemic lupus erythematosus. Arthritis Rheum, **43**: 129–134.

Rosati G (2001) The prevalence of multiple sclerosis in the world: an update. Neurol Sci, **22**: 117–139.

Rose NR (1996) Foreword — The uses of autoantibodies. In: Shoenfeld Y & Peter JB eds. Autoantibodies. Amsterdam, Elsevier, pp xxvii–xxix.

Rose NR, Hamilton RG, & Detrick B (2002) Manual of clinical laboratory immunology. Washington, DC, ASM Press.

Rosenberg AM, Semchuk KM, McDuffie HH, Ledingham DL, Cordeiro DM, Cessna AJ, Irvine DG, Senthilselvan A, & Dosman JA (1999) Prevalence of antinuclear antibodies in a rural population. J Toxicol Environ Health, **56**: 225–236.

Rosenblum MD, Olasz E, Woodliff JE, Johnson BD, Konkol MC, Gerber KA, Orentas RJ, Sandford G, & Truitt RL (2004) CD200 is a novel p53-target gene involved in apoptosis-associated immune tolerance. Blood, **103**: 2691–2698.

Rosenman KD & Zhu Z (1995) Pneumoconiosis and associated medical conditions. Am J Ind Med, **27**: 107–113.

Rosenman KD, Moore-Fuller M, & Reilly MF (1999) Connective tissue disease and silicosis. Am J Ind Med, **25**: 375–381.

Rosery H, Bergemann R, & Maxion-Bergemann S (2005) International variation in resource utilisation and treatment costs for rheumatoid arthritis: a systematic literature review. Pharmacoeconomics, **23**: 243–257.

Rossini AA, Handler ES, Mordes JP, & Greiner DL (1995) Human autoimmune diabetes mellitus: lessons from BB rats and NOD mice — Caveat emptor. Clin Immunol Immunopathol, **74**(1): 2–9.

Rowley B & Monestier M (2005) Mechanisms of heavy metal-induced autoimmunity. Mol Immunol, **42**: 833–838.

Rubin RL (1992) Autoantibody specificity in drug-induced lupus and neutrophil-mediated metabolism of lupus-inducing drugs. Clin Biochem, **25**(3): 223–234.

Rubin RL & Kretz-Rommel A (2001) A nondeletional mechanism for central T-cell tolerance. Crit Rev Immunol, **21**(1–3): 29–40.

Rubin RL, Reimer G, McNally EM, Nusinow SR, Searles RP, & Tan EM (1986) Procain-amide elicits a selective autoantibody immune response. Clin Exp Immunol, **63**(1): 58–67.

Rubin RL, Salomon DR, & Guerrero RS (2001) Thymus function in drug-induced lupus. Lupus, **10**(11): 795–801.

Rubio-Terres C & Dominguez-Gil Hurle A (2005) [Cost-utility analysis of relapsing-remitting multiple sclerosis treatment with azathioprine or interferon beta in Spain.] Rev Neurol, **40**: 705–710 (in Spanish).

Ruiz-Irastorza G, Lima F, Alves J, Khamashta MA, Simpson J, Hughes GR, & Buchanan NM (1996) Increased rate of lupus flare during pregnancy and the puerperium: a prospective study of 78 pregnancies. Am J Rheumatol, **35**: 133–138.

Ruiz-Irastorza G, Khamashta MA, Gordon C, Lockshin MD, Johns KR, Sammaritano L, & Hughes GR (2004) Measuring systemic lupus erythematosus activity during pregnancy: validation of the lupus activity index in pregnancy scale. Arthritis Rheum, **51**(1): 78–82.

Ruiz-Mendez M, Posada de la Paz M, Abian J, Calaf R, Blount B, Castro-Molero N, Philen RM, & Gelpi E (2001) Storage time and deodorization temperature influence the formation of aniline-derived compounds in denatured rapeseed oils. Food Chem Toxicol, **39**: 91–96.

Rutella S & Lemoli RM (2004) Regulatory T cells and tolerogenic dendritic cells: from basic biology to clinical applications. Immunol Lett, **94**(1–2): 11–26.

Rutgers A, Heeringa P, Damoiseaux JG, & Cohen Tervaert JW (2003) ANCA and anti-GBM antibodies in diagnosis and follow-up of vasculitic disease. Eur J Intern Med, **14**: 287–295.

Sabbatini A, Bombardieri S, & Migliorini P (1993) Autoantibodies from patients with systemic lupus erythematosus bind a shared sequence of SmD and Epstein-Barr virus-encoded nuclear antigen EBNA I. Eur J Immunol, **23**: 1146–1152.

Sabharwal P, Glaser R, Lafuse W, Varma S, Liu Q, Arkins S, Kooijman R, Kutz L, Kelley KW, & Malarkey WB (1992) Prolactin synthesized and secreted by human peripheral blood mononuclear cells: an autocrine growth factor for lymphoproliferation. Proc Natl Acad Sci U S A, **89**: 7713–7716.

Sakaguchi S (2000) Animal models of autoimmunity and their relevance to human diseases. Curr Opin Immunol, **12**(6): 684–690.

Sakaguchi S & Sakaguchi N (1989) Organ-specific autoimmune disease induced in mice by elimination of T cell subsets. V. Neonatal administration of cyclosporin A causes autoimmune disease. J Immunol, **142**(2): 471–480.

Sala M, Sunyer J, Herrero C, To-Figueras J, & Grimalt J (2001) Association between serum concentrations of hexachlorobenzene and polychlorobiphenyls with thyroid hormone and liver enzymes in a sample of the general population. Occup Environ Med, **58**(3): 172–177.

Salomon B & Bluestone JA (2001) Complexities of CD28/B7:CTLA-4 costimulatory pathways in autoimmunity and transplantation. Annu Rev Immunol, **19**: 225–252.

Sanchez-Guerrero J, Schur PH, Sergent JS, & Liang MH (1994) Silicone breast implants and rheumatic disease. Clinical, immunologic, and epidemiologic studies. Arthritis Rheum, **37**: 158–168.

Sanchez-Guerrero J, Colditz GA, Karlson EW, Hunter DJ, Speizer FE, & Liang MH (1995) Silicone breast implants and the risk of connective-tissue diseases and symptoms. N Engl J Med, **332**: 1666–1670.

Sanchez-Margalet V, Martin-Romero C, Santos-Alvarez J, Goberna R, Najib S, & Gonzalez-Yanes C (2003) Role of leptin as an immunomodulator of blood mononuclear cells: mechanisms of action. Clin Exp Immunol, **133**: 11–19.

Sanchez-Porro Valades P, Posada de la Paz M, de Andres Copa P, Gimenez Ribota O, & Abaitua Borda I (2003) Toxic oil syndrome: survival in the whole cohort between 1981 and 1995. J Clin Epidemiol, **56**: 701–708.

Sanchez-Roman J, Wichmann I, Salaberri J, Varela JM, & Nunez-Roldan A (1993) Multiple clinical and biological autoimmune manifestation in 50 workers after occupational exposure to silica. Ann Rheum Dis, **52**: 534–538.

Sanna V, Di Giacomo A, La Cava A, Lechler RI, Fontana S, Zappacosta S, & Matarese G (2003) Leptin surge precedes onset of autoimmune encephalomyelitis and correlates with development of pathogenic T cell responses. J Clin Invest, **111**: 241–250.

Sato S, Sugiyama M, Yamamoto M, Watanabe Y, Kawai T, Takeda K, & Akira S (2003) Toll/IL-1 receptor domain-containing adaptor inducing IFN-beta (TRIF) associates with TNF receptor-associated factor 6 and TANK-binding kinase 1, and activates two distinct transcription factors, NF-kappa B and IFN-regulatory factor-3, in the Toll-like receptor signaling. J Immunol, **171**(8): 4304–4310.

Sauter B, Albert ML, Francisco L, Larsson M, Somersan S, & Bhardwaj N (2000) Consequences of cell death: exposure to necrotic tumor cells, but not primary tissue cells or apoptotic cells, induces the maturation of immunostimulatory dendritic cells. J Exp Med, **191**(3): 423–434.

Savige J, Davies D, Falk RJ, Jennette JC, & Wiik A (2000) Antineutrophil cytoplasmic antibodies and associated diseases: a review of the clinical and laboratory features. Kidney Int, **57**: 846–862.

Sayeh E & Uetrecht JP (2001) Factors that modify penicillamine-induced autoimmunity in Brown Norway rats: failure of the Th1/Th2 paradigm. Toxicology, **163**(2–3): 195–211.

Schatz D, Krischer J, Horne G, Riley W, Spillar R, Silverstein J, Winter W, Muir A, Derovanesian D, Shah S, Malone J, & Maclaren N (1994) Islet cell antibodies predict insulin-dependent diabetes in United States school age children as powerfully as in unaffected relatives. J Clin Invest, **93**: 2403–2407.

Schellekens GA, Visser H, de Jong BA, van den Hoogen FH, Hazes JM, Breedveld FC, & van Venrooij WJ (2000) The diagnostic properties of rheumatoid arthritis antibodies recognizing a cyclic citrullinated peptide. Arthritis Rheum, **43**: 155–163.

Schellekens H (2003) Immunogenicity of therapeutic proteins. Nephrol Dial Transplant, **18**(7): 1257–1259.

Scheinbart LS, Johnson MA, Gross LA, Edelstein SR, & Richardson BC (1991) Procainamide inhibits DNA methyltransferase in a human T cell line. J Rheumatol, **18**: 530–534.

Schielen P, Schoo W, Tekstra J, Oostermeijer HH, Seinen W, & Bloksma N (1993) Autoimmune effects of hexachlorobenzene in the rat. Toxicol Appl Pharmacol, **122**: 233–243.

Schielen P, Van Rodijnen W, Pieters RH, & Seinen W (1995) Hexachlorobenzene treatment increases the number of splenic B-1-like cells and serum autoantibody levels in the rat. Immunology, **86**: 568–574.

Schmitt J & Papisch W (2002) Recombinant autoantigens. Autoimmun Rev, **1**: 79–88.

Schuhmann D, Kubicka-Muranyi M, Mirtschewa J, Günther J, Kind P, & Gleichmann E (1990) Adverse immune reactions to gold. I. Chronic treatment with an Au(I) drug sensitizes mouse T cells not to Au(I), but to Au(III) and induces autoantibody formation. J Immunol, **145**(7): 2132–2139.

Schuppe HC, Ronnau AC, Schmiedeberg SV, Ruzicka T, Gleichmann E, & Griem P (1998) Immunomodulation by heavy metal compounds. Clinics Dermatol, **16**: 149–157.

Schurz HH, Hill RH, Philen RM, Posada de la Paz M, Abaitua Borda I, Kilbourne EM, Bernert T, & Needham LL (1997) Analytical measurements of products of aniline and triglycerides in oil samples associated with the toxic oil syndrome. Berlin/Heidelberg, Springer Verlag.

Schwarz A, Beissert S, Grosse-Heitmeyer K, Gunzer I, Bluestone JA, Grabbe S, & Schwarz T (2000) Evidence for functional relevance of CTLA-4 in ultraviolet-radiation-induced tolerance. J Immunol, **165**(4): 1824–1831.

Schwartz M & Cohen IR (2000) Autoimmunity can benefit self-maintenance. Immunol Today, **21**(6): 265–268.

Scofield RH (1996) Autoimmune thyroid disease in systemic lupus erythematosus and Sjögren's syndrome. Clin Exp Rheumatol, **14**: 321–330.

Scott RS, McMahon EJ, Pop SM, Reap EA, Caricchio R, Cohen PL, Earp HS, & Matsushima GK (2001) Phagocytosis and clearance of apoptotic cells is mediated by MER. Nature (Lond), **411**: 207–211.

Seguin B & Uetrecht J (2003) The danger hypothesis applied to idiosyncratic drug reactions. Curr Opin Allergy Clin Immunol, **3**(4): 235–242.

Sercarz EE, Lehmann PV, Ametani A, Benichou G, Miller A, & Moudgil K (1993) Dominance and crypticity of T cell antigenic determinants. Annu Rev Immunol, **11**: 729–766.

Shah MS, Davies TF, & Stagnaro-Green A (2003) The thyroid during pregnancy: a physiological and pathological stress test. Minerva Endocrinol, **28**: 233–245.

Shaheen VM, Satoh M, Richards HB, Yoshida H, Shaw M, Jennette JC, & Reeves WH (1999) Immunopathogenesis of environmentally induced lupus in mice. Environ Health Perspect, **107**(Suppl 5): 723–727.

Sheikh A, Smeeth L, & Hubbard R (2003) There is no evidence of an inverse relationship between Th2-mediated atopy and Th1-mediated autoimmune disorders: lack of support for the hygiene hypothesis. J Allergy Clin Immunol, **111**: 131–135.

Shenker BJ, Guo TL, & Shapiro LM (1998) Low-level methylmercury exposure causes human T-cells to undergo apoptosis — evidence of mitochondrial dysfunction. Environ Res, **77**: 149–159.

Shenton JM, Chen J, & Uetrecht JP (2004) Animal models of idiosyncratic drug reactions. Chem Biol Interact, **150**(1): 53–70.

Shevach EM (2000) Regulatory T cells in autoimmunity. Annu Rev Immunol, **18**: 423–449.

Shi Y & Rock KL (2002) Cell death releases endogenous adjuvants that selectively enhance immune surveillance of particulate antigens. Eur J Immunol, **32**(1): 155–162.

Shi YF, Sahai BM, & Green DR (1989) Cyclosporin A inhibits activation-induced cell death in T-cell hybridomas and thymocytes. Nature, **339**(6226): 625–626.

Shi Y, Evans JE, & Rock KL (2003) Molecular identification of a danger signal that alerts the immune system to dying cells. Nature, **425**(6957): 516–521 [Epub 7 September 2003].

Shimada S, Yamauchi M, Takamatsu M, Uetake S, Ohata M, & Saito S (2002) Experimental studies on the relationship between immune responses and liver damage induced by ethanol after immunization with homologous acetaldehyde adducts. Alcohol Clin Exp Res, **26S**: 86–90.

Shinkai K, Nakamura K, Tsutsui N, Kuninishi Y, Iwaki Y, Nishida H, Suzuki R, Vohr HW, Takahashi M, Takahashi K, Kamimura Y, & Maki E (1999) Mouse popliteal lymph node assay for assessment of allergic and autoimmunity-inducing potentials of low-molecular-weight drugs. J Toxicol Sci, **24**(2): 95–102.

Shoenfeld Y & Isenberg D eds (1990) The mosaic of autoimmunity (The factors associated with autoimmune diseases). Amsterdam, Elsevier.

Shoenfeld Y & Rose NR (2004) Infection and autoimmunity. Amsterdam, Elsevier.

Sidransky H & Verney E (1994) Comparative studies on tryptophan binding to hepatic nuclear envelopes in Sprague-Dawley and Lewis rats. Am J Physiol, **267**: R502–R507.

Sidransky H & Verney E (1997) Mouse strain and source of L-tryptophan affects hepatic nuclear tryptophan binding. Toxicology, **118**: 37–47.

Siegmund W, Franke G, Biebler KE, Donner I, Kawellis R, Kairies M, Scherber A, & Huller H (1985) The influence of the acetylator phenotype on the clinical use of dihydralazine. Int J Clin Pharmacol Ther Toxicol, **23**: 74–78.

Silbergeld EK & Devine PJ (2000) Mercury — are we studying the right endpoints and mechanisms. Fuel Process Technol, **65**(66): 35–42.

Silman AJ & Jones S (1992) What is the contribution of occupational environmental factors to the occurrence of scleroderma in men? Ann Rheum Dis, **51**: 1322–1324.

Silman AJ, Kay A, & Brennan P (1992) Timing of pregnancy in relation to the onset of rheumatoid arthritis. Arthritis Rheum, **35**: 152–155.

Silver RM, Ludwicka A, Hampton M, Ohba T, Bingel SA, Smith T, Harley RA, Maize J, & Heyes M (1994) A murine model of the eosinophilia-myalgia syndrome induced by 1,1'-ethylidenebis(L-tryptophan). J Clin Invest, **93**: 1473–1480.

Silverman BG, Brown SL, Bright RA, Kaczmarek RG, Arrowsmith Lowe JB, & Kessler DA (1996) Reported complications of silicone gel breast implants: an epidemiologic review. Ann Intern Med, **124**: 744–756.

Silverstein MJ, Handel N, Gamagami P, Gierson ED, Furmanski M, Collins AR, Epstein M, & Cohlan BF (1992) Breast cancer diagnosis and prognosis in women following augmentation with silicone gel-filled prostheses. Eur J Cancer, **28**: 635–640.

Silverstone AE, Gavalchin J, & Gasiewicz TA (1998) TCDD, DES, and estradiol potentiate a lupus-like autoimmune nephritis in NZB × SWR (SNF$_1$) mice. Toxicologist, **42**: 403.

Sim E & Law SK (1985) Hydralazine binds covalently to complement component C4. Different reactivity of C4B gene products. FEBS Lett, **184**(2): 323–327.

Simat TJ, Kleeberg KK, Muller B, & Sierts A (1999) Synthesis, formation, and occurrence of contaminants in biotechnically manufactured L-tryptophan. Adv Exp Med Biol, **467**: 469–480.

Simopoulos AP (2002) Omega-3 fatty acids in inflammation and autoimmune diseases. J Am Coll Nutr, **21**: 495–505.

Sinigaglia F (1994) The molecular basis of metal recognition by T cells. J Invest Dermatol, **102**(4): 398–401.

Skarstein K, Wahren M, Zaura E, Hattori M, & Jonsson R (1995) Characterization of T cell receptor repertoire and anti-Ro/SSA autoantibodies in relation to sialadenitis of NOD mice. Autoimmunity, **22**(1): 9–16.

Slavin RE, Swedo JL, Brandes D, Gonzalez-Vitale JC, & Osornio-Vargas A (1985) Extrapulmonary silicosis: a clinical, morphologic, and ultrastructural study. Hum Pathol, **16**: 393–312.

Sluis-Cremer GK, Hessel PA, Hnizdo EH, Churchill AR, & Zeiss EA (1985) Silica, silicosis, and progressive systemic sclerosis. Br J Ind Med, **42**: 838–843.

Sluis-Cremer GK, Hessel PA, Hnizdo E, & Churchill AR (1986) Relationship between silicosis and rheumatoid arthritis. Thorax, **41**: 596–601.

Smith DA & Germolec DR (2000) Developmental exposure to TCDD and mercuric chloride in autoimmune-prone MRL/lpr mice. Toxicologist, **54**: 8.

Smith W & Ball GV (1980) Lung injury due to gold treatment. Arthritis Rheum, **23**: 351–354.

Sobel ES, Gianini J, Butfiloski EJ, Croker BP, Schiffenbauer J, & Roberts SM (2005) Acceleration of autoimmunity by organochlorine pesticides in (NZB × NZW)F1 mice. Environ Health Perspect, **113**(3): 323–328.

Soldan SS, Alvarez Retuerto AI, Sicotte NL, & Voskuhl RR (2003) Immune modulation in multiple sclerosis patients treated with the pregnancy hormone estriol. J Immunol, **171**: 6267–6274.

Sollid L & Thorsby E (1993) HLA susceptibility genes in celiac disease: genetic mapping and role in pathogenesis. Gastroenterology, **105**: 910–922.

Sopori M (2002) Effects of cigarette smoke on the immune system. Nat Rev Immunol, **2**: 372–377.

Sorensen J & Andersen LS (2005) The case of tumour necrosis factor-alpha inhibitors in the treatment of rheumatoid arthritis: a budget impact analysis. Pharmacoeconomics, **23**: 289–298.

Speirs C, Fielder AH, Chapel H, Davey NJ, & Batchelor JR (1989) Complement system protein C4 and susceptibility to hydralazine-induced systemic lupus erythematosus. Lancet, **1**(8644): 922–924.

Stagnaro-Green A (2002) Clinical review 152: Postpartum thyroiditis. Clin Endocrinol Metab, **87**: 4042–4047.

Staples JA, Ponsonby AL, Lim LL, & McMichael AJ (2003) Ecologic analysis of some immune-related disorders, including type 1 diabetes, in Australia: latitude, regional ultraviolet radiation, and disease prevalence. Environ Health Perspect, **111**: 518–523.

Stein EC, Schiffer RB, Hall WJ, & Young N (1987) Multiple sclerosis and the workplace: report of an industry-based cluster. Neurology, **37**: 1672–1677.

Stevens A, Ray A, Alansari A, Hajeer A, Thomson W, Donn R, Ollier WER, Worthington J, & Davis JRE (2001a) Characterization of a prolactin gene polymorphism and its association with systemic lupus erythematosus. Arthritis Rheum, **44**: 2358–2366.

Stevens A, Ray DW, Worthington J, & Davis JR (2001b) Polymorphisms of the human prolactin gene — implications for production of lymphocyte prolactin and systemic lupus erythematosus. Lupus, **10**: 676–683.

Stewart SF, Leathart JB, Chen Y, Daly AK, Rolla R, Vay D, Mottaran E, Vidali M, Albano E, & Day CP (2002) Valine–alanine manganese superoxide dismutase polymorphism is not associated with alcohol-induced oxidative stress or liver fibrosis. Hepatology, **36**: 1355–1360.

Stiller-Winkler R, Radaszkiewicz T, & Gleichmann E (1988) Immunopathological signs in mice treated with mercury compounds: I. Identification by popliteal lymph node assay of responder and nonresponder strains. Int J Immunopharmacol, **10**: 475–484.

Stolt P, Bengtsson C, Nordmark B, Lindblad S, Lundberg I, Klareskog L, Alfredsson L, & the EIRA Study Group (2003) Quantification of the influence of cigarette smoking on rheumatoid arthritis: results from a population based case–control study, using incident cases. Ann Rheum Dis, **62**: 835–841.

Stolt P, Kallberg H, Lundberg I, Sjogren B, Klareskog L, Alfredsson L, & EIRA Study Group (2005) Silica exposure is associated with increased risk of developing rheumatoid arthritis: results from the Swedish EIRA study. Ann Rheum Dis, **64**: 582–586.

Strachan DP (1989) Hay fever, hygiene, and household size. Br Med J, **299**: 1259–1260.

Stratta P, Mazzucco G, Griva S, Tetta C, & Monga G (1988) Immune-mediated glomerulonephritis after exposure to paraquat. Nephron, **48**: 138–141.

Stratta P, Messuerotti A, Canavese C, Coen M, Luccoli L, Bussolati B, Giorda L, Malavenda P, Cacciabue M, Bugiani M, Bo M, Ventura M, Camussi G, & Fubini B (2001) The role of metals in autoimmune vasculitis: epidemiological and pathogenic study. Sci Total Environ, **270**: 179–190.

Stratton K, Gable A, & McCormick MC (2001) Thimerosal-containing vaccines and neurodevelopmental disorders. Washington, DC, Institute of Medicine.

Strieder TGH, Prummel MF, Tijssen JGP, Endert E, & Wiersinga WM (2003) Risk factors for and prevalence of thyroid disorders in a cross-sectional study among healthy female relatives of patients with autoimmune thyroid disease. Clin Endocrinol, **59**: 396–401.

Sturfelt G, Hellmer G, & Truedsson L (1996) TNF microsatellites in systemic lupus erythematosus — a high frequency of the TNFabc 2-3-1 haplotype in multicase SLE families. Lupus, **5**: 618–622.

Suciu I, Drejman I, & Valeskai M (1963) Contribution to the study of the diseases caused by vinyl chloride. Med Intern, **15**: 967–978.

Susol E, Rands AL, Herrick A, McHugh N, Barrett JH, Ollier WER, & Worthington J (2000) Association of markers for TGFβ3, TGFβ2 and TIMP1 with systemic sclerosis. Rheumatology, **39**: 1332–1336.

Sutcliffe N, Clarke AE, Gordon C, Farewell V, & Isenberg DA (1999) The association of socio-economic status, race, psychosocial factors and outcome in patients with systemic lupus erythematosus. Rheumatology (Oxford), **38**(11): 1130–1137.

Suzuki A, Yamada R, Chang X, Tokuhiro S, Sawada T, Suzuki M, Nagasaki M, Nakayama-Hamada M, Kawaida R, Ono M, Ohtsuki M, Furukawa H, Yoshino S, Yukioka M, Tohma S, Matsubara T, Wakitani S, Teshima R, Nishioka Y, Sekine A, Iida A, Takahashi A, Tsunoda T, Nakamura Y, & Yamamoto K (2003) Functional haplotypes of PADI4, encoding citrullinating enzyme peptidylarginine deiminase 4, are associated with rheumatoid arthritis. Nat Genet, **34**(4): 395–402.

Suzuki S, Tourkina E, Ludwicka A, Hampton M, Bolster M, Maize J, & Silver RM (1996) A contaminant of L-tryptophan enhances expression of dermal collagen in a murine model of eosinophilia myalgia syndrome. Proc Assoc Am Physicians, **104**: 315–322.

Swanson SJ, Ferbas J, Mayeux P, & Casadevall N (2004) Evaluation of methods to detect and characterize antibodies against recombinant human erythropoietin. Nephron Clin Pract, **96**(3): c88–95.

Swygert LA, Maes EF, Sewell LE, Miller L, Falk H, & Kilbourne EM (1990) Eosinophilia-myalgia syndrome. J Am Med Assoc, **264**: 1698–1703.

Szeto C, Gillespie KM, & Mathieson PW (1999) Low-dose mercuric chloride induces resistance in Brown Norway rats to further mercuric chloride by up-regulation of interferon-gamma. Scand J Immunol, **50**(2): 195–201.

Tabuenca JM (1981) Toxic-allergic syndrome caused by ingestion of rapeseed oil denatured with aniline. Lancet, **2**: 567–568.

Takagi H, Ochoa MS, Zhou L, Helfman T, Murata H, & Falanga V (1995) Enhanced collagen synthesis and transcription by peak E: a contaminant of L-tryptophan preparations associated with the eosinophilia myalgia syndrome epidemic. J Clin Invest, **96**: 2120–2125.

Takamatsu M, Yamauchi M, Maezawa Y, Saito S, Mawyama S, & Uchikoshi T (2000) Genetic polymorphisms of interleukin-1β in association with the development of alcoholic liver disease in Japanese patients. Am J Gastroenterol, **95**: 1305–1311.

Takeuchi K, Turley SJ, Tan EM, & Pollard KM (1995) Analysis of the autoantibody response to fibrillarin in human disease and murine models of autoimmunity. J Immunol, **154**: 961–971.

Talwalkar JA & Lindor KD (2003) Primary biliary cirrhosis. Lancet, **362**(9377): 53–61.

Tamaki H, Itoh E, Kaneda T, Asahi K, Mitsuda N, Tanizawa O, & Amino N (1993) Crucial role of serum human chorionic gonadotropin for the aggravation of thyrotoxicosis in early pregnancy in Graves' disease. Thyroid, **3**: 189–193.

Tan EM, Feltkamp TEW, Smolen JS, Butcher B, Dawkins R, Fritzler MJ, Gordon T, Hardin JA, Kalden JR, Lahita RG, Maini RN, McDougal JS, Rothfield NF, Smeenk RJ, Takasaki E, Whik A, Wilson MR, & Koziol JA (1997) Range of antinuclear antibodies in "healthy" individuals. Arthritis Rheum, **40**: 1601–1611.

Taneja V & David CS (1999) HLA class II transgenic mice as models of human diseases. Immunol Rev, **169**: 67–79.

Tang L, Benjaponpitak S, DeKruyff RH, & Umetsu DT (1998) Reduced prevalence of allergic disease in patients with multiple sclerosis is associated with enhanced IL-12 production. J Allergy Clin Immunol, **102**: 428–435.

Taurog JD, Maika SD, Satumtira N, Dorris ML, McLean IL, Yanagisawa H, Sayad A, Stagg AJ, Fox GM, Le O'Brien A, Rehman M, Zhou M, Weiner AL, Splawski JB, Richardson JA, & Hammer RE (1999) Inflammatory disease in HLA-B27 transgenic rats. Immunol Rev, **169**: 209–223.

Tedeschi A & Airaghi L (2001) Common risk factors in type 1 diabetes and asthma. Lancet, **357**(9268): 1622.

Tena G (1982) Fatty acid anilides and the toxic oil syndrome. Lancet, **1**(8263): 98.

Tenenbaum SA, Rice JC, Espinoza LR, Cuéllar ML, Plymale DR, Sander DM, Williamson LL, Haïslip AM, Gluck OS, Tesser JRP, Nogy L, Stribrny KM, Bevan JA, & Garry RF (1997a) Use of antipolymer antibody assay in recipients of silicone breast implants. Lancet, **349**(9050): 449–454.

Tenenbaum SA, Rice JC, Espinoza LR, & Garry RF (1997b) Antipolymer antibodies, silicone breast implants, and fibromyalgia. Author reply. Lancet, **349**(9059): 1172–1173.

Thiele GM, Tuma DJ, Willis MS, Vidali M, Stewart SF, Rolla R, Daly AK, Chen Y, Mottaran E, Jones DE, Leatherhart JB, Day CP, & Albano E (2003) Genetic and epigenetic factors in autoimmune reactions toward cytochrome P4502E1 in alcoholic liver disease. Hepatology, **37**: 410–419.

Thomas C, Groten J, Kammuller ME, De Bakker JM, Seinen W, & Bloksma N (1989) Popliteal lymph node reactions in mice induced by the drug zimeldine. Int J Immunopharmacol, **11**(6): 693–702.

Thomas C, Punt P, Warringa R, Hogberg T, Seinen W, & Bloksma N (1990) Popliteal lymph node enlargement and antibody production in the mouse induced by zimeldine and related compounds with varying side chains. Int J Immunopharmacol, **12**(5): 561–568.

Thomson W, Harrison B, Ollier B, Wiles N, Payton T, Barrett J, Symmons D, & Silman A (1999) Quantifying the exact role of HLA-DRB1 alleles in susceptibility to inflammatory polyarthritis. Arthritis Rheum, **42**: 757–762.

Thrasher JD, Madison R, & Broughton A (1993) Immunologic abnormalities in humans exposed to chlorpyrifos: preliminary observations. Arch Environ Health, **48**(2): 89–93.

Timmer A (2003) Environmental influences on inflammatory bowel disease manifestations. Lessons from epidemiology. Dig Dis, **21**: 91–104.

Todhunter JA & Farrow MG (1998) Current scientific considerations in regard to defining a "silicone syndrome"/disease and the formation of silica from silicone. Int J Toxicol, **17**: 449–463.

Toh BH, van Driel IR, & Gleeson PA (1997) Pernicious anemia. N Engl J Med, **337**: 1441–1448.

Tomer Y (2002) Genetic dissection of familial autoimmune thyroid diseases using whole genome screening. Autoimmun Rev, **1**: 198–204.

Tomer Y, Greenberg DA, Concepcion E, Ban Y, & Davies TF (2002) Thyroglobulin is a thyroid specific gene for the familial autoimmune thyroid diseases. J Clin Endocrinol Metab, **87**: 404–407.

Tomita Y, Jyonouchi H, Engelman RW, Day NK, & Good RA (1993) Preventive action of carotenoids on the development of lymphadenopathy and proteinuria in MRL-lpr/lpr mice. Autoimmunity, **16**: 95–102.

Tonroth T & Skrifvars B (1974) Gold nephropathy prototype of membranous glomerulonephritis. Am J Pathol, **75**: 573–586.

Tournade H, Pelletier L, Pasquier R, Vial MC, Mandet C, & Druet P (1990) D-penicillamine-induced autoimmunity in Brown-Norway rats: Similarities with $HgCl_2$-induced autoimmunity. J Immunol, **144**(8): 2985–2991.

Tournade H, Guery J-C, Pasquier R, Nochy D, Hinglais N, Guilbert B, Druet P, & Pelletier L (1991) Experimental gold-induced autoimmunity. Nephrol Dial Transplant, **6**: 621–630.

References

Tremlett HL, Evans J, Wiles CM, & Luscombe DK (2002) Asthma and multiple sclerosis: an inverse association in a case–control general practice population. Q J Med, **95**: 753–756.

Trepanier LA (2004) Idiosyncratic toxicity associated with potentiated sulfonamides in the dog. J Vet Pharmacol Ther, **27**(3): 129–138.

Tsai HM (2003) Advances in the pathogenesis, diagnosis, and treatment of thrombotic thrombocytopenic purpura. J Am Soc Nephrol, **14**: 1072–1081.

Tsai HM & Lian EC (1998) Antibodies to von Willebrand factor-cleaving protease in acute thrombotic thrombocytopenic purpura. N Engl J Med, **339**: 1585–1594.

Tsankov N, Stransky L, Kostowa M, Mitrowa T, & Obreschkowa E (1990) [Induced pemphigus caused by occupational contact with Basochrom.] Derm Beruf Umbelt, **38**: 91–93 (in German).

Tsao BP (2003) The genetics of human systemic lupus erythematosus. Trends Immunol, **24**: 595–602.

Tugwell P, Wells G, Peterson J, Welch V, Page J, Davison C, McGowan J, Ramroth D, & Shea B (2001) Do silicone breast implants cause rheumatologic disorders? A systematic review for a court-appointed national science panel. Arthritis Rheum, **44**: 2477–2484.

Turner S & Cherry N (2000) Rheumatoid arthritis in workers exposed to silica in the pottery industry. Occup Environ Med, **57**(7): 443–447.

Ueda S, Wakashin M, Wakashin Y, Yoshida H, Iesato K, Mori T, Mori Y, Akikusa B, & Okuda K (1986) Experimental gold nephropathy in guinea pigs: detection of auto-antibodies to renal tubular antigens. Kidney Int, **29**: 539–548.

Ueki A, Yamaguchi M, Ueki H, Watanabe Y, Ohsawa G, Kinugawa K, Kawakami Y, & Hyodoh F (1994) Polyclonal human T-cell activation by silicate in vitro. Immunology, **82**: 332–335.

Uetrecht J (1990) Drug metabolism by leukocytes and its role in drug-induced lupus and other idiosyncratic drug reactions. Crit Rev Toxicol, **20**(4): 213–235.

United States National Institutes of Health (2000) Report of the Autoimmune Diseases Coordinating Committee. Bethesda, Maryland, United States Department of Health and Human Services, National Institutes of Health, October (http://www.niaid.nih.gov/dait/pdf/adccrev.pdf).

Vaarala O, Alfthan G, Jauhianen M, Leirsalo-Repo M, Aho K, & Palosuo T (1993) Crossreaction between antibodies to oxidized low-density lipoprotein and to cardiolipin in systemic lupus erythematosus. Lancet, **341**(8850): 923–925.

Vagenakis AG & Braverman LE (1975) Adverse effects of iodides on thyroid function. Med Clin North Am, **59**: 1075–1088.

Vaisberg MW, Kaneno R, Franco MF, & Mendes NF (2000) Influence of cholecalciferol (vitamin D3) on the course of experimental systemic lupus erythematosus in F1 (NZB×W) mice. J Clin Lab Anal, **14**: 91–96.

Vaishnaw AK, McNally JD, & Elkon KB (1997) Apoptosis in the rheumatic diseases. Arthritis Rheum, **40**: 1917–1927.

Valenti L, De Feo T, Fracanzani AL, Fatta E, Salvagnini M, Arico S, Rossi G, Fiorelli G, & Fargion S (2004) Cytotoxic T-lymphocyte antigen-4 A49G polymorphism is associated with susceptibility to and severity of alcoholic liver disease in Italian patients. Alcohol Alcohol, **39**(4): 276–280.

Vallyathan V, Shi XL, & Dalal NS (1988) ESR evidence for the hydroxyl radical formation in aqueous suspension of quartz particles and its possible significance to lipid peroxidation in silicosis. J Toxicol Environ Health, **25**: 237–245.

Van Amerongen BM, Dijkstra CD, Lips P, & Polman CH (2004) Multiple sclerosis and vitamin D: an update. Eur J Clin Nutr, **58**: 1095–1109.

Vandebriel RJ, Meredith C, Scott MP, van Dijk M, & van Loveren H (2000) Interleukin-10 is an unequivocal Th2 parameter in the rat, whereas interleukin-4 is not. Scand J Immunol, **52**: 519–524.

van der Pol W & van de Winkel JG (1998) IgG receptor polymorphisms: risk factors for disease. Immunogenetics, **48**(3): 222–232.

Vanderpump MP, Tunbridge WM, French JM, Appleton D, Bates D, Clark F, Grimley Evans J, Hasan DM, Rodgers H, Tunbridge F, & Young ET (1995) The incidence of thyroid disorders in the community: a twenty-year follow-up of the Whickham Survey. Clin Endocrinol (Oxf), **43**: 55–68.

VandeVord PJ, Gupta N, Wilson RB, Vinuya RZ, Schaefer CJ, Canady AI, & Wooley PH (2004) Immune reactions associated with silicone-based ventriculo-peritoneal shunt malfunctions in children. Biomaterials, **25**: 3835–3860.

van Loveren H, Vos JG, Germolec D, Simeonova PP, Eijkemanns G, & McMichael AJ (2001) Epidemiologic associations between occupational and environmental exposures and autoimmune disease: Report of a meeting to explore current evidence and identify research needs. Int J Hyg Environ Health, **203**: 483–495.

van Vliet E, Uhrberg M, Stein C, & Gleichmann E (1993) MHC control of IL-4-dependent enhancement of B cell Ia expression and Ig class switching in mice treated with mercuric chloride. Int Arch Allergy Immunol, **101**(4): 392–401.

van Zijverden M, van der Pijl A, Bol M, van Pinxteren FA, de Haar C, Penninks AH, van Loveren H, & Pieters R (2000) Diesel exhaust, carbon black, and silica particles display distinct Th1/Th2 modulating activity. Toxicol Appl Pharmacol, **168**(2): 131–139.

Varga J, Maul GG, & Jimenez SA (1992) Autoantibodies to nuclear lamin C in the eosinophilia-myalgia syndrome associated with L-tryptophan ingestion. Arthritis Rheum, **35**: 106–109.

Varga J, Li L, & Jimenez S (1993) Increased type I collagen gene expression in L-tryptophan associated eosinophilia-myalgia syndrome skin fibroblasts. J Rheumatol, **20**: 1303–1308.

Verdier F, Virat M, & Descotes J (1990) Applicability of the popliteal lymph node assay in the Brown-Norway rat. Immunopharmacol Immunotoxicol, **12**(4): 669–677.

Vergani D & Mieli-Vergani G (2003) Autoimmune hepatitis. Autoimmunol Rev, **2**: 241–247.

Verge CF, Gianani R, Kawasaki E, Yu L, Pietropaolo M, Jackson RA, Chase HP, & Eisenbarth GS (1996) Prediction of type I diabetes in first-degree relatives using a combination of insulin, GAD, and ICA512bdc/IA-2 autoantibodies. Diabetes, **45**: 926–933.

Vermeire S, Noman M, Van Assche G, Baert F, Van Steen K, Esters N, Joossens S, Bossuyt X, & Rutgeerts P (2003) Autoimmunity associated with anti-tumor necrosis factor alpha treatment in Crohn's disease: a prospective cohort study. Gastroenterology, **125**: 32–39.

Vestergaard P (2002) Smoking and thyroid disorders — a meta-analysis. Eur J Endocrinol, **146**: 153–156.

Via CS, Shustov A, Rus V, Lang T, Nguyen P, & Finkelman FD (2001) In vivo neutralization of TNF-alpha promotes humoral autoimmunity by preventing the induction of CTL. J Immunol, **167**: 6821–6826.

Vial T, Choquet-Kastylevsky G, & Descotes J (2002) Adverse effects of immuno-therapeutics involving the immune system. Toxicology, **174**(1): 3–11.

Vicario JL, Serrano-Rios M, San Andres F, & Arnaiz-Villena A (1982) HLA-DR3, DR4 increase in chronic stage of Spanish oil disease. Lancet, **1**(8266): 276.

Vidali M, Stewart SF, Rolla R, Daly AK, Chen Y, Mottaran E, Jones DEJ, Leathart JB, Day CP, & Albano E (2003) Genetic and epigenetic factors in autoimmune reactions toward cytochrome P4502E1 in alcoholic liver disease. Hepatology, **37**: 410–419.

Viitala K, Makkonen K, Israel Y, Lehtimaki T, Jaakkola O, Koivula T, Blake JE, & Niemela O (2000) Autoimmune responses against oxidant stress and acetaldehyde-derived epitopes in human alcohol consumers. Alcohol Clin Exp Res, **24**: 1103–1109.

Villard-Mackintosh L & Vessey MP (1993) Oral contraceptives and reproductive factors in multiple sclerosis incidence. Contraception, **47**: 161–168.

Vincent A, Palace J, & Hilton-Jones D (2001) Myasthenia gravis. Lancet, **357**: 2122–2128.

Vingerhoets AJ, Assies J, Goodkin K, van Heck GL, & Bekker MH (1998) Prenatal diethylstilbestrol exposure and self-reported immune-related diseases. Eur J Obstet Gynecol Reprod Biol, **77**: 205–209.

Vogel A, Strassburg CP, Obermayer-Straub P, Brabant G, & Manns MP (2002) The genetic background of autoimmune polyendocrinopathy–candidiasis–ectodermal dystrophy and its autoimmune disease components. J Mol Med, 80: 201–211.

von Herrath MG & Harrison LC (2003) Antigen-induced regulatory T cells in autoimmunity. Nat Rev Immunol, 3(3): 223–232.

von Hertzen LC (2000) Puzzling associations between childhood infections and the later occurrence of asthma and atopy. Ann Med, 32: 397–400.

von Schmiedeberg S, Fritsche E, Ronnau AC, Specker C, Golka K, Richter-Hintz D, Schuppe HC, Lehmann P, Ruzicka T, Esser C, Abel J, & Gleichmann E (1999) Polymorphisms of the xenobiotic-metabolizing enzymes CYP1A1 and NAT-2 in systemic sclerosis and lupus erythematosus. Adv Exp Med Biol, 455: 147–152.

Vos JG & Moore JA (1974) Suppression of cellular immunity in rats and mice by maternal treatment with 2,3,7,8-tetrachlorodibenzo-p-dioxin. Int Arch Allergy Appl Immunol, 47: 777–794.

Vos JG, van Logten MJ, Kreeftenberg JG, & Kruizinga W (1979a) Hexachlorobenzene-induced stimulation of the humoral response in rats. Ann NY Acad Sci, 320: 535–550.

Vos JG, van Logten MJ, Kreeftenberg JG, Steerenberg PA, & Kruizinga W (1979b) Effect of hexachlorobenzene on the immune system of rats following combined pre- and postnatal exposure. Drug Chem Toxicol, 2: 61–76.

Vos JG, Brouwer GMJ, van Leeuwen FXR, & Wagenaar S (1983) Toxicity of hexachlorobenzene in the rat following combined pre- and post-natal exposure: comparison of effects on immune system, liver and lung. In: Parke DV, Gibson GG, & Hubbard R eds. Immunotoxicology. London, Academic Press, pp 219–235.

Wang C & Crapo LM (1997) The epidemiology of thyroid disease and implications for screening. Endocrinol Metab Clin North Am, 26(1): 189–218.

Wang J, Zheng L, Lobito A, Chan FK, Dale J, Sneller M, Yao X, Puck JM, Straus SE, & Leonardo MJ (1999a) Inherited human caspase 10 mutations underlie defective lymphocyte and dendritic cell apoptosis in autoimmune lymphoproliferative syndrome type II. Cell, 98: 47–58.

Ward DL & Bing-You RG (2001) Autoimmune thyroid dysfunction induced by interferon-alpha treatment for chronic hepatitis C: screening and monitoring recommendations. Endocr Pract, 7: 52–58.

Waterman SJ, El-Fawal HAN, & Snyder CA (1994) Lead alters the immunogenicity of two neural proteins: a potential mechanism for the progression of lead-induced neurotoxicity. Environ Health Perspect, 102: 1052–1056.

Watts RA, Lane SE, Bentham G, & Scott DG (2000) Epidemiology of systemic vasculitis: a ten-year study in the United Kingdom. Arthritis Rheum, 43(2): 414–419.

Ways SC, Mortola JF, Zvaifler NJ, Weiss RJ, & Yen SSC (1987) Alterations in immune responsiveness in women exposed to diethylstilbestrol in utero. Fertil Steril, 48: 193–197.

Weatherill AR, Stang BV, O'Hara K, Koller LD, & Hall JA (2003) Investigating the onset of autoimmunity in A.SW mice following treatment with "toxic oils". Toxicol Lett, **136**: 205–216.

Weaver JL, Chapdelaine JM, Descotes J, Germolec D, Holsapple M, House R, Lebrec H, Meade J, Pieters R, Hastings KL, & Dean JH (2005) Evaluation of a lymph node proliferation assay for its ability to detect pharmaceuticals with potential to cause immune-mediated drug reactions. J Immunotoxicol, **2**: 11–20.

Weiner JA, Nylander M, & Berglund F (1990) Does mercury from amalgam restorations constitute a health hazard? Sci Total Environ, **99**: 1–22.

Weiss RA, Madaio MP, Tomaszewski JE, & Kelly CJ (1994) T cells reactive to an inducible heat shock protein induce disease in toxin-induced interstitial nephritis. J Exp Med, **180**: 2239–2250.

Weissman DN, Hubbs AF, Huang SH, Stanley CF, Rojanasakul Y, & Ma JK (2001) IgG subclass responses in experimental silicosis. J Environ Pathol Toxicol Oncol, **20**(Suppl 1): 67–74.

Weltzien HU, Moulon C, Martin S, Padovan E, Hartmann U, & Kohler J (1996) T cell immune responses to haptens. Structural models for allergic and autoimmune reactions. Toxicology, **107**(2): 141–151.

Wester L, Koczan D, Holmberg J, Olofsson P, Thiesen HJ, Holmdahl R, & Ibrahim S (2003) Differential gene expression in pristane-induced arthritis susceptible DA versus resistant E3 rats. Arthritis Res Ther, **5**(6): R361–R372.

Westman P, Leirisalo-Repo M, Partanen J, & Koskimies S (1996) A comparative study of HLA genes in HLA-B27 positive ankylosing spondylitis and HLA-B27 positive peripheral reactive arthritis. Arthritis Rheum, **39**(6): 943–949.

Whitekus MJ, Santini RP, Rosenspire AJ, & McCabe MJ Jr (1999) Protection against CD95-mediated apoptosis by inorganic mercury in Jurkat T cells. J Immunol, **162**: 7162–7170.

Wick G, Brezinschek HP, Hala K, Dietrich H, Wolf H, & Kroemer G (1989) The obese strain of chickens: an animal model with spontaneous autoimmune thyroiditis. Adv Immunol, **47**: 433–500.

Williams DF (1996) Silicon, silicone, and silica: the importance of the right ending. Med Device Technol, **7**(1): 7–11.

Willis MS, Klassen LW, Tuma DJ, Sorrell MF, & Thiele GM (2002) Adduction of soluble proteins with malondialdehyde–acetaldehyde (MAA) induces antibody production and enhances T-cell proliferation. Alcohol Clin Exp Res, **26**: 94–106.

Willis MS, Thiele GM, Tuma DJ, & Klassen LW (2003) T cell proliferative responses to malondialdehyde–acetaldehyde haptenated protein are scavenger-receptor mediated. Int Immunopharmacol, **3**: 1381–1399.

Willison HJ & Yuki N (2002) Peripheral neuropathies and anti-glycolipid antibodies. Brain, **125**: 2591–2625.

Wilson RB, Gluck OS, Tesser JRP, Rice JC, Meyer A, & Bridges AJ (1999b) Antipolymer antibody reactivity in a subset of patients with fibromyalgia correlates with severity. J Rheumatol, **26**: 402–407.

Wilson RH, McCormick WE, Tatum CF, & Creech JL (1967) Occupational acroosteolysis: report of 31 cases. J Am Med Assoc, **201**: 577–581.

Wilson WA, Gharavi AE, Koike T, Lockshin MD, Branch DW, Piette JC, Brey R, Derksen R, Harris EN, Hughes GR, Triplett DA, & Khamashta MA (1999a) International consensus statement on preliminary classification criteria for definite antiphospholipid syndrome: report of an international workshop. Arthritis Rheum, **42**: 1309–1311.

Winer JB (2001) Guillain Barre syndrome. Mol Pathol, **54**: 381–385.

Wingard DL & Turiel J (1988) Long-term effects of exposure to diethylstilbestrol. West J Med, **149**: 551–554.

Woeber KA (1991) Iodine and thyroid disease. Med Clin North Am, **75**: 169–178.

Wong FS, Dittel BN, & Janeway CA Jr (1999) Transgenes and knockout mutations in animal models of type 1 diabetes and multiple sclerosis. Immunol Rev, **169**: 93–104.

Wooley PH & Whalen JD (1991) Pristane-induced arthritis in mice. III. Lymphocyte phenotypic and functional abnormalities precede the development of pristane-induced arthritis. Cell Immunol, **138**(1): 251–259.

Wooley PH, Griffin J, Panayi GS, Batchelor JR, Welsch KI, & Gibson TJ (1980) HLA-DR antigens and toxic reaction to sodium aurothiomalate and D-penicillamine in patients with rheumatoid arthritis. N Engl J Med, **303**: 300–302.

Wooley PH, Sud S, Whalen JD, & Nasser S (1998) Pristane-induced arthritis in mice: V. Susceptibility to pristane-induced arthritis is determined by the genetic regulation of the T cell repertoire. Arthritis Rheum, **41**(11): 2022–2031.

Woolf AD & Pfleger B (2003) Burden of major musculoskeletal conditions. Bull World Health Organ, **81**: 646–656.

Woosley RL, Drayer DE, Reidenberg MM, Nies AS, Carr K, & Oates JA (1978) Effect of acetylator phenotype on the rate at which procainamide induces antinuclear antibodies and the lupus syndrome. N Engl J Med, **298**: 1157–1159.

Wraith DC, Goldman M, & Lambert PH (2003) Vaccination and autoimmune disease: what is the evidence? Lancet, **362**(9396): 1659–1666.

Wulferink M, Gonzalez J, Goebel C, & Gleichmann E (2001) T cells ignore aniline, a prohapten, but respond to its reactive metabolites generated by phagocytes: possible implications for the pathogenesis of toxic oil syndrome. Chem Res Toxicol, **14**(4): 389–397.

Wulferink M, Dierkes S, & Gleichmann E (2002) Cross-sensitization to haptens: formation of common haptenic metabolites, T cell recognition of cryptic peptides, and true T cell cross-reactivity. Eur J Immunol, **32**(5): 1338–1348.

Xu D, Thiele GM, Beckenhauer JL, Klassen LW, Sorrell MF, & Tuma DJ (1998) Detection of circulating antibodies to malondialdehyde–acetaldehyde adducts in ethanol-fed rats. Gastroenterology, **115**: 686–692.

Yamamoto K (2003) Pathogenesis of Sjogren's syndrome. Autoimmunol Rev, **2**: 13–18.

Yamauchi M, Maezawa Y, Mizuhara Y, Ohata M, Hirakawa J, Nakajima H, & Toda G (1995) Polymorphisms in alcohol metabolizing enzyme genes and alcoholic cirrhosis in Japanese patients: a multivariate analysis. Hepatology, **22**: 1136–1142.

Yang JM, Hildebrandt B, Luderschmidt C, & Pollard KM (2003) Human scleroderma sera contain autoantibodies to protein components specific to the U3 small nucleolar RNP complex. Arthritis Rheum, **48**(1): 210–217.

Yee LJ, Kelleher P, Goldin R, Marshall S, Thomas HC, Alberti A, Chiaramonte M, Braconier J-H, Hall AJ, & Thursz MR (2004) Antinuclear antibodies (ANA) in chronic hepatitis C virus infection: correlates of positivity and clinical relevance. J Viral Hepat, **11**(5): 459–464.

Yen JH, Chen CJ, Tsai WC, Tsai JJ, Ou TT, & Liu HW (1999) HLA-DMA and HLA-DMB genotyping in patients with systemic lupus erythematosus. J Rheumatol, **26**: 1930–1933.

Yin M, Wheeler MD, Kono H, Bradford BU, Gallucci RM, Luster MI, & Thurman RG (1999) Essential role of tumor necrosis factor α in alcohol-induced liver injury in mice. Gastroenterology, **117**: 942–952.

Yoshida S & Gershwin ME (1993) Autoimmunity and selected environmental factors of disease induction. Semin Arthritis Rheum, **22**: 399–419.

Yu J, Yu L, Bugawan TL, Erlich HA, Barriga K, Hoffman M, Rewers M, & Eisenbarth GS (2000) Transient antiislet autoantibodies: infrequent occurrence and lack of association with "genetic" risk factors. J Clin Endocrinol Metab, **85**: 2421–2428.

Yucesoy B, Vallyathan V, Landsittel DP, Simeonova P, & Luster MI (2002) Cytokine polymorphisms in silicosis and other pneumoconioses. Mol Cell Biochem, **234/235**(1–2): 219–224.

Yu-Lee LY, Luo G, Moutoussamy S, & Finidory J (1998) Prolactin and growth hormone signal transduction in lymphohemopoetic cells. Cell Mol Life Sci, **54**: 1067–1075.

Yung R, Johnson K, & Richardson B (1995) New concepts in the pathogenesis of drug-induced lupus. Lab Invest, **73**: 746–759.

Yung R, Powers D, Johnson K, Amento E, Carr D, Laing T, Yang J, Chang S, Hemati N, & Richardson B (1996) Mechanism of drug-induced lupus. II. T cells overexpressing lymphocyte function-associated antigen 1 become autoreactive and cause a lupuslike disease in syngenic mice. J Clin Invest, **97**(12): 2866–2871.

Yung R, Chang S, Hemati N, Johnson K, & Richardson B (1997) Mechanisms of drug-induced lupus. IV. Comparison of procainamide and hydralazine with analogs in vitro and in vivo. Arthritis Rheum, **40**(8): 1436–1443.

Yurino H, Ishikawa S, Sato T, Akadegawa K, Ito T, Ueha S, Inadera H, & Matsushima K (2004) Endocrine disruptors (environmental estrogens) enhance autoantibody production by B1 cells. Toxicol Sci, **81**:139–147.

Zandman-Goddard G, Blank M, Ehrenfeld M, Gilburd B, Peter J, & Schoenfeld Y (1999) A comparison of autoantibody production in asymptomatic and symptomatic women with silicone breast implants. J Rheumatol, **26**: 73–77.

Zangrilli JG, Mayeno AN, Vining V, & Varga J (1995) 1,1'-Ethylidenebis[L-tryptophan], an impurity in L-tryptophan associated with eosinophilia-myalgia syndrome, stimulates type I collagen gene expression in human fibroblasts in vitro. Biochem Mol Biol Int, **37**: 925–933.

Zella JB & DeLuca HF (2003) Vitamin D and autoimmune diabetes. J Cell Biochem, **88**: 216–222.

Zenarola P, Gimma A, & Lomuto M (1995) Systemic contact dermatitis from thimerosal. Contact Dermatitis, **32**: 107–123.

Zhang SM, Willett WC, Hernán MA, Olek MJ, & Ascherio A (2000) Dietary fat in relation to risk of multiple sclerosis among two large cohorts of women. Am J Epidemiol, **152**: 1056–1064.

Zhang SM, Hernán MA, Olek MJ, Spiegelman D, Willett WC, & Ascherio A (2001) Intakes of carotenoids, vitamin C, and vitamin E and MS risk among two large cohorts of women. Neurology, **57**: 75–80.

Zhou Y, Gsicombe R, Huang D, & Lefvert AK (2002) Novel genetic association of Wegener's granulomatosis with the interleukin-10 gene. J Rheumatol, **29**: 317–320.

Ziegler AG, Hummel M, Schenker M, & Bonifacio E (1999) Autoantibody appearance and risk for development of childhood diabetes in offspring of parents with type 1 diabetes: the 2-year analysis of the German BABYDIAB Study. Diabetes, **48**: 460–468.

RESUME

L'autoimmunité se caractérise par une réaction des cellules (lymphocytes T autoréactifs) ou des produits (autoanticorps) du système immunitaire de l'organisme contre ses propres antigènes (autoantigènes). Elle peut constituer un élément de la réponse immunitaire physiologique (« autoimmunité naturelle ») ou être provoquée par un processus pathologique susceptible de déboucher sur des anomalies cliniques (« maladies autoimmunes »). Des maladies autoimmunes nombreuses et diverses peuvent se produire mais toutes se caractérisent par une réponse immunitaire inadaptée ou excessive vis-à-vis des autoantigènes conduisant à un état inflammatoire chronique ainsi qu'à une destruction ou à une dysfonction tissulaires. On connaît aujourd'hui plus de soixante maladies qui ont une étiologie autoimmune avérée ou fortement suspectée.

On croit généralement que ces maladies sont relativement rares, mais les estimations montrent que la prévalence globale des maladies autoimmunes est élevée (3 à 5 % de la population générale), d'où leur importance pour la santé publique. En raison des difficultés que soulèvent le diagnostic ainsi que la conception et la normalisation des études épidémiologiques relatives à ces affections, il est possible qu'en fait, leur prévalence soit sous-estimée. Les données épidémiologiques montrent néanmoins que la prévalence de certaines d'entre elles est en augmentation dans les pays très industrialisés, ce qui ne peut s'expliquer uniquement par l'amélioration du diagnostic. Par ailleurs, on est de plus en plus fondé à penser que des mécanismes autoimmunitaire pourraient jouer un rôle dans un grand nombre d'autres maladies (l'athérosclérose, par exemple).

Les maladies autoimmunes sont multifactorielles. Elles peuvent apparaître, se développer et progresser sous l'action de facteurs intrinsèques (par ex. des facteurs génétiques ou hormonaux ou encore l'âge) comme de facteurs environnementaux (par ex. une infection, le régime alimentaire, des médicaments ou des substances chimiques présentes dans l'environnement). On pense que les facteurs environnementaux jouent un rôle crucial dans l'augmentation de leur prévalence. Chez un hôte génétiquement réceptif, ces facteurs environnementaux peuvent amorcer, faciliter ou exacerber directement le processus immunitaire pathologique, provoquer des mutations au niveau des gènes codant pour les facteurs immunorégulateurs ou encore modifier la tolérance immunitaire ou les voies régulatrices ou effectrices.

Les troubles autoimmunitaires provoqués par des médicaments ou autres troubles de type autoimmunitaire, constituent, au même titre que les phénomènes d'hypersensibilité, un grave sujet de préoccupation et ils sont souvent à l'origine du retrait de certains médicaments du marché ou de restrictions dans leur utilisation. L'allergie systémique est un syndrome encore mal compris que l'on estime souvent être de nature isosyncrasique, mais qui pourrait être de nature allergique ou autoimmune. On a appris beaucoup de choses au sujet des mécanismes qui sont à la base des maladies autoimmunes autosyncrasiques en étudiant les phénomènes auto-immunitaires résultant d'une exposition à des substances thérapeutiques. Par ailleurs, plusieurs flambées ponctuelles de maladies autoimmunes dues à une exposition environnementale à des produits comme l'huile espagnole toxique ou le L-tryptophane ont fait notablement avancer nos connaissances.

On possède maintenant une somme importante de données épidémiologiques selon lesquelles il existe un lien entre l'exposition professionnelle à la poussière de silice cristalline (quartz) et le risque de plusieurs maladies autoimmunes généralisées (en particulier la sclérodermie généralisée, le lupus érythémateux disséminé, la polyarthrite rhumatoïde et la vasculite disséminée des petits vaisseaux). Les études épidémiologiques tendent également à confirmer le rôle de l'exposition professionnelle aux solvants dans l'apparition de la sclérodermie généralisée, mais il n'y a pas encore véritablement de consensus quant au type d'exposition ou de substance chimique qui seraient en cause ni sur le point de savoir si cette corrélation vaut aussi pour d'autres maladies. Le tabagisme est incriminé dans l'étiologie de certaines maladies autoimmunes (comme la maladie de Graves ou la polyarthrite rhumatoïde), notamment chez les fumeurs actuels, mais cette association paraît faible ou inexistante dans le cas d'autres affections. Pour faire progresser notre connaissance de la pathogénèse des maladies autoimmunes, il est nécessaire de compléter l'expérimentation par des recherches sur l'effet de ces agents ou d'autres agents physiques ou chimiques en utilisant des voies d'exposition correspondant à celles des sujets humains sur leur lieu de travail ou dans un environnement pollué. Alors qu'il existe nombre d'études sur la silice, les solvants et le tabagisme, les données épidémiologiques relatives au rôle des dioxines, des pesticides ou des métaux lourds dans l'apparition ou l'évolution des maladies autoimmunes sont relativement rares.

Un certain nombre de travaux ont également été consacrés à l'influence des facteurs alimentaires sur les maladies autoimmunes. Il s'agit là d'un vaste domaine de recherche portant sur l'apport calorique, certains types de nutriments ou d'aliments ou encore sur les suppléments diététiques. La maladie coeliaque est un exemple de maladie autoimmune clairement liée à l'alimentation dans laquelle la réponse immunitaire à certaines protéines du blé, de l'orge et du seigle produit des anticorps dirigés contre la transglutaminase tissulaire qui ont pour de provoquer des lésions au niveau de la muqueuse de l'intestin grêle.

Il est tout à fait probable que les infections jouent un rôle dans nombre de maladies autoimmunes, même si l'agent infectieux et le mécanisme de son action pathogène varient d'une affection à l'autre. La plupart des hypothèses qui ont été émises au sujet du rôle de l'infection dans l'autoimmunité supposent que celle-ci est directement en cause, alors qu'elle pourrait n'être qu'un facteur prédisposant. L'action des agents infectieux pourrait s'expliquer par une sorte de « mimétisme moléculaire » dû à une homologie séquentielle avec certaines protéines endogènes, mais ils pourraient aussi jouer le rôle d' « amorces » par une stimulation non spécifique / polyclonale de facteurs immunitaires tels que les cytokines ou les molécules de co-stimulation. L'état d'hygiène, dans la mesure où il conduit à l'élimination des stimuli infectieux, pourrait intervenir dans l'autoimmunité. Par leur interaction avec les agents infectieux, certaines substances chimiques pourraient également jouer un rôle, mais c'est un domaine qui reste insuffisamment étudié.

Il existe diverses méthodes pour mettre en évidence une formation excessive d'anticorps ou d'autoanticorps chez un sujet humain ou un animal de laboratoire à la suite d'une exposition environnementale. En revanche, il n'y a guère de tests qui permettent de déterminer dans quelle mesure certains produits chimiques ou facteurs environnementaux sont susceptibles de provoquer des maladies autoimmunes ou d'aggraver une maladie autoimmune existante.

On dispose d'un grand nombre de modèles animaux qui sont principalement utilisés pour étudier les mécanismes à la base des certaines maladies autoimmunes et les possibilités de les traiter. Les facteurs étiologiques utilisés avec ces divers modèles sont la prédisposition génétique, l'induction du processus pathologique au moyen d'antigènes spécifiques (la plupart du temps en association avec un adjuvant) ou l'exposition à un agent infectieux. Les modèles de maladie autoimmune chimio-induite sont plus rares. Par ailleurs, les études toxicologiques habituelles ne recherchent généralement pas les effets autoimmunogènes ou allergéniques des substances à expertiser, pour une part du fait qu'elles utilisent des animaux exogames et que les paramètres intéressants ne sont pas pris compte. En outre, les observations aberrantes sont généralement éliminées, alors qu'en fait elles pourraient être l'indication d'effets immunitaires idiosyncrasiques inattendus.

On ne dispose pas d'une stratégie générale pour évaluer le pouvoir autoimmunogène des substances chimiques, mais le test du ganglion poplité représente une méthode prometteuse. Il s'agit d'un modèle animal simple et robuste qui peut être utilisé pour établir un lien direct entre une réaction lymphocytaire ganglionnaire et l'application locale d'un produit chimique potentiellement immunogène. Toutefois, s'il peut se révéler prédictif dans le cas du pouvoir sensibilisateur d'un agent donné, ce test ne l'est pas forcément dans le cas du pouvoir autoimmunogène et ne correspond pas à une voie d'exposition systémique.

Le fardeau sanitaire et financier que représentent les maladies autoimmunes montre combien il est important d'en évaluer le risque. Pour évaluer le risque d'autoimmunité liée à des agents physiques ou chimiques il faut prendre en compte les données épidémiologiques disponibles, la nature du danger, les relations dose-réponse tirées d'études sur l'animal et sur des sujets humains ainsi que les données relatives au mode d'action des agents en cause ou encore les facteurs de sensibilité. Au final, cette démarche pourrait permettre de calculer plus facilement le coût des maladies autoimmunes liées à une exposition à des agents physiques ou chimiques. Pour l'instant, l'évaluation du risque inhérent aux agents que l'on suspecte d'induire une autoimmunité, de provoquer des maladies autoimmunes ou encore de les exacerber, bute sur le fait que l'on ne dispose pas des informations appropriées et que l'on manque notamment de modèles animaux validés. En raison de la charge que ces maladies représentent au niveau des individus et de la population, l'évaluation du risque relatif à ces pathologies est particulièrement importante.

RESUMEN

La autoinmunidad se caracteriza por la reacción de células (linfocitos T autorreactivos) o productos (autoanticuerpos) del sistema inmunitario frente a los antígenos del propio organismo (autoantígenos). Puede formar parte de la respuesta inmunitaria fisiológica ("autoinmunidad natural") o tener una inducción patológica, que con el tiempo puede llevar a la aparición de anomalías clínicas ("enfermedades autoinmunitarias"). Se pueden producir numerosas enfermedades autoinmunitarias diferentes, pero todas ellas se caracterizan por una respuesta inmunitaria inapropiada o excesiva frente a antígenos, cuyo resultado es una inflamación crónica, destrucción de los tejidos y/o disfunción. Hasta el momento, hay más de 60 enfermedades con una etiología autoinmunitaria demostrada o con una fuerte sospecha.

En general, se supone que las enfermedades autoinmunitarias son relativamente poco frecuentes. Sin embargo, cuando se combinan todas estas enfermedades, la prevalencia estimada es alta (3-5% de la población general), lo cual pone de manifiesto su importancia para la salud pública. Debido a las dificultades de diagnóstico y de formulación y normalización de los estudios epidemiológicos, los datos disponibles son limitados, y en realidad se puede haber subestimado la prevalencia. No obstante, hay pruebas epidemiológicas de una prevalencia creciente de determinadas enfermedades autoinmunitarias en países muy industrializados, que no se puede atribuir solamente a un diagnóstico mejor. Además, se tienen cada vez más pruebas de que los mecanismos autoinmunitarios pueden influir en otras muchas enfermedades (la aterosclerosis por ejemplo).

Las enfermedades autoinmunitarias son multifactoriales. Hay factores intrínsecos (por ejemplo, la genética, las hormonas, la edad) y factores ambientales (por ejemplo, las infecciones, la alimentación, los medicamentos, la química ambiental) que pueden contribuir a la inducción, desarrollo y progresión de estas enfermedades. Se considera que los factores ambientales tienen una responsabilidad importante en su creciente prevalencia. La actuación de los factores ambientales en un huésped genéticamente susceptible puede iniciar, facilitar o exacerbar directamente el proceso inmunitario patológico, inducir mutaciones en genes que codifican factores de inmunorregulación o modificar la tolerancia inmunitaria o las vías de los efectores reguladores e inmunitarios.

Los trastornos y la hipersensibilidad autoinmunitarios o análogos inducidos por medicamentos son motivo de una gran preocupación y con frecuencia la razón de la retirada de medicamentos del mercado o de la restricción de su utilización. La alergia sistémica no se conoce bien y a menudo se considera idiosincrásica, pero puede tener un carácter alérgico o autoinmunitario. Se ha aprendido mucho acerca de los mecanismos de las enfermedades autoinmunitarias idiosincrásicas estudiando los fenómenos autoinmunitarios derivados de la exposición a productos terapéuticos. Además, se han observado varios brotes de "fuentes puntuales" de enfermedades autoinmunitarias debidos a exposiciones ambientales a sustancias químicas, como el aceite tóxico en España y el L-triptófano, que han permitido mejorar nuestros conocimientos de manera sustancial.

Hay ahora pruebas epidemiológicas abundantes de la asociación entre la exposición ocupacional al polvo de sílice cristalino (cuarzo) y el riesgo de varias enfermedades autoinmunitarias sistémicas (en particular, la esclerosis sistémica, el lupus eritematoso sistémico, la artritis reumatoide y la vasculitis sistémica de los vasos pequeños). Los estudios epidemiológicos también respaldan la existencia de una función de la exposición ocupacional a disolventes en la aparición de la esclerosis sistémica, pero no hay un consenso claro sobre las exposiciones específicas o los tipos de sustancias químicas involucradas y si esta asociación se extiende a otras enfermedades. Algunas enfermedades autoinmunitarias (por ejemplo, la enfermedad de Graves, la artritis reumatoide) se han asociado con el consumo de tabaco, en particular en los fumadores habituales, pero con otras enfermedades sólo se han observado asociaciones débiles o nulas. Se necesitan otras investigaciones experimentales en las que se examinen los efectos de éstos y otros agentes químicos y físicos utilizando vías de exposición pertinentes a la experiencia humana en los entornos ocupacionales o en la contaminación ambiental para mejorar nuestros conocimientos acerca de la patogénesis de las enfermedades autoinmunitarias. A diferencia de los estudios disponibles relativos al sílice, los disolventes y el hábito de fumar, son relativamente escasos los datos epidemiológicos sobre el efecto de las dioxinas, los plaguicidas o los metales pesados en la aparición o progresión de las enfermedades autoinmunitarias.

Hay también algunas investigaciones sobre la influencia de factores de la alimentación en las enfermedades autoinmunitarias. Se trata de un sector amplio que incluye la ingesta calórica, nutrientes y alimentos específicos y complementos alimentarios. La enfermedad celíaca es un ejemplo de enfermedad autoinmunitaria con una clara vinculación con la alimentación, en la cual una respuesta inmunitaria a proteínas específicas del trigo, la cebada y el centeno produce anticuerpos dirigidos contra la transglutaminasa de los tejidos, provocando daños en la mucosa del intestino delgado.

Es muy probable que las infecciones desempeñen una función en muchos trastornos autoinmunitarios, aunque el agente infeccioso y el mecanismo mediante el cual provoca la enfermedad pueda diferir de un trastorno a otro. La mayoría de las hipótesis que relacionan la infección con la autoinmunidad suponen que desempeña una función causal directa, aunque simplemente puede servir como factor de predisposición. Los agentes infecciosos pueden desempeñar una función debido a la homología de secuencias con proteínas endógenas, que da lugar a un "mimetismo molecular", y también pueden actuar como agentes de "reactivación" debido a la estimulación no específica/policlonal de factores inmunitarios como las citoquinas y las moléculas coestimuladoras. Las condiciones de higiene, derivadas de una ausencia de estímulos infecciosos, pueden tener efectos en la autoinmunidad. Los agentes químicos pueden desempeñar una función importante en la interacción con las infecciones, esfera que ha sido escasamente estudiada.

Hay diversos métodos para detectar un aumento de la formación de anticuerpos y la presencia de anticuerpos en las personas y los animales de experimentación tras la exposición ambiental. En cambio, no hay pruebas fácilmente disponibles que permitan medir el potencial de las sustancias químicas o los factores ambientales para producir enfermedades autoinmunitarias o aumentar las existentes.

Hay un gran número de modelos animales que se han utilizado fundamentalmente para investigar mecanismos básicos y posibilidades terapéuticas para determinadas enfermedades autoinmunitarias. La etiología en los distintos modelos se basa en la predisposición genética, la inducción con antígenos específicos (la mayor parte en combinación con un coadyuvante) o la inoculación de prueba de agentes infecciosos. Los modelos de enfermedades autoinmunitarias de inducción química son menos comunes. Además, los efectos autoinmunogénicos y alergénicos de los compuestos no se suelen identificar en los estudios de toxicidad normales, en parte porque se utilizan animales exogámicos y los parámetros pertinentes no se estudian. Además, los valores atípicos se suelen descartar de los experimentos, mientras que en realidad son éstos los que pueden indicar efectos inmunitarios inesperados e idiosincrásicos.

Se carece de una estrategia general para evaluar el potencial de autoinmunogenicidad de las sustancias químicas. Un método prometedor es la valoración de los ganglios linfáticos poplíteos. Consiste en un modelo de prueba en animales sencillo y sólido que se puede utilizar para vincular reacciones directas de nódulos de linfocitos con la aplicación local de sustancias químicas potencialmente inmunoactivas. Sin embargo, estas valoraciones pueden predecir el potencial de sensibilización, pero no necesariamente el de autoinmunogenicidad de los agentes y no representan una vía sistémica de exposición.

La carga para la salud y los costos elevados de las enfermedades autoinmunitarias resaltan su importancia con respecto a una evaluación del riesgo. En la evaluación del riesgo de autoinmunidad asociado con agentes químicos o físicos se deben considerar los datos epidemiológicos disponibles, la identificación del peligro y los datos de la relación dosis-respuesta derivados de estudios realizados en animales y personas, los datos relativos al mecanismo de acción y los factores de susceptibilidad. El proceso de evaluación del riesgo puede ayudar a calcular en último término el costo de las enfermedades autoinmunitarias asociadas con la exposición a agentes químicos y físicos. En la actualidad, la evaluación del riesgo para agentes sospechosos de inducir o exacerbar la autoinmunidad o las enfermedades autoinmunitarias tropieza con la dificultad de la ausencia de información apropiada, en particular modelos animales validados. Debido a la carga de las enfermedades autoinmunitarias a nivel individual y colectivo, la evaluación del riesgo con respecto a este grupo de enfermedades adquiere una importancia especial.

www.ingramcontent.com/pod-product-compliance
Ingram Content Group UK Ltd.
Pitfield, Milton Keynes, MK11 3LW, UK
UKHW021315180426
11947UKWH00015B/1234